ULTRASOUND
for
Congenital Fetal Anomalies

ULTRASOUND
for
Congenital Fetal Anomalies

Editor

Sonal Panchal MD (Radiology)
Consultant Ultrasound Specialist
Dr Nagori's Institute for Infertility and IVF
Ahmedabad, Gujarat, India
Professor
Dubrovnik International University
Dubrovnik, Croatia
Academic Director
Ian Donald Inter-University School of
Medical Ultrasound, India

Foreword

Chaitanya Nagori

JAYPEE

JAYPEE BROTHERS MEDICAL PUBLISHERS

The Health Sciences Publisher

New Delhi | London

Jaypee Brothers Medical Publishers (P) Ltd

Headquarters
EMCA House
23/23-B, Ansari Road, Daryaganj
New Delhi 110 002, India
Landline: +91-11-23272143, +91-11-23272703
+91-11-23282021, +91-11-23245672
E-mail: jaypee@jaypeebrothers.com

Corporate Office
Jaypee Brothers Medical Publishers (P) Ltd.
4838/24, Ansari Road, Daryaganj
New Delhi 110 002, India
Phone: +91-11-43574357
Fax: +91-11-43574314
E-mail: jaypee@jaypeebrothers.com

Overseas Office
JP Medical Ltd.
83, Victoria Street, London
SW1H 0HW (UK)
Phone: +44-20 3170 8910
E-mail: info@jpmedpub.com

EU GPSR Authorised Representative
Logos Europe, 9 rue Nicolas Poussin
17000, La Rochelle, France
Phone: +33 (0) 6 67 93 73 78
E-mail: Contact@logoseurope.eu

Website: www.jaypeebrothers.com
Website: www.jaypeedigital.com

Inquiries for bulk sales may be solicited at: jaypee@jaypeebrothers.com

Ultrasound for Congenital Fetal Anomalies

First Edition: 2017

Reprint: **2026**

ISBN 978-93-5270-088-2

Printed at Replika Press Pvt. Ltd.

CONTRIBUTORS

Ashok Khurana MBBS MD
Trained at the HERLEV Hospital, Denmark
The Ultrasound Lab
New Delhi, India

BS Ramamurthy MBBS DMRD DNB MD
Srinivasa Ultrasound Scanning Centre
Bengaluru, Karnataka, India

Binodini Mahendra Chauhan MD (OBG)
Fellowship Fetal Medicine
Consultant, Fetal Medicine
Fetal Medicine Centre
Honorary Fetal Medicine Consultant
Government Medical College
Surat, Gujarat, India

Chaitanya Nagori MD DGO
Director
Dr Nagori's Institute for Infertility and IVF
Ahmedabad, Gujarat, India

Pavithra M Vengetesh MS (OG) DGO DNB(OG)
Fellow in Fetal Medicine
Coimbatore, Tamil Nadu, India

S Boopathy Vijayaraghavan MD DMRD
Consultant
Diagnostic Radiology and
Fetal Medicine
SONOSCAN: Ultrasonic Scan Centre
Coimbatore, Tamil Nadu, India

Sanjay Vasoya MD
Patel X-ray and Sonography Clinic
Surat, Gujarat, India

Sathiya Senthil MBBS RDMS MSc (Ultrasonography)
Consultant in Fetal Medicine
SONOSCAN: Ultrasonic Scan Centre
Coimbatore, Tamil Nadu, India

Sonal Panchal MD (Radiology)
Consultant Ultrasound Specialist
Dr Nagori's Institute for Infertility and IVF
Ahmedabad, Gujarat, India

Professor
Dubrovnik International University
Dubrovnik, Croatia

Academic Director
Ian Donald Inter-University School of
Medical Ultrasound
India

KV Sridevi MS (OBG) RCOG (UK)
Fellow Fetal Medicine
Consultant
Fetal Medicine and OBG Imaging
Pinnacle Hospital and Pinnacle Women's
Imaging Centre
Visakhapatnam, Andhra Pradesh, India

FOREWORD

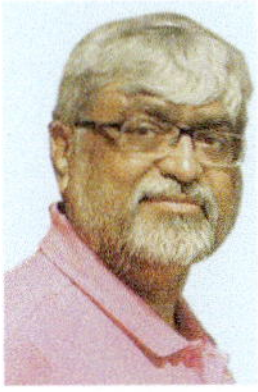

It gives me a pleasure to preview this book *Ultrasound for Congenital Fetal Anomalies* edited by Sonal Panchal. It is designed for clear understanding of the ultrasound findings of all common fetal abnormalities, with a clear 'to-the-point' approach. The initial chapters explaining the normal anatomy of the fetus and also clear description about the correct methodology of scanning and measurements, makes the understanding of the abnormal ultrasound findings more precise. The book also discusses the prognosis and management strategies of most lesion, making it a complete book for quick reference of the obstetric ultrasound practitioner.

Chaitanya Nagori MD DGO
Director
Dr Nagori's Institute for Infertility and IVF
Ahmedabad, Gujarat, India

PREFACE

This book is designed to lead the path from ultrasound findings to precise diagnosis of congenital fetal anomalies. It describes the correct method of assessment of each fetal part both qualitatively and quantitatively. Role of all ultrasound modalities (B mode, Doppler, 3D and 3D power Doppler) are discussed here. For all pathologies, an overview of therapeutic guidelines and counseling tips are also discussed. It will surely be a useful book for obstetricians and radiologists for ultrasound diagnosis of congenital fetal abnormalities.

Sonal Panchal

ACKNOWLEDGMENTS

I am sincerely grateful to each one who has contributed to make this book perfect. Two persons require a special acknowledgment, Dr KV Sridevi and Dr Sanjay Vasoya. They have stood by me and have supported and helped me to fill up the gaps, that were so difficult to, for the completion of the book. I acknowledge the support from Dr Ashok Khurana, Dr BS Ramamurthy and Dr Boopathy Vijayaraghavan, for their very relevant and up-to-date contributions. My special thanks to Dr Chaitanya Nagori, who has always supported and encouraged me as friend, philosopher and guide.

CONTENTS

1
CHAPTER

Normal and Abnormal Embryo

Chaitanya Nagori, Sonal Panchal

INTRODUCTION

The earliest phase of human life is the embryo and the fetus from fertilization till the end of the first trimester. This is a highly dynamic phase consisting of several developmental and evolutionary processes. This complex process was earlier studied only by observing the lab specimens of aborted fetuses. Development of high resolution transvaginal ultrasound especially with volume scan technology has brought a revolution in the study of embryo.

These scans are done with intracavitary (transvaginal) probes with frequencies varying from 5-12 MHz.

Early pregnancy can be assessed even before the sac appears. It is known that the blastocyst implants in the endometrium, five days after the fertilization of the ovum in the fallopian tube, i.e. approximately 18th to 20th day of the 28 days cycle. With implantation the progesterone secretion is enhanced from corpus luteum and this is reflected as increased blood flow to the corpus luteum. The receptive organ to this progesterone and proteolytic and other factors is the endometrium. It thickens due to the decidual reaction. New blood vessels develop to provide nutritional support to the embryo.

On ultrasound these changes are represented as:

- 2D US
  - Asymmetrical endometrial thickening. (one of the endometrial is more thickened as compared to other because of implanting embryo
  - Corpus luteum **(Figure 1)**.
- Color Doppler
  - Corpus luteum vascularity with low RI <0.5 **(Figure 2A)**.
  - High velocity, low resistance trophoblastic flow (PSV >6) in the thickened endometrial lip. This is typically described as a comet sign by Honemeyer et al. **(Figure 2B)**.[1]
- 3D US
  - Asymmetrical endometrial thickening is more evident on 3D US, with thickened part showing increase echogenecity due to decidual reaction and increased vascularity **(Figure 3)**.

Endometrial thickness of <6 mm, non-hyperechogenic endometrium with scanty vascularity in midluteal phase are negative predictors of conception.

Embryo is a very fast growing structure and therefore its anatomy changes every day or may be even faster. It is understood that

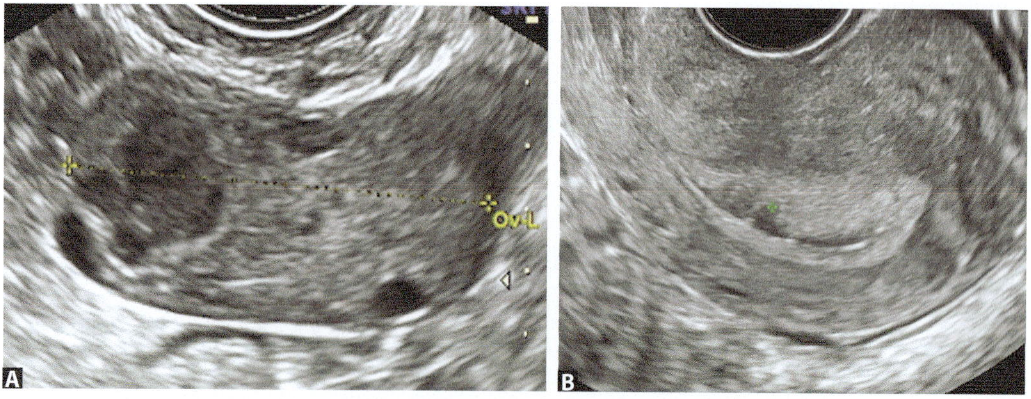

Figure 1: Corpus luteum and asymmetrical endometrium on B-mode (brightness mode)

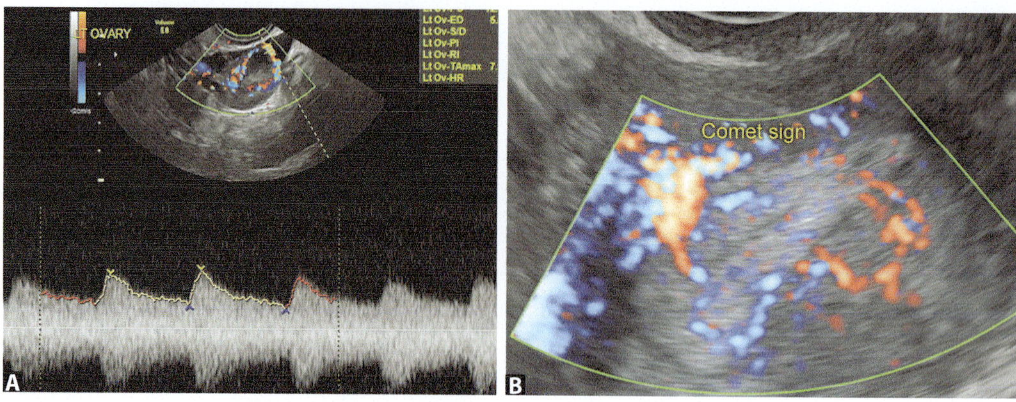

Figure 2: Corpus luteum and comet sign in endometrium

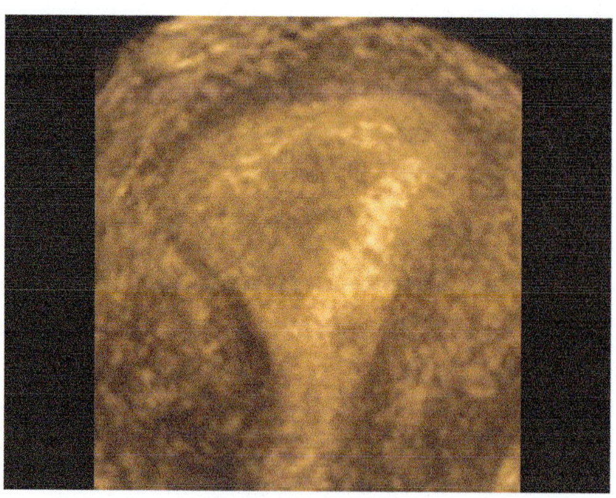

Figure 3: 3D US: Possibly conception cycle: midluteal phase

scans can not be done or findings cannot be described so often. Therefore changes in the embryo are described week to week.

Scans are done during early pregnancy for:

- Confirmation of pregnancy
- Confirm location of pregnancy
- Early detection of multiple gestation
- Assessment of progress of pregnancy
- Evaluation of abnormal early pregnancy.

CONFIRMATION OF PREGNANCY

Presence of gestational sac can be confirmed in the endometrial cavity as early as four weeks and 3–4 days by transvaginal scan and is diagnostic of pregnancy. Gestational sac is a round/oval anechoic structure with thick hyperechoic margins eccentrically placed in the endometrium **(Figure 4)**.

This echogenic margin is because of decidual reaction and is known as double

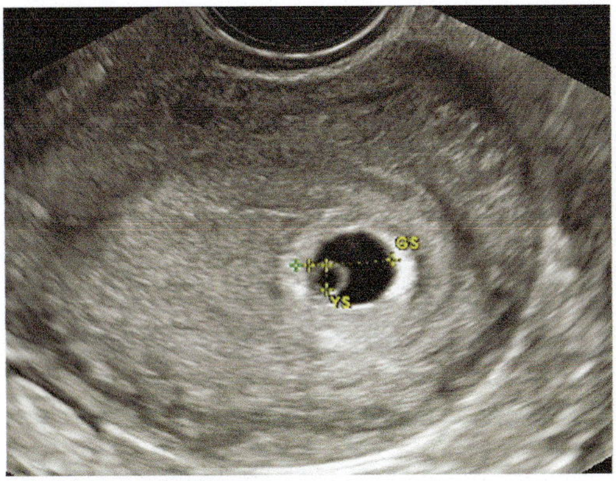

Figure 4: True gestational sac

Table 1: Difference between true sac and pseudosac

Features	*True sac*	*Pseudosac*
Situation	Eccentric in endocavity	Central in endocavity
Margins	Double decidual ring	No hyperechoic ring
With uterine peristalsis	No change in shape	Changes shape
On Doppler	Peripheral vascular ring	No peripheral vascularity

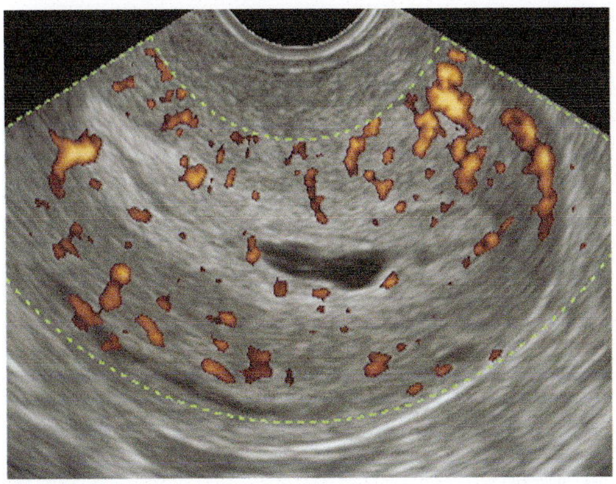

Figure 5: Pseudo sac

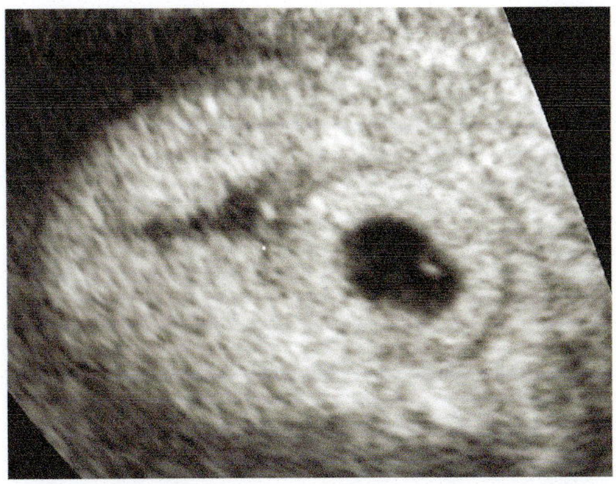

Figure 6: Residual endometrial cavity

decidual ring sign. The true gestational sac must be differentiated from pseudosac **(Figure 5)**, that may often be seen in patients with ectopic pregnancies and the differentiating points are given in **Table 1**.

β hCG is the earliest and the first marker for confirmation of pregnancy and gestational sac must be detected in the endometrial cavity on transvaginal scan when β hCG levels are >1000 IU/mL. In absence of which, an abnormal pregnancy must be suspected. At appearance, gestational sac is 2–3 mm in diameter. It grows at the rate of 1 mm/day and at 7 weeks it occupies 1/3rd of endometrial cavity. As it is implanted in one of the endometrial leaves, the endometrial cavity still persists till the sac grows large enough to abut the cavity. This residual cavity may be seen till 7 weeks and fluid seen surrounding the sac till this time should be first considered as a residual cavity, rather than perisac bleeding **(Figure 6)**.

A gestational sac that is not circular, does not have thick echogenic margins, appears late and does not show peripheral vascularity, is considered abnormal and carries a bad prognosis for pregnancy **(Figure 7)**. Choirionic thickness of atleast 3 mm is considered a sign of healthy pregnancy.

CONFIRM LOCATION OF GESTATIONAL SAC

Normally, the gestational sac is implanted in the fundal area **(Figure 8)**. Gestational sac that is implanted at any other location, is considered abnormal or ectopic.

Gestational sac that is implanted low **(Figure 9)** in the endometrial cavity, though

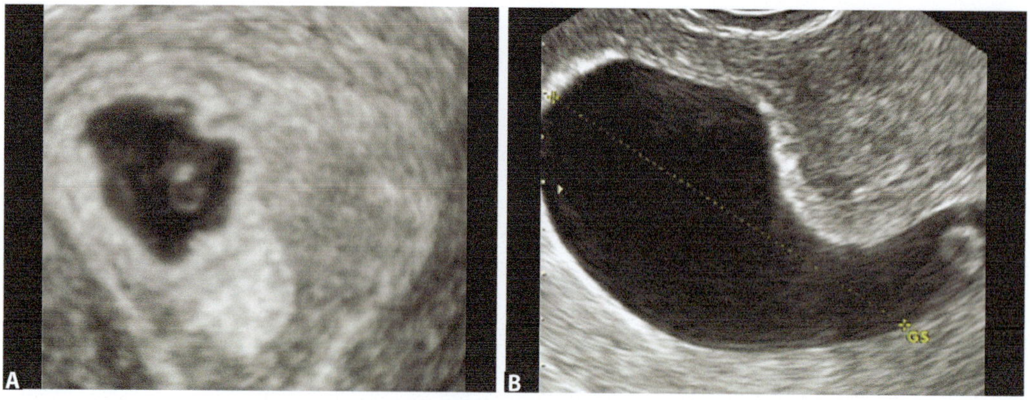

Figure 7: Irregular gestational sac and a large gestational sac

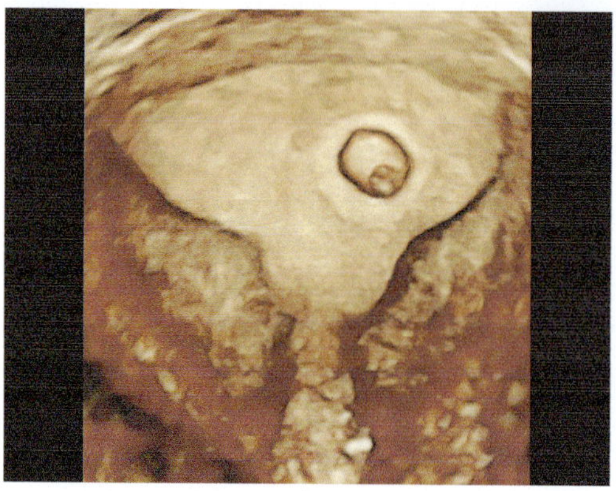

Figure 8: Normally implanted gestational sac

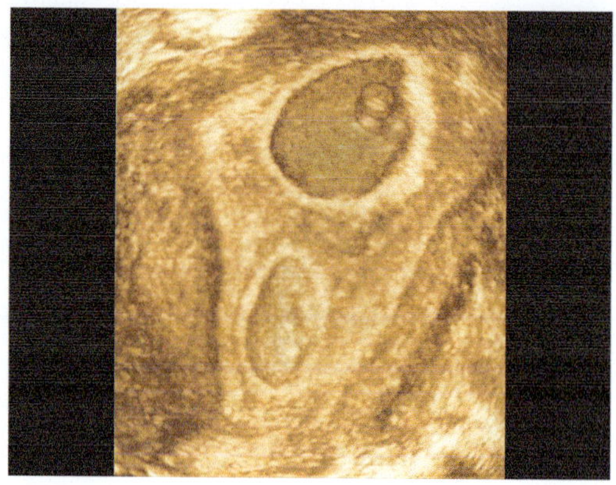

Figure 9: Low implanted sac in a twin pregnancy

may not be called ectopic but has increased chance of abortion.

Other locations of gestational sac in uterine cavity that are not considered normal are angular and interstitial pregnancy. Gestational sac in angle usually cannot grow beyond 8 weeks and can lead to serious complications. Interstitial part of the tube is covered by myometrium and cannot distend beyond 6-7 weeks. Differentiation between two is also important.

In interstitial pregnancy, sac is seen >1 cm lateral from the lateral edge of the endometrial cavity and is surrounded only by a thin layer of myometrium. Where as an angular pregnancy, medially is in continuity with the endometrium, but lateral to the gestational sac, no endometrial mantle is seen **(Figure 10)**.

Gestational sac may also implant in the cervix and is known as cervical pregnancy and is typically seen as ballooning of the cervix and hour glass shape of the uterus **(Figure 11)**.

Cervical pregnancy can be differentiated from abortion in process of abortion by its eccentric location in the cervical canal and surrounding vascularity. Rarely gestational sac may implant in a uterine scar of previous surgery also. This is known as a scar pregnancy. Scar pregnancies are more often seen now than earlier probably because of increased number of ceasarean pregnancies than earlier. These pregnancies typically do not show any endometrium surrounding the sac.

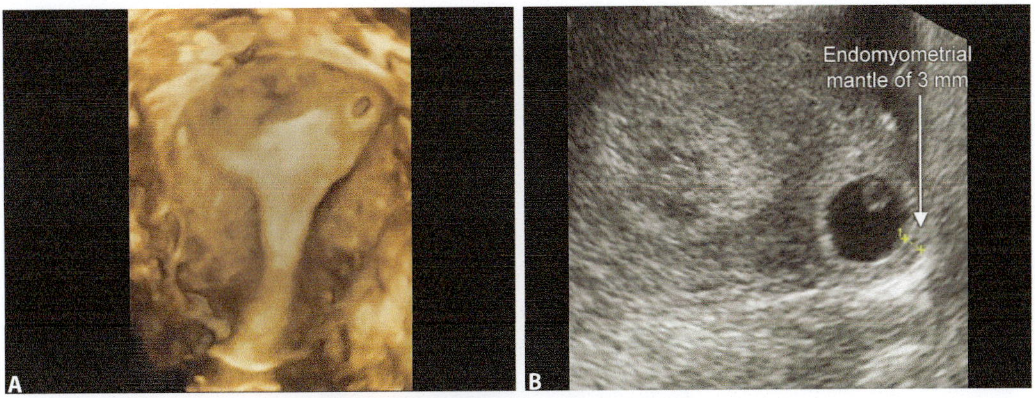

Figure 10: Angular pregnancy and interstitial pregnancy

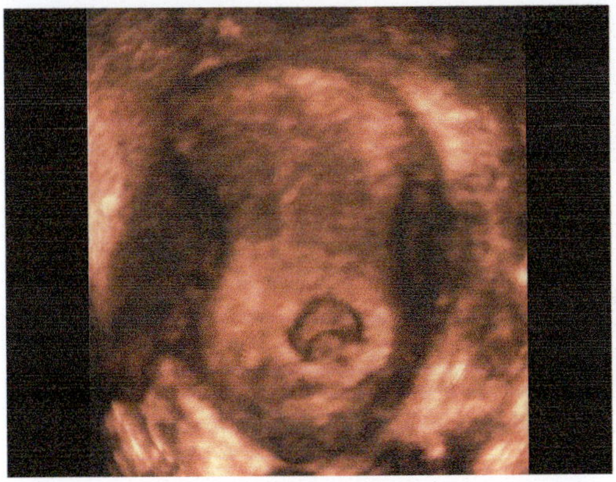

Figure 11: Cervical pregnancy

Abnormal locations of pregnancy, that are extrauterine are in the tube, ovary or free in the peritoneal cavity. Tubal ectopics are the commonest of all ectopic pregnancies.

Typically presentation of a patient with ectopic pregnancy is a history of missed period with raised β-hCG levels, though lower than expected for the time of gestation with either fainting attacks, dizziness or acute lower abdominal pain. Some patients may also present with spotting.

The ultrasound diagnostic signs are:

- *Tubal ectopic*
  - No intrauterine gestational sac with symmetrical endometrial cavity **(Figure 12A)**
  - Adnexal mass with peripheral low resistance vascularity with or without gestational sac, which is tender on probe pressure **(Figure 12B)**
  - Ipsilateral active corpus luteum
  - Free fluid in pelvis.
- *Ovarian ectopic* **(Figure 13)**
  - No intrauterine gestational sac with symmetrical endometrial cavity
  - Anechoic circular gestational sac in ovary with typical hyperechoic decidual reaction like rim, with peripheral vascularity
  - This can be differentiated from a corpus luteum only by its hyperechoic rim
  - It must be remembered that ovarian ectopic pregnancies are extremely rare and are often over diagnosed.
- *Abdominal/peritoneal ectopic* **(Figure 14)**
  - No intrauterine gestational sac with symmetrical endometrial cavity
  - Gestational sac is seen lying free outside uterus, tubes or ovaries
  - It is usually surrounded by fluid
  - Location of the gestational sac in these cases can not be related to ovaries or adnexa
  - Is very difficult to locate as it can be placed anywhere in the peritoneal cavity.

It must be remembered that ectopic pregnancy may coexist with intrauterine pregnancy and is known as heterotopic pregnancy.

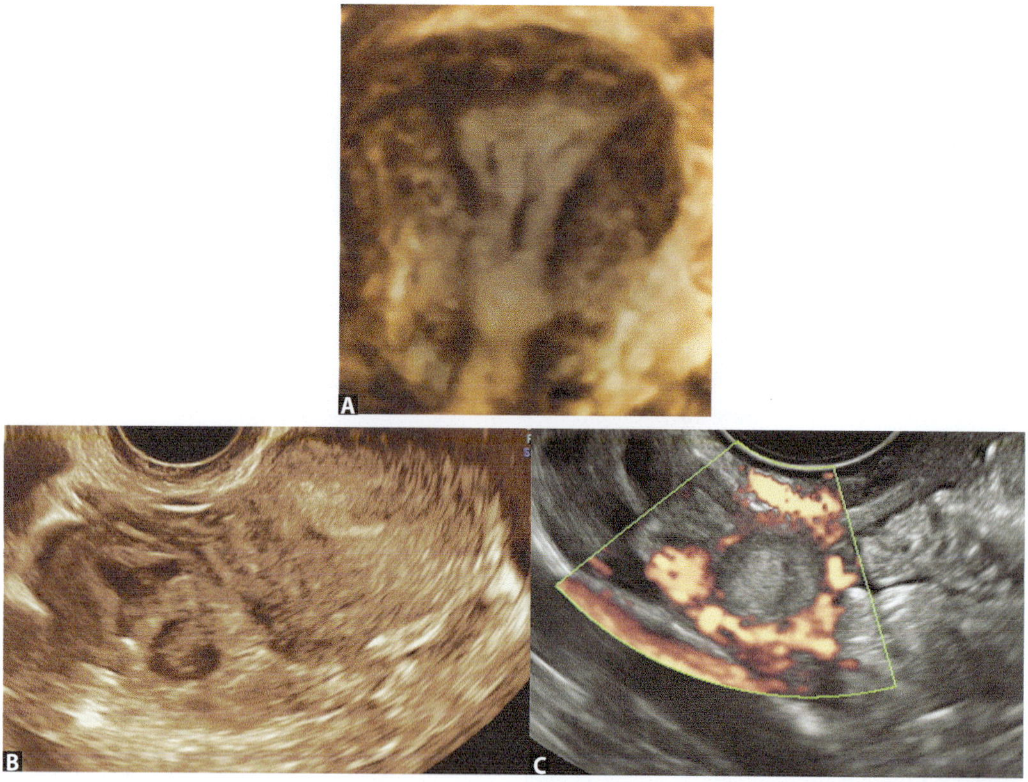

Figure 12: (A) Symmetrical endometrial cavity: Equal thickness of either endometrial leaf; (B and C) Tubal ectopic pregnancy

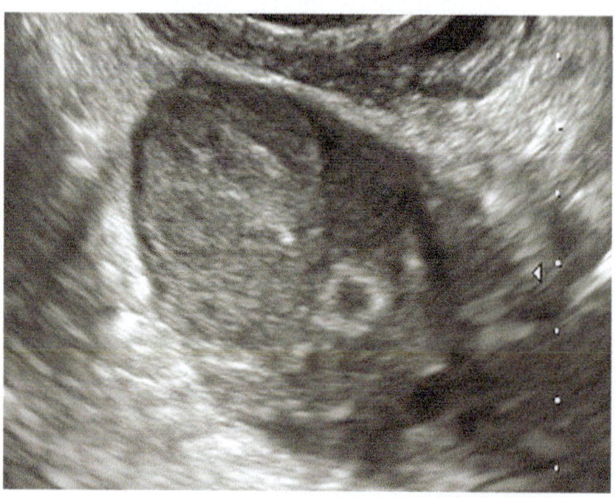

Figure 13: Ovarian ectopic pregnancy

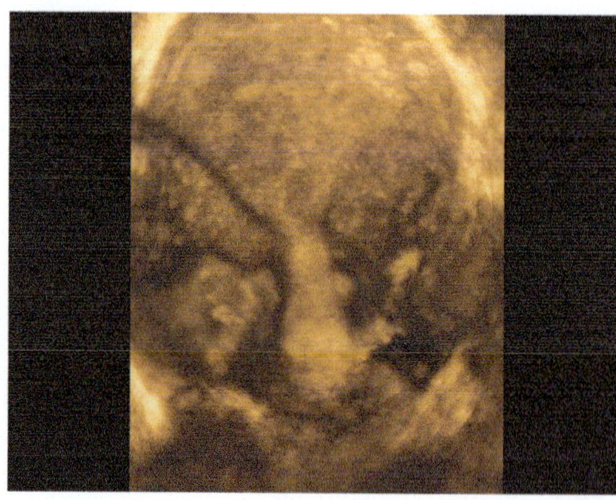

Figure 14: Abdominal ectopic pregnancy

EARLY DETECTION OF MULTIPLE GESTATION

Multiple gestations have much higher complication rate than singleton pregnancy. The complication rate and management are different for monochorionic and dichorionic, and monoamniotic and diamniotic pregnancies. It is therefore essential to confirm the chorionicity and amnionicity of any multiple gestation. This can be best done at 6–8 weeks of pregnancy. This is the time when gestational sacs are small and therefore individual sac margins can be confidently identified **(Figure 15)**. Without mentioning the chorionicity and amnionicity, no report of multiple gestation is to be considered complete.

GROWTH AND PROGRESS OF PREGNANCY

Growth of pregnancy is assessed by increase in the size of gestational sac or fetal pole and appearance of new structures. Gestational sac, yolk sac, amniotic sac and fetal pole, all have a definite time of appearance and pace of growth. These growth rates are very precise in first trimester and do not have genetic or individual variation. Abnormalities of these can be signs of abnormal prognosis of pregnancy. The technique for these measurements therefore should be standardized.

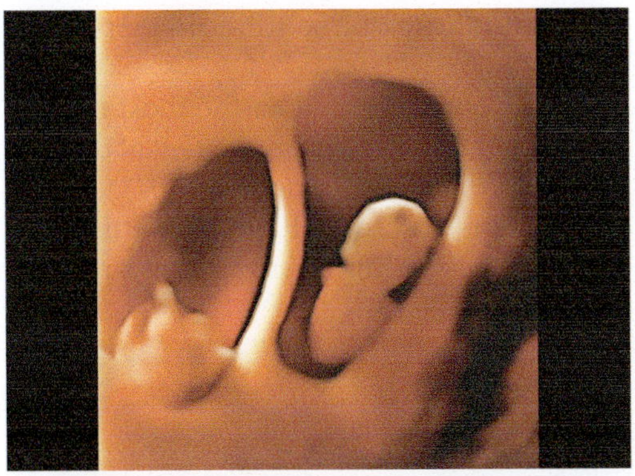

Figure 15: Multiple gestations: Dichorionic diamniotic twins

Gestational Sac (Figure 16A)

- Measured from inner edge to inner edge.
- Always take a mean of three orthogonal diameters.
- Volume is now considered more reliable
- Gestational sac volume can be assessed best by 3D ultrasound and VOCAL/Sono AVC (automated volume calculation) software and is especially required when the gestational sac is not round **(Figure 16B)**.

Yolk sac appears toward the end of the fourth week or when gestational sac is 10 mm in diameter. Fetal pole must be seen when gestational sac is 15 mm in diameter.

Yolk Sac

It has nutritive, metabolic, endocrine, immunological and hematopoietic functions.

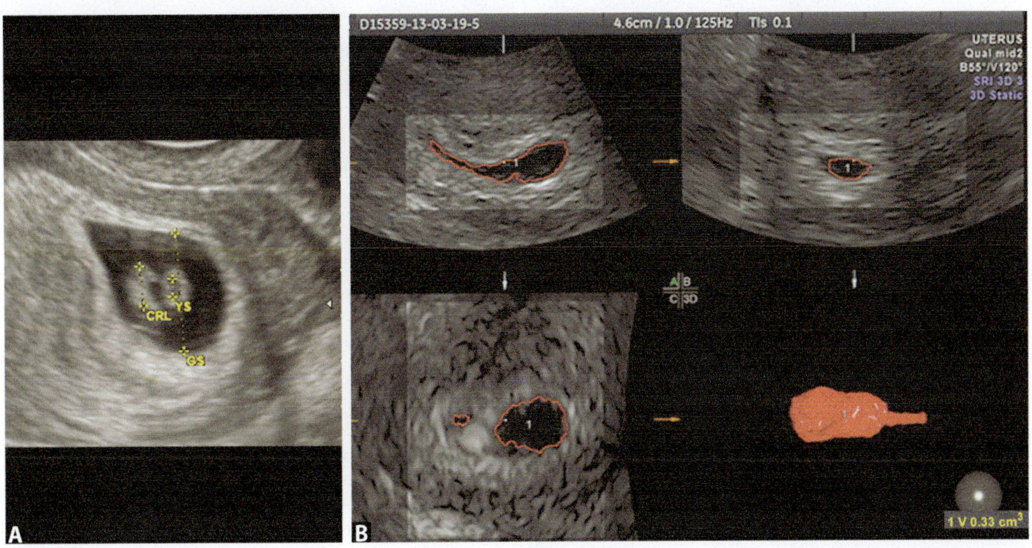

Figure 16: (A) Measuring gestational sac, yolk sac and CRL (crown rump length); (B) Sono AVC calculation gestational sac volume

It must be seen after 7-8 days of visualization of the gestational sac. It is a confirmatory sign of true gestational sac.

- Measured inner wall to inner wall
- Increases 0.1 mm/day till 10 weeks—max. 5-6 mm.

Yolk sac is an indicator of poor outcome of pregnancy if it is **(Figure 17)**

- Too small yolk sac <2 mm
- Too large yolk sac >6 mm
- Thick walled yolk sac
- Irregular yolk sac
- Solid yolk sac.

It was only 3D ultrasound which made possible to see the yolk sac surface and recognized it as a structure having honeycomb surface instead of a smooth one **(Figure 18)**.

Yolk sac volume by 3D US along with its vascularity have been found to be predictive of pregnancy outcome by Kupesic et al.[2]

Fetal Pole

Fetal pole is the structure to follow the appearance of yolk sac. Detection of the fetal pole is actually by visualization of the cardiac activity. By transvaginal ultrasound fetal cardiac activity can be detected at 5-6 weeks approximately, when the fetal pole appears like a linear structure by the side of the yolk sac of approximately 1-2 mm in length. Its length is measured from end to end and grows at a rate of 1 mm/day. Size to date discrepancy of up to 5 days can be considered to be within normal limits. Difference in CRL of >7 mm of normal indicates three times higher risk of aneuploidy.

CRL is considered to be the most reliable measure parameter for assessment of the fetal age. It is a reliable parameter till 10–11 weeks. Beyond this gestational age, the fetus has a tendency to flex on its trunk and so crown

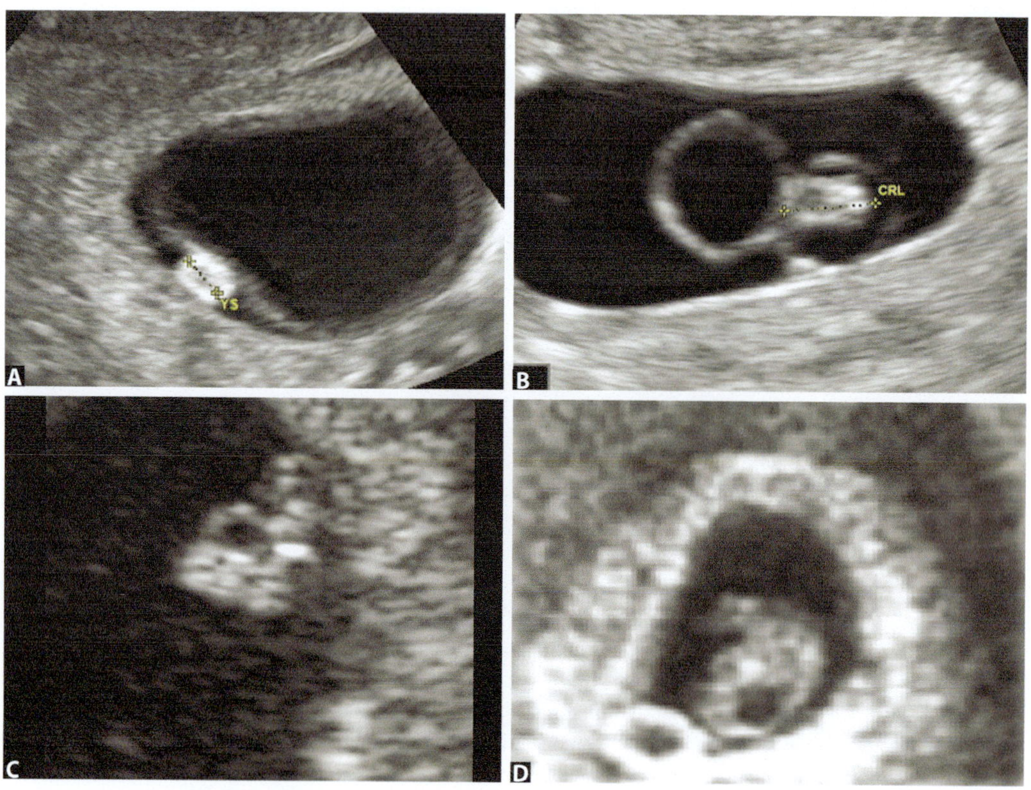

Figure 17: Solid, large, thick walled and irregular yolksac (clockwise)

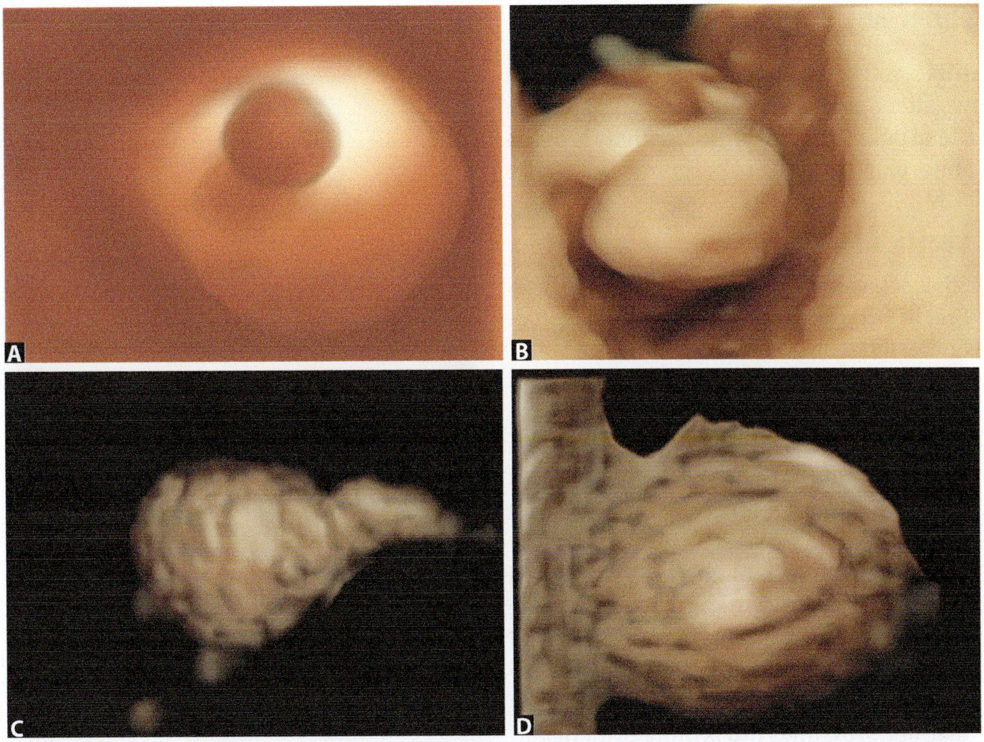

Figure 18: Progressive changes in yolk sac as embryo develops

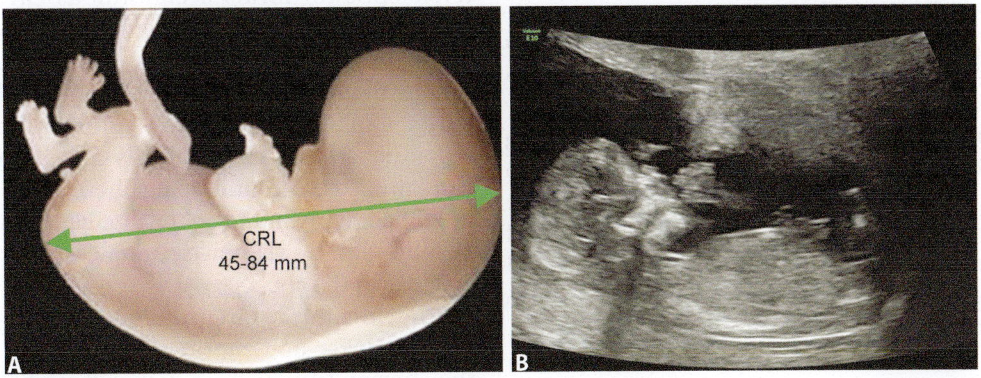

Figure 19: Measuring crown rump length

rump length can not be then considered a reliable parameter of assessment of gestational age. The gestational age is therefore decided based on CRL in the first trimester and it must be remembered that the gestational age once decided in the first trimester, it should then not be changed. This is of special importance when the patient is not sure of dates or when IUGR is suspected in the later trimesters.

Being of such importance therefore CRL must be measured with due standardization. When the fetus is not flexed, in the mid-sagittal section and end to end. Midsagittal section is confirmed by absence of visualization of any of the fetal lower limbs in the image and if the upper limbs are seen these are only the distal part of the upper limbs which are usually in front of the fetal chest as this is a very common habitus of the fetus at this gestational age **(Figure 19)**.

CARDIAC ACTIVITY

Cardiac activity must always be seen at all times after 6 weeks of pregnancy. Appearance of a fetal pole, without cardiac activity is a sign of abnormal (nonviable) pregnancy.

Normal Heart Rate

- 5th week—slow like peristalsis—60-80/min
- End of 5th week—100/min
- End of 6th week—105-130/min
- 9 weeks—160-170 / min, then 120-160/min
- Heart rate of >200/min is termed as tachycardia and <100/min is termed as bradycardia in the first trimester, though it is known that in the later pregnancy this limit is 120-160 bpm.

Persistently abnormal heart rate has a bad prognosis and late appearance of cardiac activity also indicates pregnancy with bad prognosis. Irregular cardiac rhythm is also a sign of cardiac arrhythmia and high risk of cardiac abnormalities but is more evident and considered of more importance in 2nd and 3rd trimesters of pregnancy.

3D power Doppler can be used to visualize the areas of developing intervillous circulation. 3D power Doppler allows to study the turgescent blood vessels withstanding from the surface of the yolk sac and also to study the evolution from embryovitelline to embryoplacental circulation. Study of both the intervillous and embryoplacental circulation can also be used prognostically to know the pregnancy outcome.

Structures then to appear by completion of each following week after 5 weeks are as follows:

SIX WEEKS (FIGURE 20)

Fetal pole with cephalic and caudal poles. Shape of the embryo now is a round bulky head and thin body, with no limb buds, but long omphalomesentric duct. Amniotic membrane is seen initially dorsally and then covering the embryo. Aortic and umbilical blood flows are now seen.

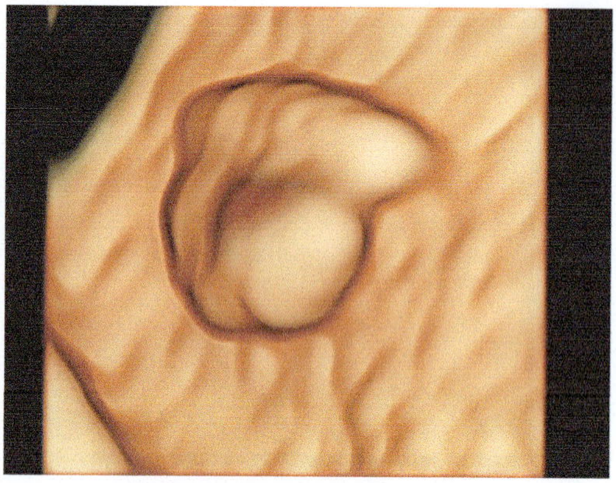

Figure 20: Six weeks pregnancy

SEVEN WEEKS (FIGURE 21)

Spine and limb buds appear. Brain vesicles are now seen. Lateral ventricles appear like round vesicles and diencephalons (future third ventricle) runs posteriorly. Medial telencephalon forms a continuous cavity between two lateral ventricles. Foramen of Munro is wide and height of diencephalons is more than mesencephalon. Mesencephalic cavity, a tube like structure is future sylvian aqueduct, which lies aneriorly and points caudally. Two cerebral hemispheres can be identified. Early intracerebral circulation can also be seen by 3D power Doppler. Head is flexed over the chest.

Chorion now start differentiating into Chorion leave and chorion frondosum. It is the chorion frundosum which will form the future placenta. Amniotic membrane is now is visible.

Amniotic Membrane

Seen when CRL is 5-7 mm.

In early pregnancy, when its size is equal to yolksac, it shows like double bleb sign. Amniotic sac grows at a rate of 1 mm/day and fuses with chorion at about 14 weeks.

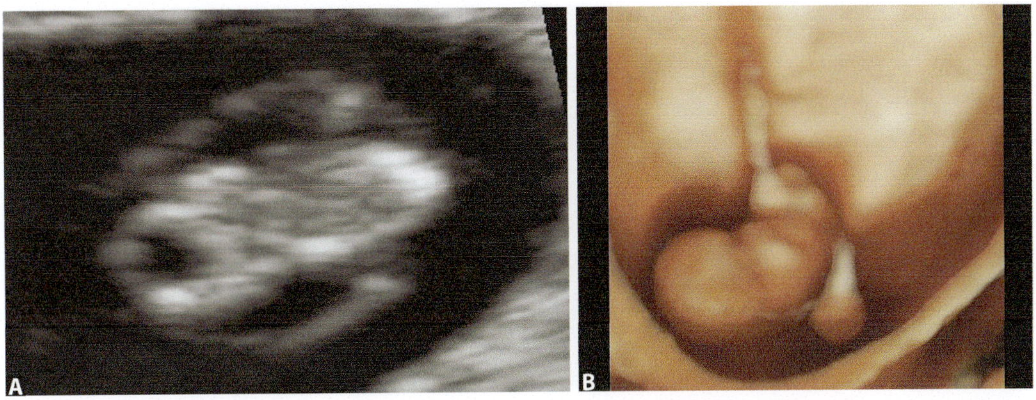

Figure 21: Seven weeks embryo showing rhombencephalon and limb buds

If it doesn't fuse it may suggest a higher risk of chromosomal abnormality.

Normal US at eight weeks of pregnancy is a positive prognostic sign for a normal pregnancy outcome.

EIGHT WEEKS (FIGURE 22)

The trunk of the fetus strainghtens. Limb buds are seen as elongated projections ending with thicker areas (future hands and feet). Movements of the limb buds can also be seen towards to end of 8th week. Head flexion decreases as the ventricular system of the brain expands. Future 4th ventricle can now be visualized. Brain structure can now be seen clearly.[3] Two distinct hemispheres with deepening of the rhombencephalic cavity. It now takes a pyramid like shape with central deepening of pontine flexures as peak of the pyramid.[4]

3D power Doppler now allows visualization of entire fetal circulation, including cerebral circulation.Physiological umbilical hernia starts appearing towards the end of the week, but becomes visible on ultrasound only in the subsequent week of gestation.

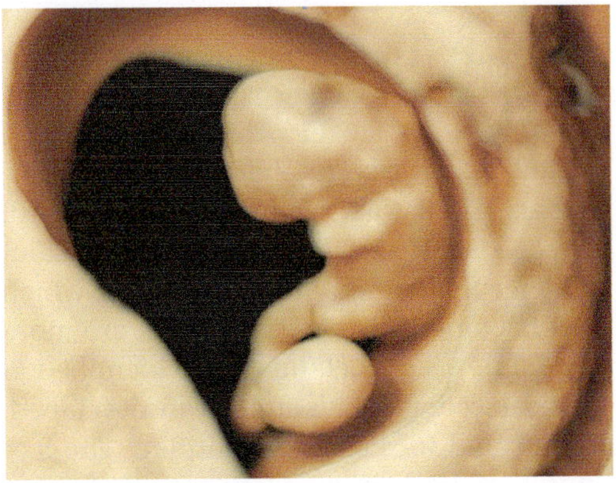

Figure 22: Eight weeks embryo

NINE WEEKS (FIGURE 23)

Spine can now be seen along its entire length and neck and coccygeal prominence become evident. Omphalocele is well seen at ninth week. Elbows and knees can be identified and feet approach the midline. Lateral ventricles enlarge. Thallamic growth narrows down the anterior part of the third ventricle. Beyond CRL of 25 mm, a gap is seen between rhombencephalon and mesencephalon, due to growing cerebellum. Diencephalon starts narrowing in its upper anterior part. On axial section, falx and choroid plexuses can be identified.

At this stage, 3D can fairly clearly show fetal facial images.[5] 3D power Doppler shows circle of Willis and choroids plexus vessels (***See* Figure 6**). Cranial venous system also can now be identified. Umbilical cord circulation can be clearly demonstrated with both arterial and venous pulsations.

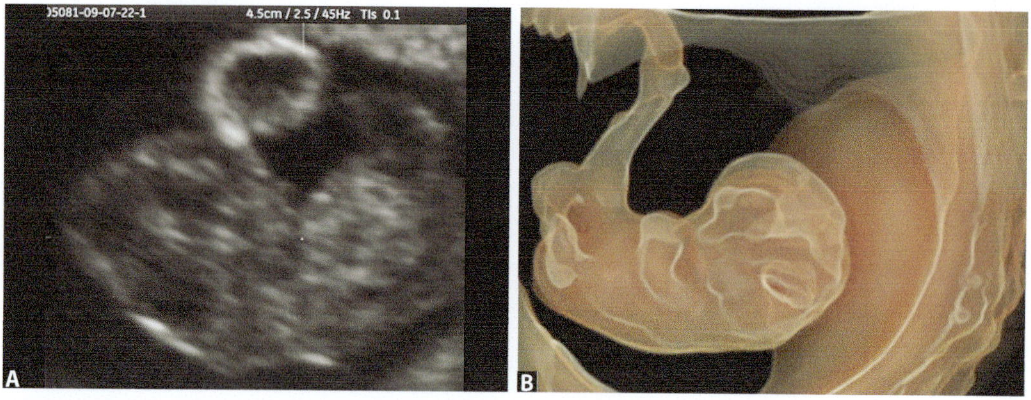

Figure 23: Nine weeks embryo showing prosen-, mesen- and rhomben-cephalon, strainghtened trunk and developing limb buds

TEN WEEKS (FIGURE 24)

Facial details—nose, orbits, maxilla and mandible can be seen. Abdominal organs like stomach, kidneys and bladder can be identified. *Three cerebral vesicles*—rhombencephalon, mesencephalon and prosencephalon, which start becoming visible in 9th week are more evident now. Cerebellum can be identified in the axial section. Hands and feet are developed. Fingers and toes can be identified. The feet approach the midline. Ossification of spine starts.

Power Doppler may show aorta and carotids also.

ELEVEN WEEKS

Culvarial ossification starts. Choroid plexus and falx are seen and on axial plain gives a typical butterfly appearance. Spinal column is now clearly seen.Facial sturctures- nose, orbits and jaws are easily identified. Abdominal organs are clearly seen. Physiological omphalocoele disappears latest by 11 weeks and 4 days.

TWELVE WEEKS (FIGURE 25)

Detailed facial structure—nose, eyes, ears, lips, premature skull bones with sutures in between, details of abdominal organs, limbs including not only fingers and toes but individual phalanges and detailed cerebral and cerebellar anatomy can be seen. Four chamberd heart can be seen. 3D power Doppler demonstrates complete fetal vasculature.

THIRTEEN WEEKS

The face is well defined. Facial features can be identified. Each vertebrae and IV disc can be identified. Diaphragm can be clearly visualized along with all abdominal organs. Umbilical hernia has already disappeared by this gestational age. Four chamber heart, out flow tracts and three vessel view can be seen in at least 40–50% of fetuses on transvaginal scan.

There are abnormalities that can be suspected or even at times diagnosed early in the first trimester.

These include:

- *Acrania* **(Figure 26)**: Cranial vault ossification starts at 10 weeks and is complete by the end of 12th week. Acrania is lack of skull bone development. This leads to abnormal head shape as the developing brain tissue is directly exposed to amniotic fluid. This can be diagnosed as early as 10 weeks of gestation. Brain when exposed to amniotic fluid, it is destroyed and results in anencephaly.

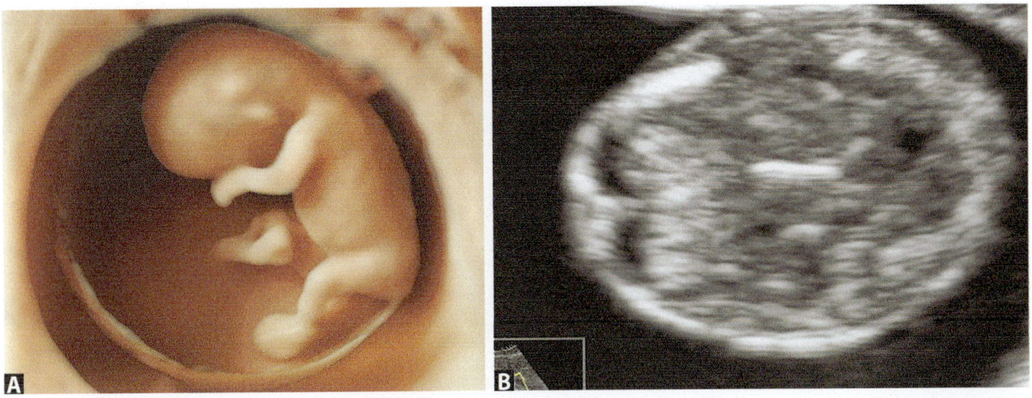

Figure 24: 10 weeks pregnancy

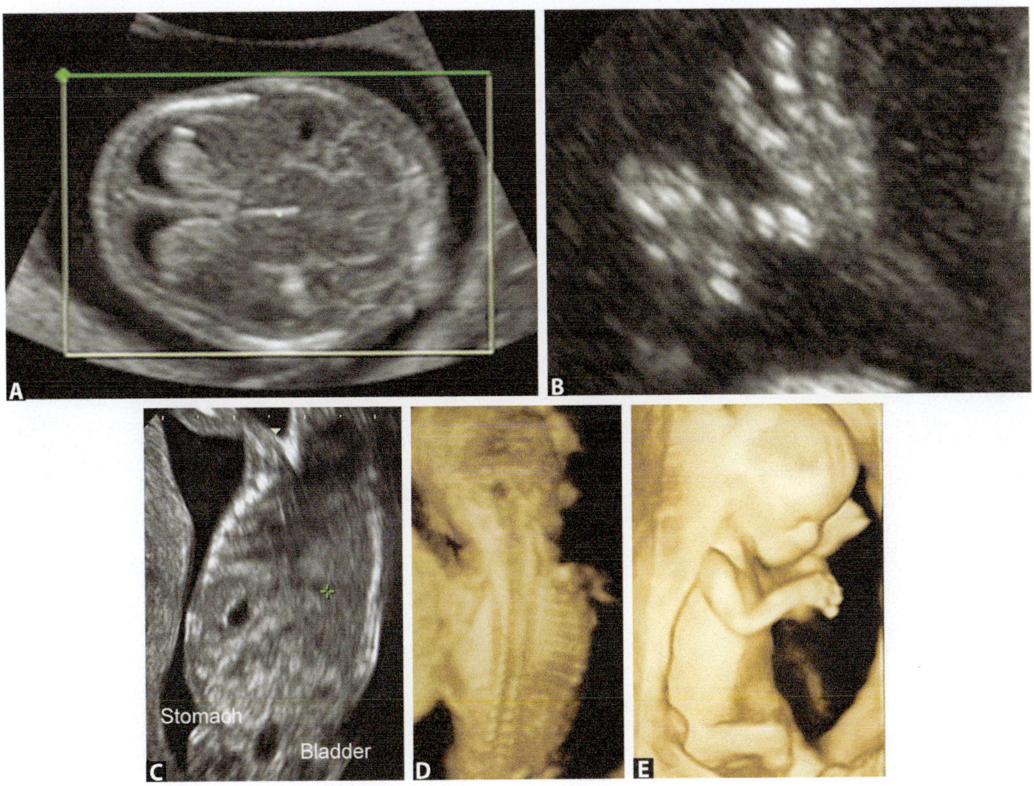

Figure 25: Anatomical details of 12 weeks fetus

- *Encephalocele*: This is deficient development of the neural tube posteriorly, leading to herniation of meninges and sometimes brain tissue also.
  Partial failure of closure of cephalic end of neural tube and lack of neurocranium results in exencephaly.
- *Holoprosencephaly* **(Figure 27)**: Cessation of cleavage of prosencephaly leads to holoprosencephaly, which may be lobar, semilobar or alobar depending on the stage of arrest. This results in absence of development of falx. It has been discussed earlier that falx can be seen at all times after

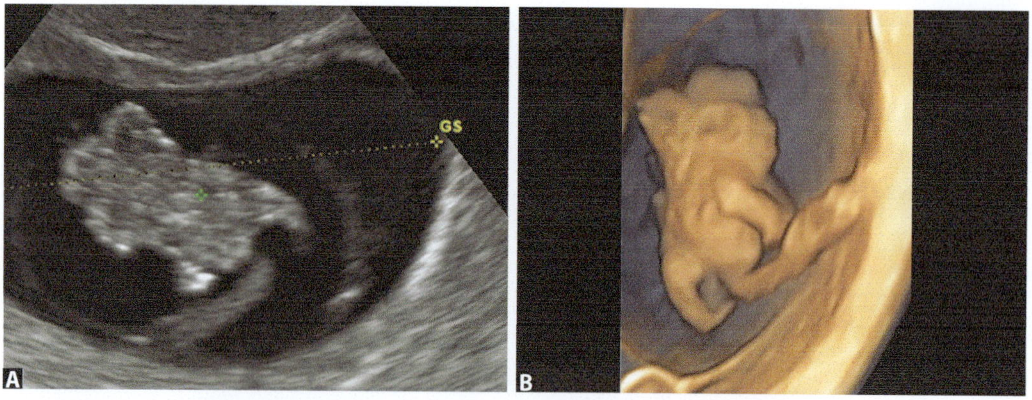

Figure 26: Acrania-irregular head shape due to absence of culvarium

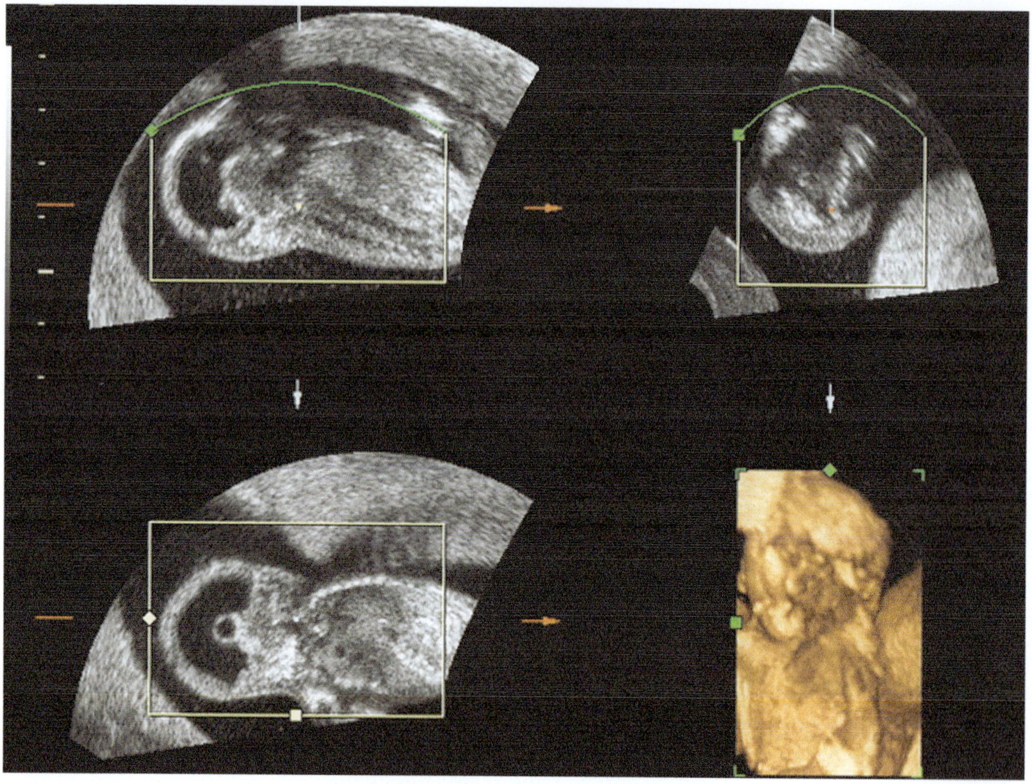

Figure 27: Holoprosencephaly

completion of 9th week. If it is not seen beyond 10th week, holoprosencephaly must be suspected. Apart from fused thalami and basal ganglia there are several facial defects like cleft lip, palate, hypotelorism, cyclopia, arhinia with proboscis associated especially with alobar holoprosencephaly.

- *Iniencephaly*: It is a persistent hyper-extension habitus of the fetus, typically described as a star gazing fetus **(Figure 28)**.
- *Major limb abnormalities* **(Figure 29)**: All limb buds appear at 8 weeks and by the end of 10 weeks, all the segments of all four limbs are formed. Complete or partial absence of

any of the limbs can be detected at all times after 10 weeks. Severe limb abnormalities like phocomelia, sirenomelia, and even club foot can be diagnosed as early as 12 weeks of pregnancy. Bone dysplasias like achondroplasia can be also diagnosed by 12 weeks but are better demonstrated with 3D ultrasound as it shows the entire fetus in a single image and therefore the disproportion is easy to demonstrate.

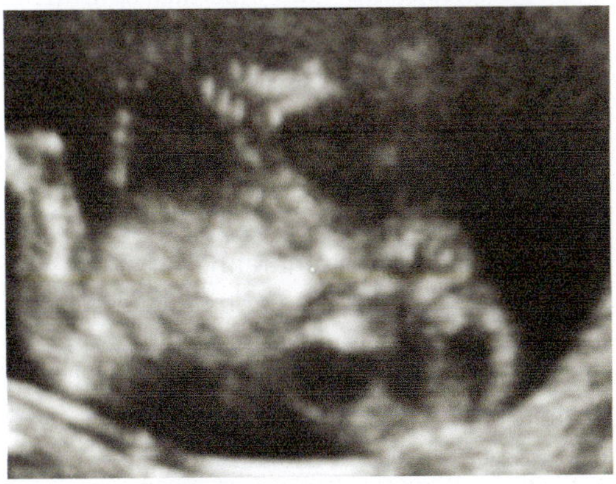

Figure 28: Iniencephaly

- *Situs abnormalites*: Situs inversus is complete reverse position of all fetal organs: a mirror image, where heart, aorta and stomach are on right side and liver, gall bladder and IVC are on left side. Situs solitus with dextrocarida is when the abdominal organs and the aorta have a normal position but the heart is on the left side. Situs inversus with levocardia, when all abdominal organs and aorta are on opposite side than what they should be in but the heart is in the normal position on left side. As heart and stomach are developed and are evident at 10 weeks, their position can be checked and situs abnormalities can be diagnosed in first trimester.

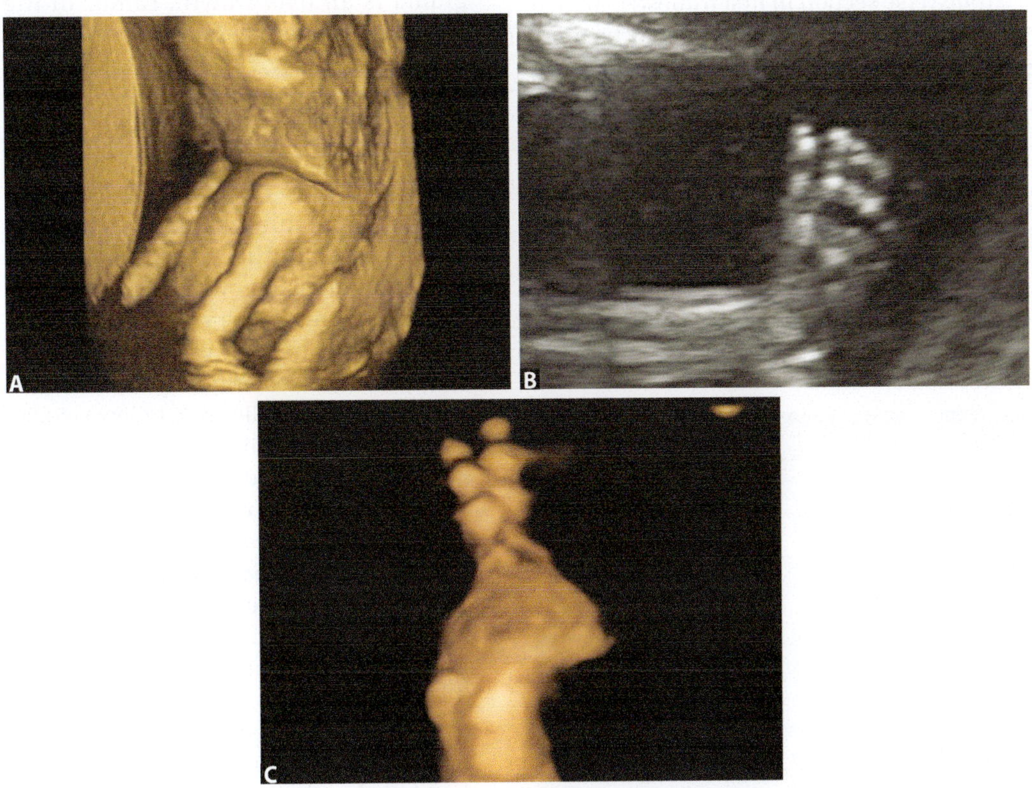

Figure 29: Major limb abnormalities

- *Major cardiac abnormalities*: By 11 weeks, four chamber heart is formed and can be seen clearly on transvaginal scan. Major cardiac abnormalities like single ventricle, truncus arteriosus, etc. can be diagnosed on first trimester scans.
- *Major spinal defects*: Ossification centers of the spine are formed at the end of 10 weeks. Major spinal defects, multiple vertebral abnormalities, hemivertebrae, etc. can be diagnosed on first trimester scans.
- *Facial anomalies*: Maxilla and palate can be reliably studied as early as 11 weeks by axial section as well as coronal section (premaxillary triangle) **(Figure 30)**.
  Early diagnosis of median cleft syndrome is possible in which the frontal bones and nasal bones are largely separated with hypertelorism, flat nasal bridge, rudimentary nostrils and other facial abnormalities.[6] Palate can be best studied by TUI of face in transverse section in first trimester, though later in pregnancy rendering may be more helpful. Lips may be better visualized in anterior coronal sections and rendered image. Abnormalities like facial cleft, micrognathia, nasal abnormalities and eye abnormalities like anophthalmia, can all be seen by 3D ultrasound, as early as late first trimester. Genetic syndromes are often diagnosed by craniofacial dysmorphism.
- *Abdominal wall defects*: Herniation of the bowel loops through the anterior abdominal wall at the base of the umbilical cord—omphalocele is a physiological phenomenon from 9th to 11th week. Even during that period a omphalocele neck of larger than 7 mm or an omphalocoele that is larger than the actual fetal abdominal circumference is pathological. This size assessment is more precise by 3D ultrasound rather than 2D US **(Figure 31)**. An omphalocele which projects beyond 11 weeks, may contain liver or bowel and depending on this content the fetus may have a lower or higher risk of chromosomal abnormality respectively. This differentiation is easy by Doppler, depending on hepatic vessels are seen in the abdomen or in the omphalocele. Gastroschisis is another abdominal wall defect which has attachment of the umbilical cord by the side of the defect in abdominal wall.

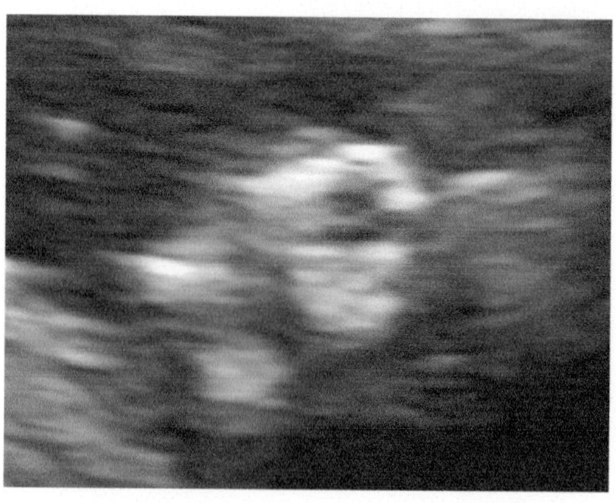

Figure 30: Normal premaxillary triangle

- *Chorioangioma* **(Figure 32)**: Chorioangioma is an overgrowth, tumor of the chorionic tissue. These can be seen very early in pregnancy, 7–8 weeks of pregnancy. Small chorioangiomas do not affect the pregnancy, but larger ones may lead to circulatory failures in fetus.
- *Vesicular mole* **(Figure 33)**: Another chorionic lesion, vesicular mole is a common lesion. High β-hCG levels with absent gestational sac with thick echogenic endometrium, that has small anechoic areas is diagnostic of vesicular mole. In early phases, vascularity may not be picked up on Doppler studies due to low velocity flow. Only when it becomes invasive, it disrupts the endometriomyometrial junction and then is usually large enough to show abundant low resistance vascularity.
- *Miscellaneous abnormalities*: Umbilical cord cyst is another not so uncommon lesion, that can be picked up in first trimester, but is not clinically significant **(Figure 34)**.
  Single umbilical artery is also now not given significant clinical importance.
  Amniotic bands also can be picked up by the end of the first trimester. These may

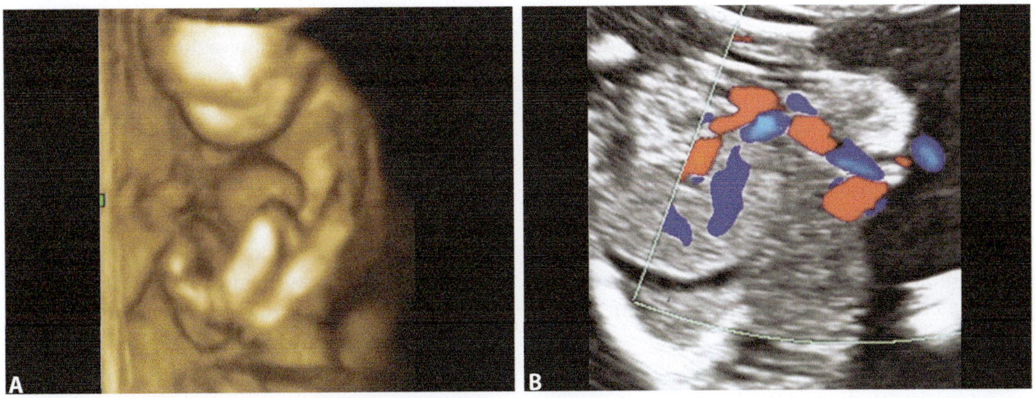

Figure 31: Omphalocele and gastroschisis

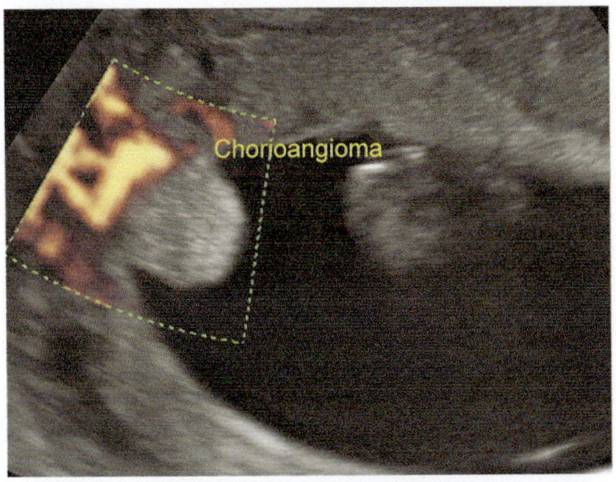

Figure 32: Chorioangioma

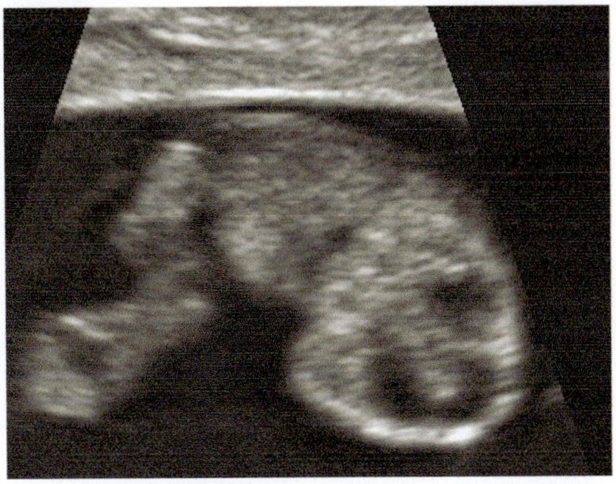

Figure 34: Umbilical cord cyst

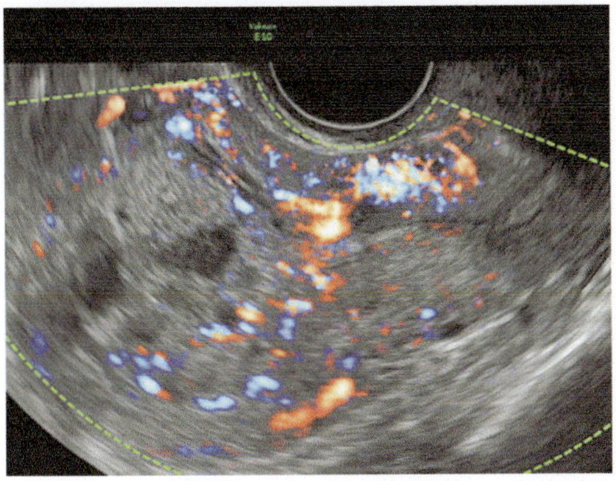

Figure 33: Vesicular mole

at times lead to amputation like major consequences in later pregnancy, often times these may not be of any significance. Of course ultrasound plays a major role for diagnosis of chromosomal abnormalities in the first trimester. The dedicated scan is known as a nuchal scan or a genetic scan or 11-13+6 weeks scan, but that will be discussed in chapter 3.

Detailed and careful systematic scanning technique can therefore help in early diagnosis of several fetal abnormalities. Volume ultrasound is very informative for first trimester scanning.

REFERENCES

1. Honemeyer U, Kurjak A, Monni G. Normal and abnormal early pregnancy. Donald School Textbook of Ultrasound in Obstetrics and Gynecology, Jaypee Brothers Medical Publishers (P) Ltd. 2008;2:pp.106-29.

2. Kupesic S, Kurjak A, Ivancic-Kosuta M. Volume and vascularity of yolk sac studied. three dimensional ultrasound and colour Doppler. J Perinat Med. 1999;27:91-6.
3. Blaas H-G, Eik-Nis SH, Kiserud T, Berg B, Angelson B, Olstad B. Three dimensional imaging of the brain cavities in human embryos. Ultrasound Obstet Gynecol. 1995;5:228-32.
4. O'Rahilly R, Mueller F. Ventricular system and choroids plexuses of the human brain during the embryonic period proper. Am J Anat. 1990;189:285-302.
5. Merz E, Weber G, Bahlmann F, Miric-Tesanic D. Application of transvaginal and abdominal three-dimensional ultrasound for detection or exclusion of fetal malformations of fetal face. Ultrasound Obstet Gynecol. 1997;9: 237-43.
6. Sieurs E, Goncalves LF, Jhonson A, Espinoza J, Devers P, Chalworapongsa T, et al. First trimester ultrasonic findings in a fetus with frontonasal malformation. The Journal of Maternal-fetal and neonatal medicine. 2004; 16:187-97.

2
CHAPTER

Normal Fetal Anatomy in Second Trimester

Chaitanya Nagori, Sonal Panchal

INTRODUCTION

Second trimester scan is done for detailed structural assessment of the fetus. It carries the importance almost equal to the 11–13+6 weeks scan. This scan is usually done between 18–20 weeks and maximum up to 22 weeks. The optimum time period of doing this scan may vary a little in different parts of the world depending on the local rules for permission of legal abortions.

At this gestational age most fetal structures are already functional and therefore a detailed scan at this time is planned. More over the bones are also not too dense at this stage to obstruct the view of the soft tissues of the fetus. Though usually this scan is not done before 18 weeks, it may be planned at 16–18 weeks especially for fetuses at a higher risk of abnormalities. This group may include those with abnormal ultrasound findings or abnormal biochemical markers in the first trimester, fetuses of mothers with previous abnormal babies, old age mothers, etc.

As mentioned earlier this scan is done to assess the complete fetal anatomy and a systematic approach is required. It is ideal to move from crown to feet or feet to crown in any fetus, so that no part of the body would be left out. But it is known that fetus is moving and sometimes may be very active to allow to assess the intended part of its body. Therefore when doing fetal assessment one has to be opportunistic and start with imaging the part of the fetal body that is readily seen. In this case, it might be possible to skip or forget to image and assess certain parts of the fetal body, therefore it is best to make a checklist of the sections and measurements of the fetal body required and confirm that all the items on the checklist are assessed before the scan is declared complete.

A list of sections suggested by fetal medicine foundation, UK and most authentic workers in the field, for this scan is as follows:

HEAD AND FACE

Axial Sections

- Transventricular plane
- Transthallamic plane
- Transcerebellar plane
- Transorbital plane
- Maxillary plane.

Coronal Pane

- Lips
- Lenses.

Midsagittal Plane

- Nasal bone, frontomaxillary facial angle.

TRUNK

Axial Sections

Thorax

- Four chamber heart
- RVOT
- LVOT
- Three vessel trachea view.

Abdomen

- Stomach section for abdominal circumference
- Kidneys
- Umbilical cord insertion
- Sacrum transverse.

Sagittal Plane

- Spine
- Bladder
- Aortic arch—optional
- Ductus arch—optional.

Coronal Plane

- Spine.

Limbs

- All four limbs, all three segments
- Sagittal leg and foot
- Forearm with hand.

It is very essential that all these sections are imaged in a standardized manner to be reliable and comparable, with least interobserver and intra-observer variations. It is also important for optimal anatomical analysis and also for the measurements (biometry) that are to be used for assessment of fetal growth or prediction of any abnormalities of the fetus. To minimize the errors in anatomical details and measurements, it is also essential that the image is optimized and area of interest must be in the center of the screen and sufficient zoom should be used so that the image covers at least 2/3rd of the screen.

So let us discuss the details of each of these sections and the fetal anatomy that these demonstrate.

HEAD

Axial sections

These sections are usually easiest to achieve especially in a singleton fetus.

Transventricular Plane

This plane cuts through the ventricles as shown in figure as line 'A' **(Figure 1)**. The optimum section must show posterior horns of lateral ventricles, choroid plexus, lateral sulcus, falx, cavum septum and anterior horns of lateral ventricles **(Figure 2)**. The oval shape of the skull vault is seen in this section and the culvarial thickness should be symmetrical all around and not more than 3 mm in second trimester. Thicker culvarial thickness and especially asymmetrical may suggest an oblique section.

Thalami must not be seen in this section, as this section cuts higher up in the head. This is an ideal plane for assessment of the ventricles and choroid plexus. The abnormalities that can be picked up on this section are ventriculomegaly, hydrocephalus, choroid plexus cysts, holoprosencephaly, corpus callosal defects, skull vault defects, abnormal skull shape like brachy- or dolicocephaly **(Figures 3)**.

Transthallamic Plane (line B in the Figure 1)

This plane cuts through the thalamus. The optimum section must show the thallami,

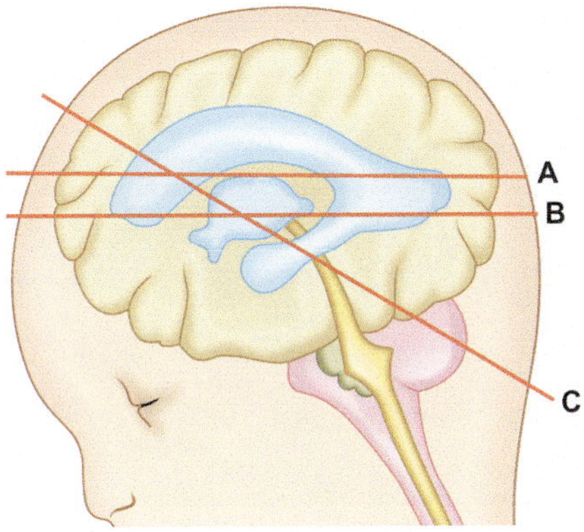

Figure 1: Diagram showing the three basic axial section of the head: (A) Transventricular section; (B) Transthallamic section; (C) Transcerebellar section

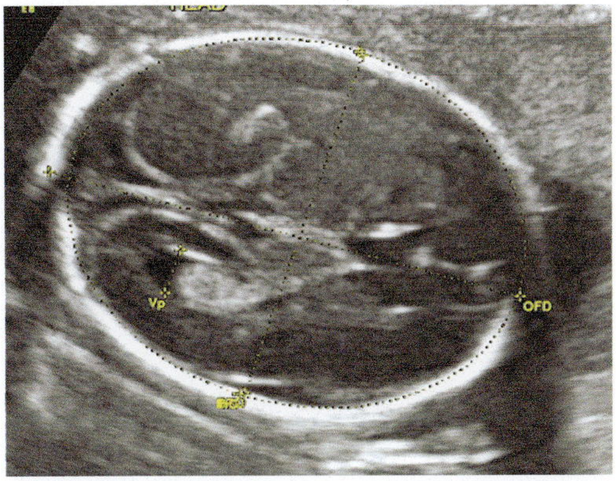

Figure 2: Transventricular section of the fetal head showing falx, cavum septum pellucidum, choroid plexuses in posterior horns of lateral ventricles

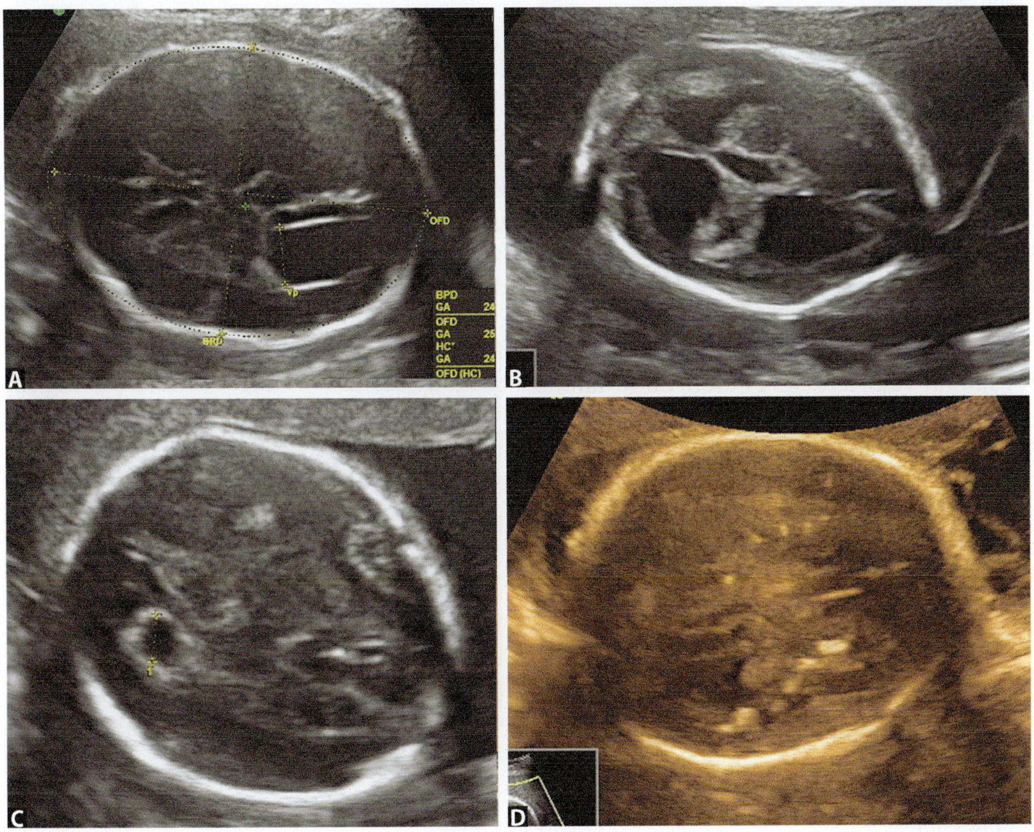

Figures 3A to D

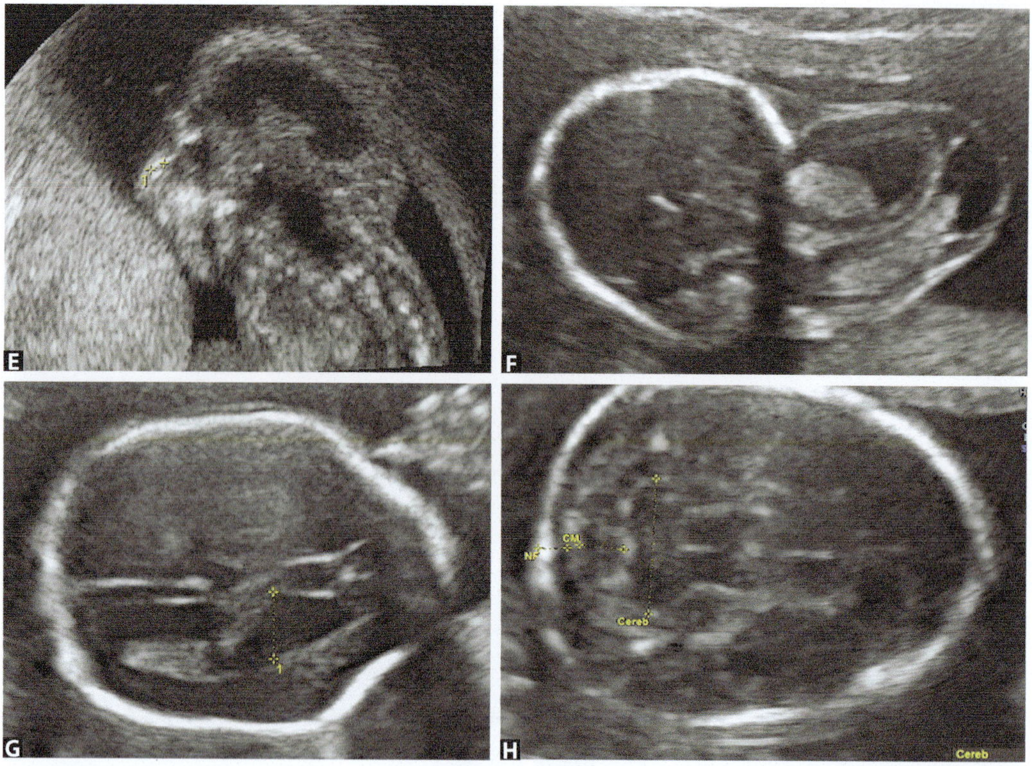

Figures 3E to H

Figure 3: (A) Ventriculomegaly; (B) Hydrocephalus; (C) Choroid plexus cyst; (D) Ventricular calcifications; (E) Anencephaly; (F) Exencephaly; (G) Lemon skull; (H) Brachycephaly

cavum septum pellucidum, anterior horns of lateral ventricle, falx cerebri and lateral sulcus. It also shows hippocampal gyrus, posterolateral to the thallami **(Figure 4)**. The complete oval skull vault should be seen, with symmetrical skull thickness all around and it should not be more than 3mm. This plane must not show cerebellum or orbits. This plane shows abnormalities of cavum septum pellucidum and corpus callosum, midline shift if present, is evident on this plane. Absence of lateral sulcus is an earliest indicator of lissencephaly. Coronal sutures can be identified in this plane and therefore abnormalities like craniostenosis can be diagnosed.

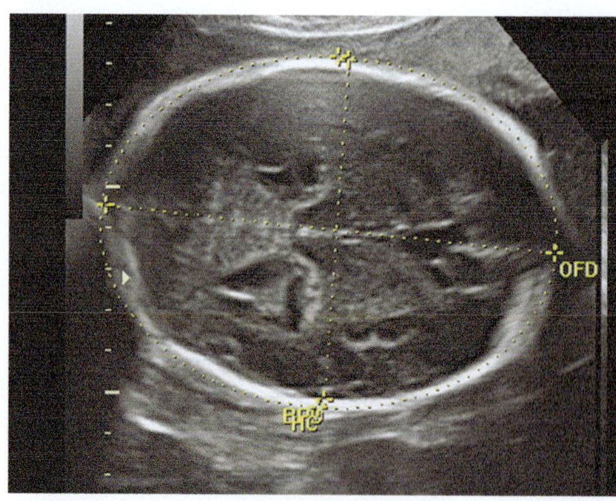

Figure 4: Transthallamic section showing falx, cavum septum pellucidum

Cavum septum pellucidum: Cavum septum is a cavity in the midline inferior to the corpus callosum. It is visible at 16 weeks and obliterates near term. This means it must always be visualized between 18 and 37

weeks, which means when BPD of between 44–88 mm.

Both of these above mentioned planes can be used for the quantitative assessment of the head. This consists of biparietal diameter (BPD), occipitofrontal diameter (OFD), and head circumference (HC) **(Figure 5)**. Though conventionally these were measured in transthallamic plane, the recent trend is to measure these in transventricular plane. Transventricular plane is also used to assess the ventricular diameter.

There is also a suggestion that transthallamic plane may be omitted from the routine protocol of second trimester targeted scan. But another consideration is that in the late trimester as the brain matter develops, there is compression on the ventricles and ventricular size decreases. This might at times make identification of ventricles difficult and therefore transventricular plane may be difficult to obtain. In this case if head parameters were measured in transventricular plane during 2nd trimester scan, its comparison for growth assessment might become difficult or less accurate in 3rd trimester.

Biparietal Diameter

This measurement is taken perpendicular to falx cerebri, at the broadest part of the oval

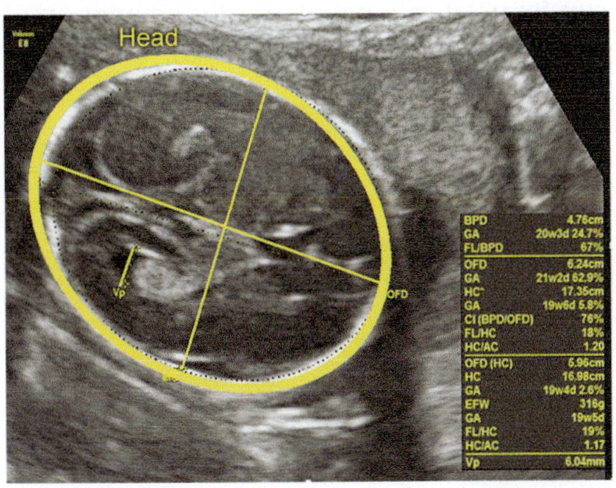

Figure 5: Transventricular section of the head showing the assessment of biparietal diameter (BPD), occipitofrontal diameter (OFD), head circumference (HC) and ventricular width

skull vault, this is usually at the mid-point between the frontal and the occipital end of the oval skull vault as seen in this axial section. The measurement is taken from outer margin of the proximal parietal bone to the inner margin of the distal parietal bone.

Biparietal diameter increases by:

- 3 mm/wk till 30 wks
- 1.5 mm/wk 30–38 wks
- 1 mm/wk after 38 wks
- Nil at 42 wks.

IUGR is suspected if growth rate is decreased by <5th percentile. There is a high chance of error when the measurements are between 5th and 10th percentile.

Sensitivity of BPD is considered as only 45% at 34–36 wks for prediction of gestational age. Though its sensitivity for growth assessment is much higher in earlier pregnancy. As such as the pregnancy advances the genetic factors play a role in controlling the growth pattern and so with advancing pregnancy the accuracy of growth assessment with all biometric parameters decrease. This measurement is not much affected by placental insufficiency or nutritional deprivation and so is more reliable than abdominal circumference, though it is variable with change in skull shape, like brachycephaly or dolichocephaly. In such cases it is considered reliable only when CI is 70–85% (CI : BPD/OFD × 100). As long as the CI is within normal limits, the head shape is considered normal. But when CI is <70 or >85, these are indicators of pathologically abnormal head shape.

Head Circumference

It is measured on the outer edges of culvarium, not the scalp, on the same plane as BPD. It is the better predictor of gestational age as compared to other commonly used predictors.

This parameter is not affected by change in head shape as long as CI is within limits (70–85). Its sensitivity is 52% and specificity is 80% for prediction of age in the third trimester.

It is altered in Trisomy 18 -where the head is strawberry shaped or in craniosynostosis.

Depending on the head parameters, the IUGR can be classified as:

- Type I (symmetrical)—Below-2SD (standard deviation) in early pregnancy and remains parallel to the normal growth curves
- Type II (asymmetrical)—Falls below line after 30 weeks, and therefore it cuts across the normal growth curves
- Type III—Intermediate pattern when there is early deviation of the growth curves, usually in the second trimester.

Ventricular Atrium Diameter

It is the measurement of the size of the lateral ventricles. It is measured at the level of parieto-occipital sulcus, perpendicular to the medial ventricular wall and not perpendicular to the midline. Calipers are placed inside the ventricular walls **(Figure 6)**.

The lateral ventricle to hemisphere ratio decreases from 70% at 18–20 weeks to 30% at 28–29 weeks and remains steady there after. In second and third trimester, it measures 6–8 mm, 8–10 mm is borderline ventriculomegaly and > 10 mm is ventriculomegaly. Ventricular diameter of up to 10 mm is treated expectantly, if it is a solitary finding. Larger ventricular diameters may be considered as a soft marker for chromosomal abnormality. Ventricular diameter of 10–12 mm is ventriculomegaly and >15 mm with increased pressure is called hydrocephalus and may be associated thinning of skull vault and widening of sutures. It is also a marker of abnormal cerebral development. This may require in utero or immediate postnatal treatment of the fetus.

Transcerebellar Plane (Line C on the Figure 1)

This section passes through the cerebellar hemispheres. It is obtained by angulating the probe towards fetal back from the transthallamic plane. Optimum transcerebellar section will show the cerebellar hemispheres, cisterna magna, falx cerebri, septum pellucidum and also cuts through the thalamus. Lateral sulcus also extends to this level. As for the previous two sections, the skull vault should be seen as a complete oval outline and should be symmetrical. Orbits should not be seen on this section. Cerebellar hypoplasia, megacisterna magna, Dandy walker's syndrome and variant, Blake's pouch cyst are the lesions, diagnosed on this section **(Figure 7)**.

Cerebellum: It is measured from outer to outer margin of the cerebellum on transcerebellar section. Transverse cerebellar diameter increases by 1 mm every week from 14 to 21 weeks. Diameter corresponds to the weeks of gestation in second trimester and is not affected by IUGR. Therefore in cases of severe IUGR it can be used as a parameter for estimation of correct gestational age **(Figure 8)**.

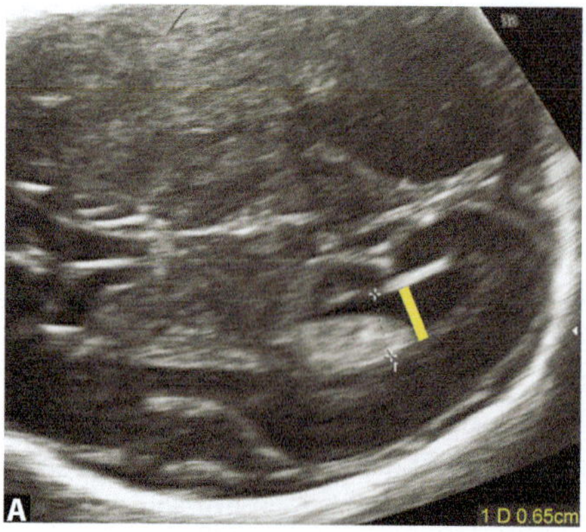

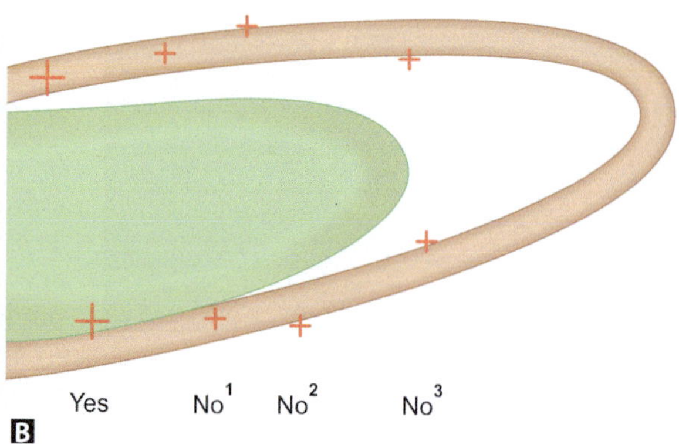

Figure 6: Ultrasound image and diagram showing assessment of ventricular width

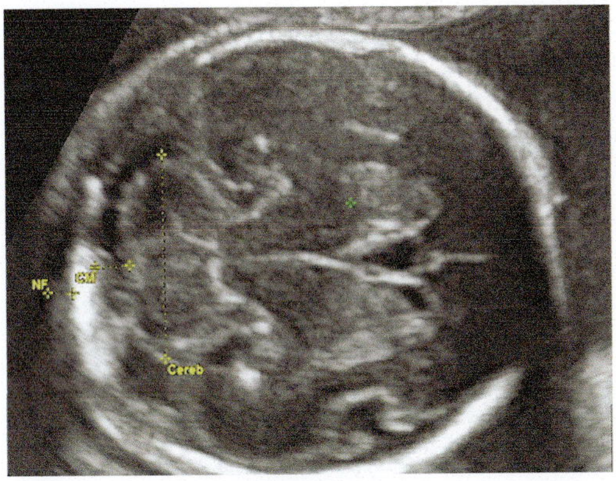

Figure 7: Transcerebellar section of fetal head showing falx, cavum septum pellucidum, thalamus, cerebellum, cisterna magna and nuchal fold

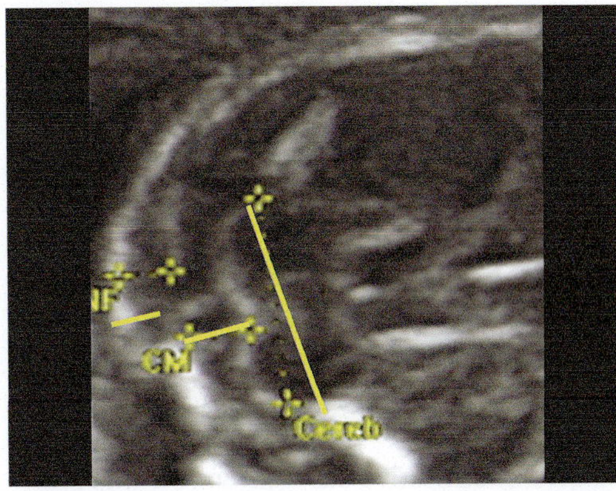

Figure 8: Transcerebellar section of the head (magnified view) showing measurements of cerebellum, cisterna magna and nuchal fold thickness

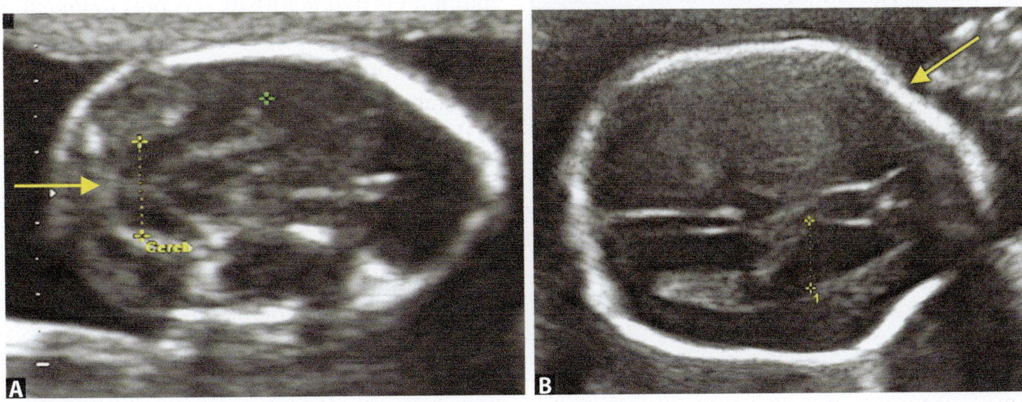

Figure 9: (A) Obliteration of the posterior concavity of the cerebellum due to open spinal canal defect making cerebellum look like a banana; (B) Collapsing of the frontal bones due to open spinal canal defect make the culvarial shape look like a lemon skull

Cisterna magna: It is measured from posterior margin of cerebellar vermis to the anterior margin of overlying occipital bone **(see Figure 8)**. Cisterna magna is traversed by thin septa and this is a normal appearance. These represent remnants of the walls of Blake's pouch. These are markers of development of roof of rhombencephalon.

It measures 2–10 mm but is slightly more in dolicocephaly. It is enlarged in cerbellar pathologies, especially in vermian pathologies, like vermian hypoplasia, Dandy walker's malformations or variants but in neural canal defects when cerebellum is pulled caudally and cistern magna is obliterated. This is known as 'banana sign' of cerebellum. This is also associated with collapsed frontal bones and makes the skull shape like a lemon and is called' lemon sign' **(Figure 9)**.

Though major open spinal canal defects can be suspected as early as the 11–13+6 weeks scan. Intracranial translucency is seen in the midsagittal section of 11–14 weeks fetus **(Figure 10)**. This should have a minimum diameter of 2 mm at this gestational age. If it is decrease, it indicates posterior displacement of posterior fossa structures due to spinal canal defect.

Transorbital Plane

This plane cuts through the middle of the orbits. It is obtained by slight angulation of the probe towards fetal anterior aspect. It shows both bony orbits in transverse section with nasal bones in between. It might cut through the upper part of the thalamus, but should not show the cerebellum. Bony orbits on this plane show lens—one in each orbit and may also show the artery posterior to it **(Figure 11A)**.

The quantitative assessment on this plane includes the binocular diameter, interocular diameter and ocular diameter **(Figure 11B)**.

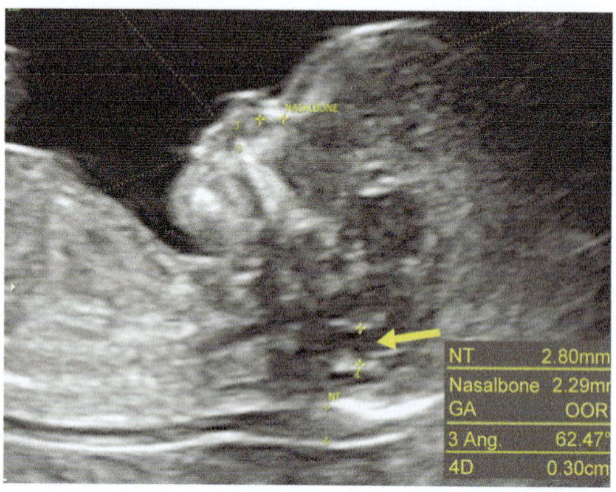

Figure 10: Midsagital section of 11–14 weeks fetus showing intracranial translucency

Binocular diameter is measured as the largest distance from lateral inner wall of one orbit to the lateral inner wall of another orbit. Interocular diameter is measured as broadest diameter from medial inner bony wall of one orbit to medial inner bony wall of another orbit. Ocular diameter is measured as broadest diameter of orbit from medial inner bony wall to lateral inner bony wall. Interocular distance and ocular diameter are almost equal always. This plane is used to diagnose abnormalities of the orbits like hypotelorism, hypertelorism, single orbit, anophthalmia.

Increased interocular diameter is hypertelorism and decreased interocular diameter is hypotelorism. It is best to take the measurements when the fetus is facing the probe. Though lenses are best seen when the fetal face is not towards the probe but on one of the sides.

Plane of Maxilla

This plane is just slightly caudal to the transorbital plane. This plane shows the tooth line of maxilla. This plane is best achieved in a fetal position where the fetus faces the probe. It is used to exclude maxillary abnormalities like cleft palate. The soft tissues seen anterior to the maxilla is the upper lip and so it is one

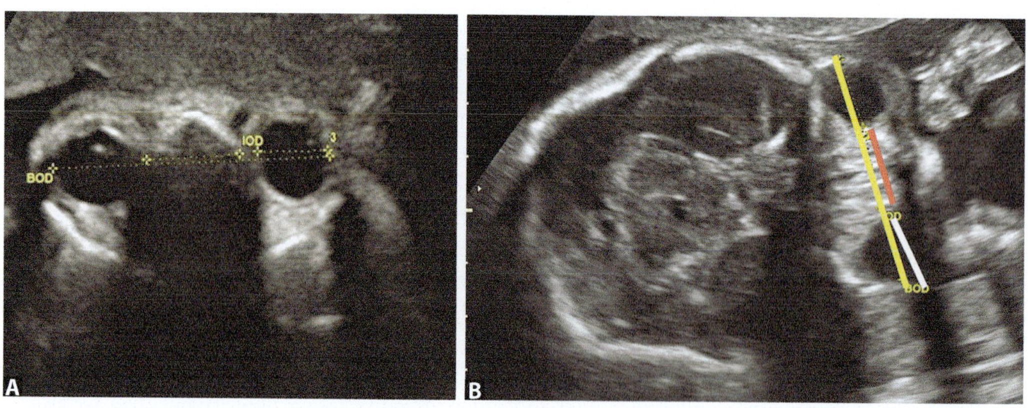

Figure 11: (A) Transorbital section showing both orbits with lenses; (B) Transorbital section showing the binocular (yellow), interocular (red) and ocular diameters (white)

of the views suggested for diagnosis of cleft lip and palate **(Figure 12)**.

HEAD: CORONAL SECTION

Lips (Figure 13)

From the previous plane 90° rotation of the probe shows coronal or sagittal plane. If sagittal plane is seen on this rotation, lift up the probe to place it on one of the sides of the maternal abdomen to see the coronal plane. Move the probe then towards anterior aspect of the fetus and this will show the tip of the nose/nostrils, upper lip and the lower lip. This plane is used for diagnosis of cleft lip. Fetuses with cleft lip may also show asymmetry of the nostrils which may be seen on this section as well.

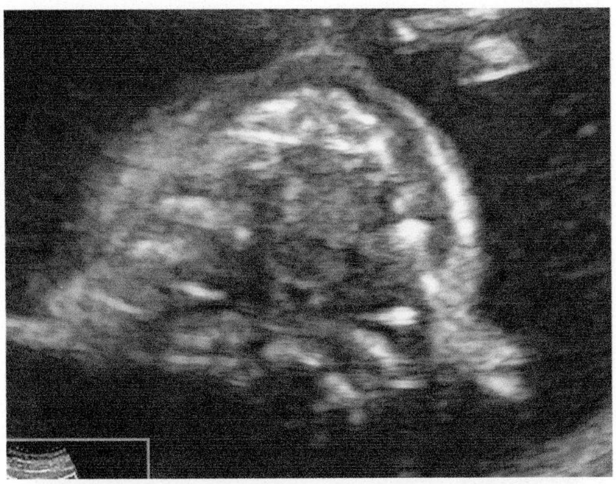

Figure 12: Maxilla in transverse section

Midsagital Plane

This plane is same as the midsagittal plane taken for nuchal translucency on nuchal scan. A true plane will show the tip of the nose, maxilla in sagittal section as a bold line and not as a triangle, nasal bone, mandible is seen as a dot, frontal process of maxillary bone is not seen between nasal bone and maxilla. Because of the ossification of the frontal bone, brain anatomy is not much seen on this section at this stage of pregnancy. This plane is obtained in a fetal position when the fetus is preferably facing the probe. Nasal bone length and fronto-maxillary-facial angle are the two measurements taken on this plane **(Figure 14)**. Nasal bone length is measured end to end. Frontomaxillary facial angle is measured by drawing one line on the superior surface of the maxilla and the other line is a line joining anterior-superior end of maxilla to the nasion.

Nasion is the point where the nasal bone is attached to the frontal bone. Frontomaxillary facial angle is 66.6°–89.5° in normal fetus with a mean of 78.5°. The trisomy 21 fetuses because of the flat face or a flat nasal bridge, this angle is increased to 75.4° to 104°, with a mean of 88.7°. Even a rotation of the fetal face of 2–3° can lead to a measurement error of

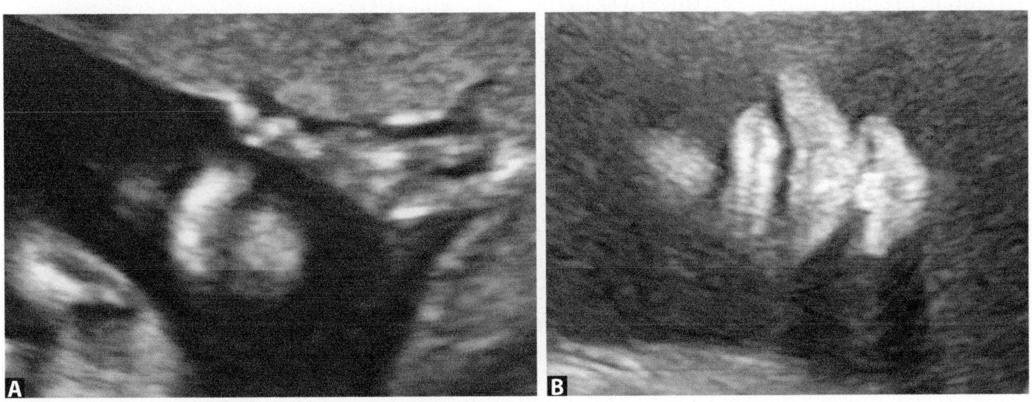

Figure 13: Nostrils, upper lip, lower lip and chin seen in coronal section

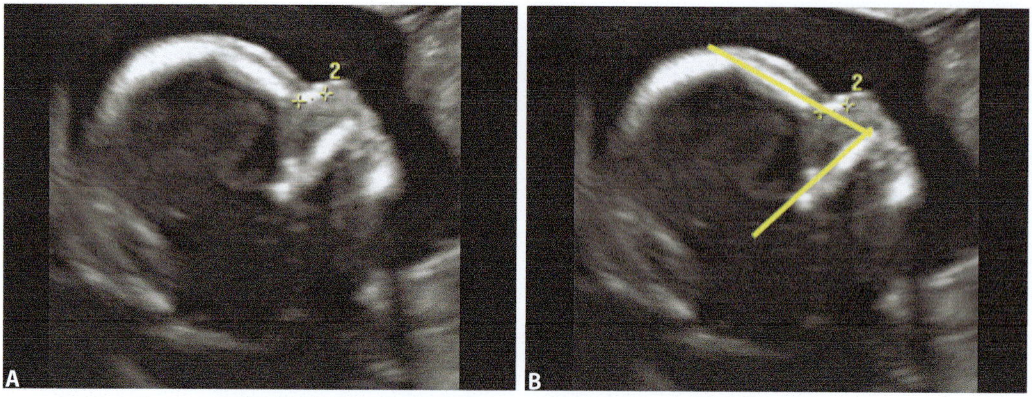

Figure 14: Midsagittal section of the head showing nasal bone assessment in figure on the left (A) and frontomaxillary-facial angle assessment in figure on the right (B)

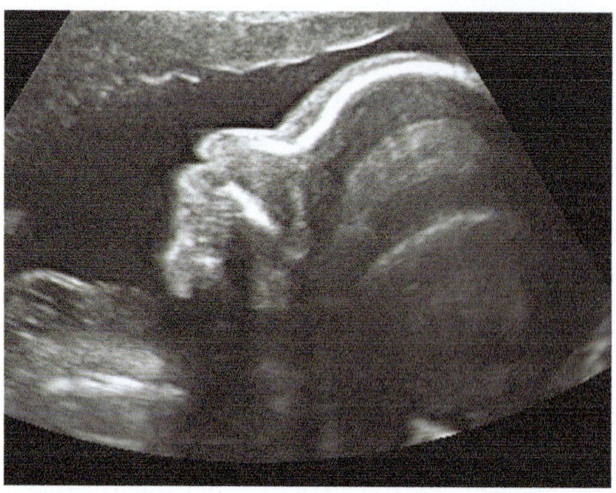

Figure 15: Midsagittal section of the head showing a small receeding chin- micrognathia

5-15°. Therefore a correct fetal position is very essential. Prenasal thickness (thickness of the skin anterior to the nasion) is also assessed now as one of the markers for trisomy 21.

It is this section which will also demonstrate micrognathia **(Figure 15)**. This can also quantitatively assessed. Cephalometric analysis by prenatal sonography can be performed to study the anteroposterior jaw relationship. We think that this procedure could be useful to improve prenatal diagnosis of retrognathism in high-risk pregnancies.[1] Inferior facial angle (IFA) and the frontal nasomental angle have been used on stored gray scale images to objectively establish the diagnosis. The mean values for IFA and frontal nasomental angle were 44.8° and 123.3°, respectively.[2]

TRUNK

Axial Sections: Chest

Four Chamber View of Heart (Figure 16)

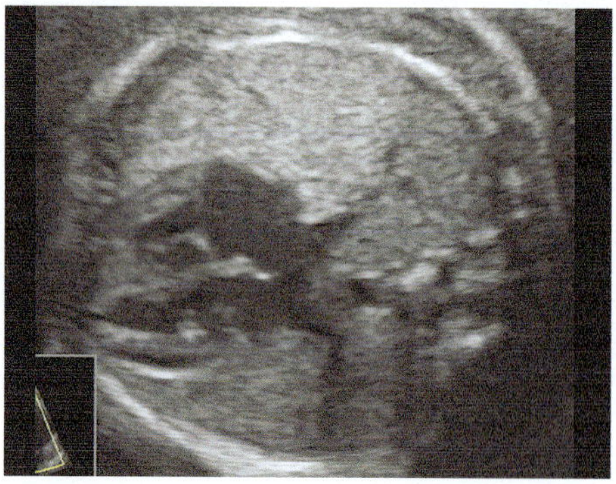

Figure 16: Four-chamber view of the heart

Left Ventricular Outflow Tract (Figure 17)

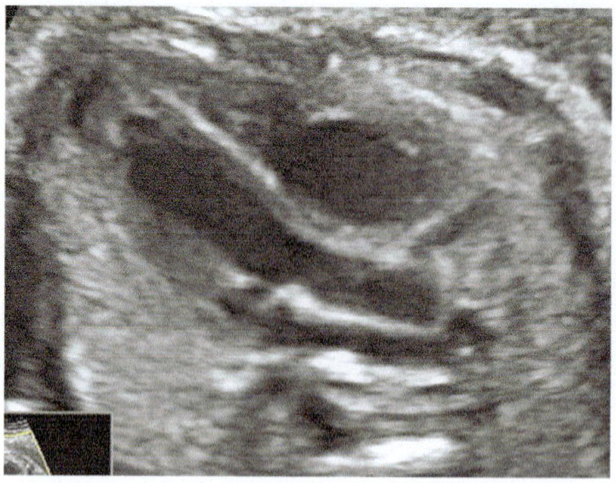

Figure 17: Left ventricular outflow tract

Right Ventricular Outflow Tract (Figure 18)

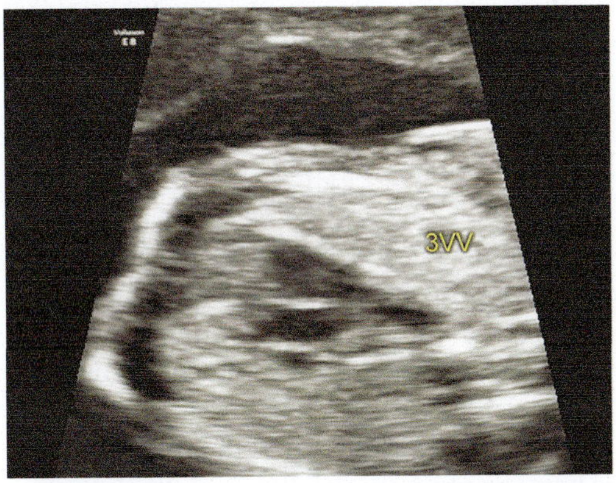

Figure 18: Right ventricular outflow tract

Three Vessel View (Figure 19)

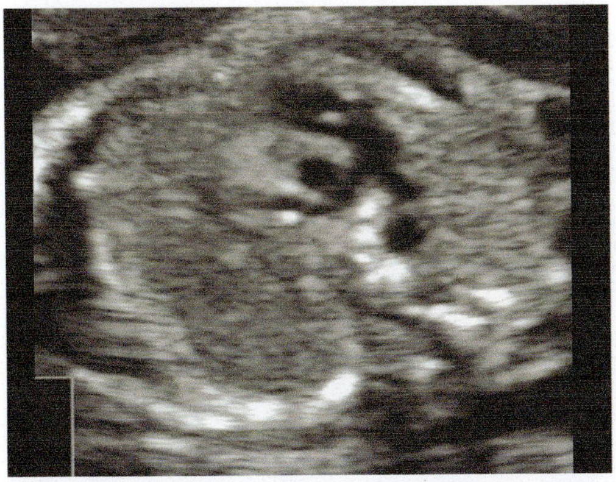

Figure 19: Three-vessel view

The above mentioned four planes **(Figures 16 to 19)** will be discussed in detail in the chapter 7 of this book.

Axial sections: Abdomen

- Section through stomach
- Section through renal pelves
- Section through umbilical cord attachment
- Section through sacrum (transverse sacrum section).

SECTION THROUGH THE STOMACH FOR ABDOMINAL CIRCUMFERENCE

As mentioned this section passes through the stomach and entry of umbilical vein to DV seen as a J with curve of the J concave towards fetal right **(Figure 20)**. The ribs cover the contour symmetrically on both sides. This ensures it is a true transverse section and the section is achieved during fetal apnea. Kidneys must not be seen on this plane.

Abdominal circumference is measured on the outer margin of this section. Most accurate is the smallest measurement. It shows linear rise till 36 weeks of 11–12 mm per week and fall thereafter. It is the first measurement to show alteration in IUGR. This is the single

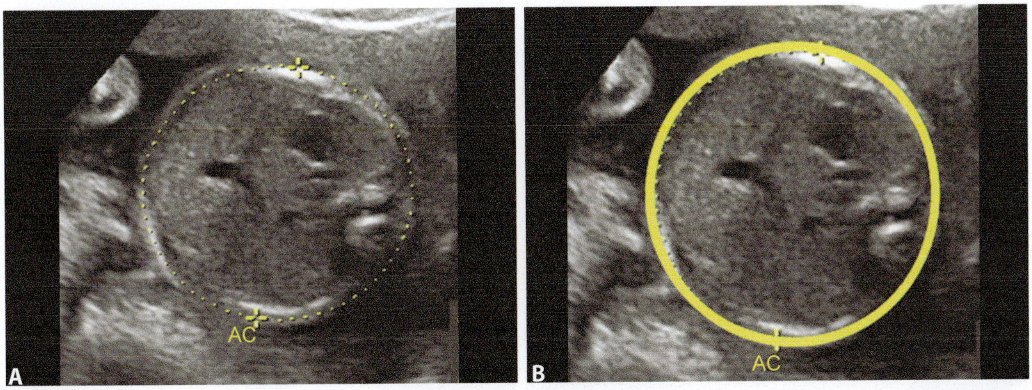

Figure 20: Axial section of the abdomen showing stomach and mid-third of the vein mentioned in the text above. Figure on the right side shows (B) the same plane with the measurement of abdominal circumference

most sensitive measure of fetal growth and so it is better to measure accurately, than to add other parameters.

UMBILICAL CORD INSERTION PLANE

This plane is a true transverse plane again and is caudal to the abdominal circumference plane. It is at the level where the umbilical cord enters the fetal abdomen.

This plane may be imaged on B mode or with Doppler **(Figure 21)**. Doppler has an advantage of showing the entry of cord vessels into fetal abdomen more clearly. This plane helps to exclude abnormalities like omphalocele and gastroschisis **(Figure 22)**.

Alternatively, some workers would prefer to demonstrate the cord vessels with the urinary bladder, to confirm the presence of two umbilical arteries.

RENAL PELVIS PLANE

This plane is caudal to the plane of cord insertion and it cuts the abdomen through both renal pelves. This plane should not include the stomach shadow and should be symmetrical and circular. This plane is used to measure the diameter of the renal pelvis. It is best to obtain this section with the fetus in a position with spine anterior or spine posterior. The renal pelvis diameter is measured

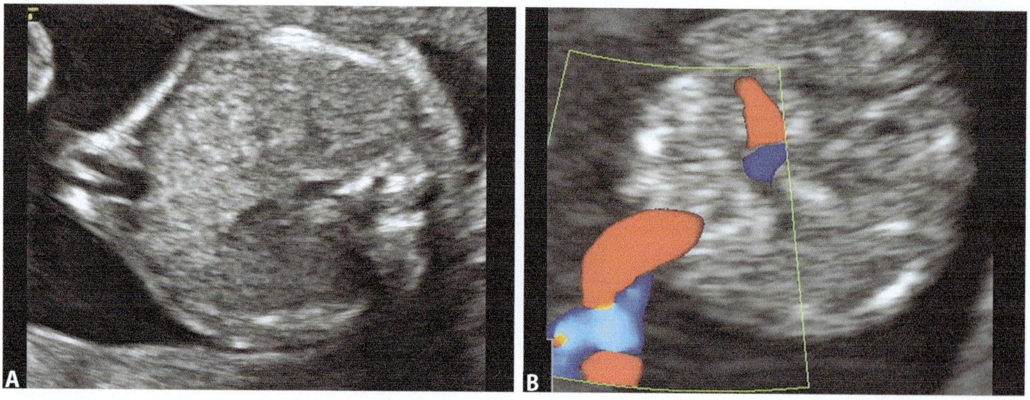

Figure 21: Axial section of the abdomen showing insertion of the umbilical cord. Figure on the left (A) shows B mode and figure on the right (B) shows color Doppler demonstration of the same

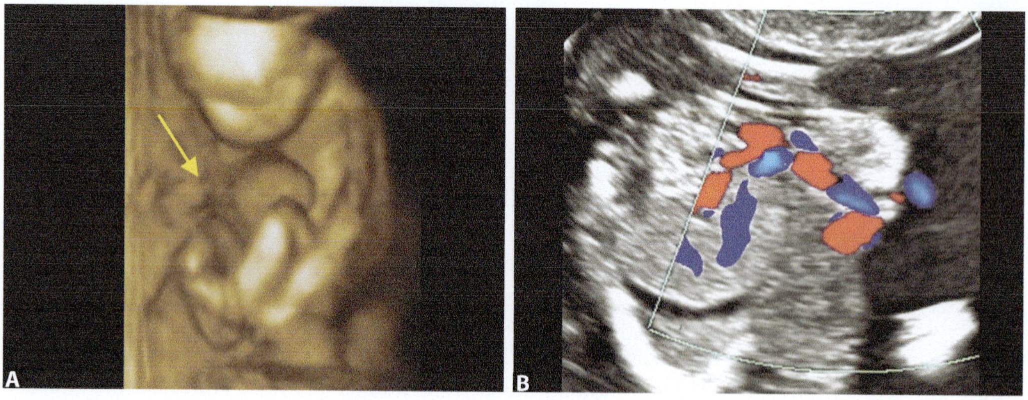

Figure 22: Figure on the left side (A) shows omphalocele with the umbilical cord arising from the dome of the herniation, figure on the right side (B) is gastroschisis where the cord is seen arising from the side of the herniation in color Doppler

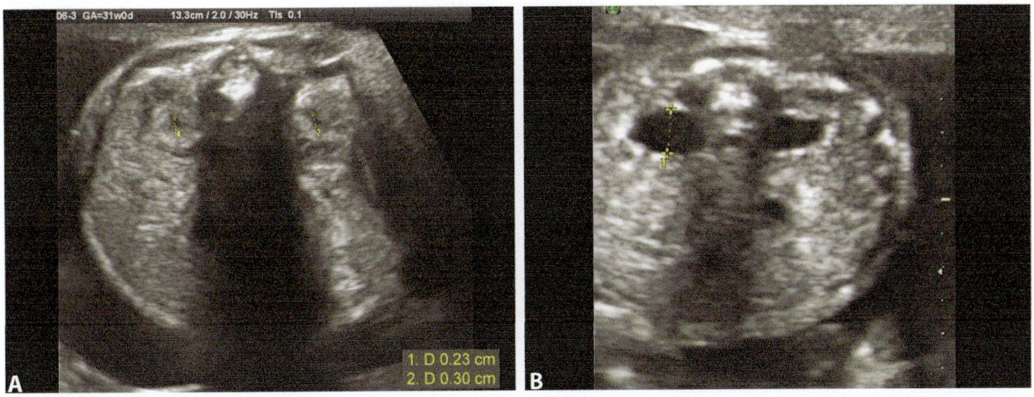

Figure 23: Both figures show transverse section of the abdomen at the level of renal pelvis. Figure on the right side (B) shows assessment of renal pelvic diameter

anteroposteriorly, from inner margin to inner margin **(Figure 23)**.

Normal measurements:

- 16–20 weeks, 4 mm
- 20–30 weeks, 5 mm
- 30–40 weeks, 7 mm.

Dilated renal pelvis may be indicative of chromosomal abnormality. There may also be an obstructive lesion in the ureter or bladder leading to dilatation of renal pelvis and may be unilateral or bilateral.

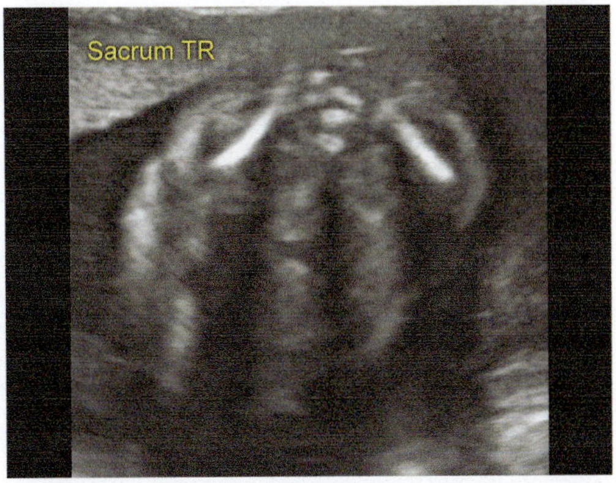

Figure 24: Axial section of the pelvis or transverse section of sacrum

TRANSVERSE SACRAL PLANE (FIGURE 24)

This is the lowest transverse section through the fetal trunk. Two iliac bones are seen with three ossification centers of the sacrum seen in the center. This helps to confirm absence of spina bifida or open sacral defects at the level of the sacrum.

TRUNK: ABDOMEN

Midsagittal Section (Figure 25)

This section is taken to assess the spine on sagittal section. It is seen as two parallel lines of echogenic dots (ossification centers). It is essential to establish the continuity of the overlying skin. It is also important to observe the whole spine, establish the continuity and also to confirm tapering of ossification centers of the sacrum. Though chiefly aimed to assess the spine this plane also shows the bladder, especially if the fetal spine is posterior.

Coronal Plane

A posterior coronal plane section is essential to observe the whole spine in coronal section **(Figure 26)**. At the level of vertebral bodies, it is seen as a single line of ossification centers and at the transverse process level it appears like two parallel lines. Widening of the distance between two lines may be indicative of spina bifida or open spinal canal. Both lines if do not make pairs of ossification centers, it may be indicative of hemivertebrae. On this

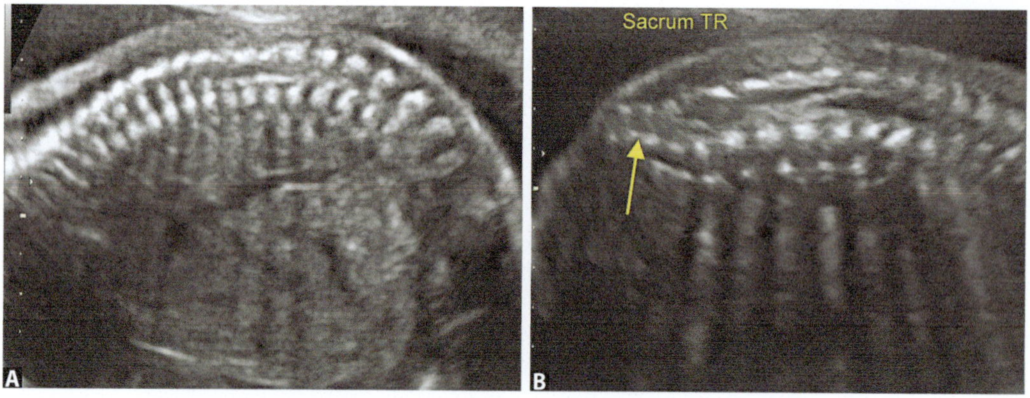

Figure 25: Midsagittal section of the trunk showing spine in sagittal plane, Figure A shows the cervicothoracic and upper lumber spine and; Figure B shows lumbosacral spine. Arrow shows the sacral tapering

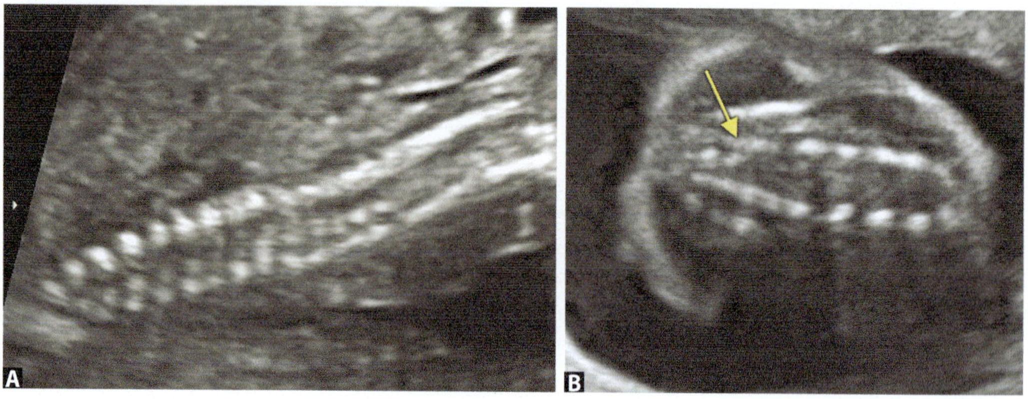

Figure 26: Coronal section of the spine showing transverse processes of vertebral bodies. Image on left (A) shows thoracolumbar spine and image on right (B) shows lumbosacral spine with sacral tapering (arrow)

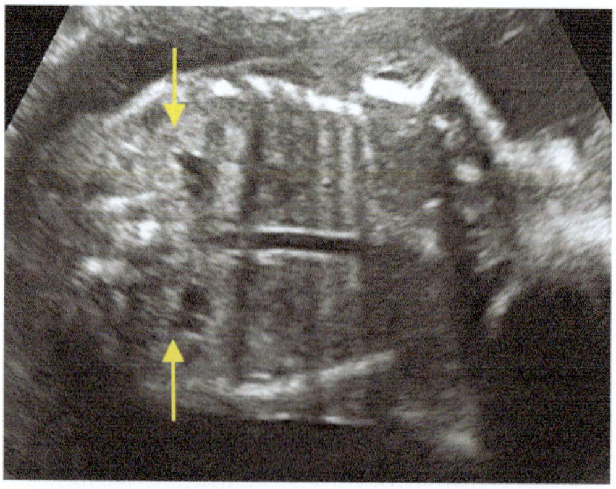

Figure 27: Coronal section of the abdomen, showing renal pelves on both the sides (arrow)

plane it is essential to establish the tapering of ossification centers of the sacral spine. The vertebral body plane, which is a slightly anterior to this plane, may also show kidneys in coronal plane.

Seeing kidneys in this plane is especially important for diagnosis of renal parenchymal disorders and renal dysplasias **(Figure 27)**.

LIMBS

It is essential to document the presence of all four limbs and all three segments of all the limbs. It is best to demonstrate both forearms

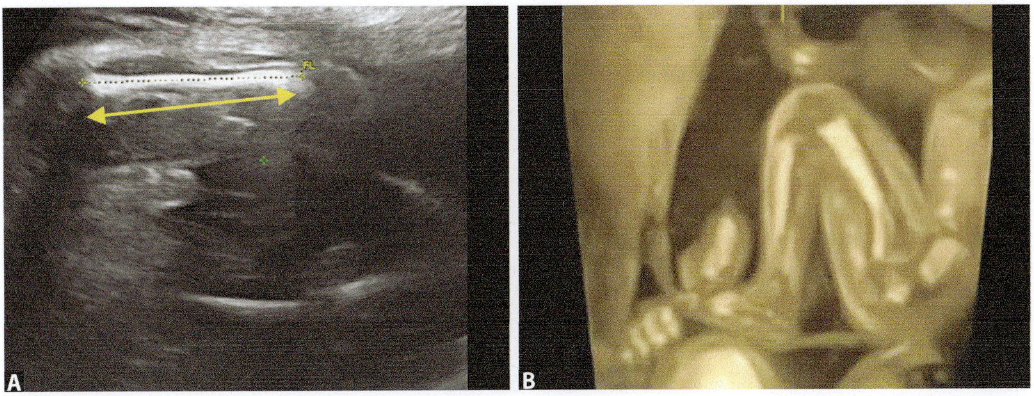

Figure 28: Image on the left side (A) shows the femur and its longitudinal measurement and image on the right side (B) shows the full lower limb. The special attention is towards the normal relationship of leg to foot

and hands in a single image and both legs and feet in a single image to establish both limbs have been assessed.

In leg and forearm, presence of two long bones must be documented. Relation of foot to leg and forearm to hand must be established. Long bones must be measured from end to end, **(Figure 28)** excluding the epiphysis. Though counting fingers and toes may be done, it is not mandatory for the detailed 2nd trimester scan. If an open hand can be demonstrated is an image which would be of significance **(Figure 29)**.

When measuring the femur length, long axis of femur should be aligned with the transducer and only osseous part of diaphysis and metaphysis is measured. Femur grows at a rate of 3 mm/week from 14 to 27 weeks and 1 mm/ week in third trimester.

It shows moderate curvature from 18 weeks onwards giving a typical 'golf club' like appearance. It is not affected in asymmetrical IUGR, but is affected in symmetrical IUGR. But as compared to femur length only, FL/AC has been considered to be more reliable. This is so because, independent of gestational age the ratio remains constant after 22 weeks. Its sensitivity is 63%, and positive predictive value is 30% for IUGR.

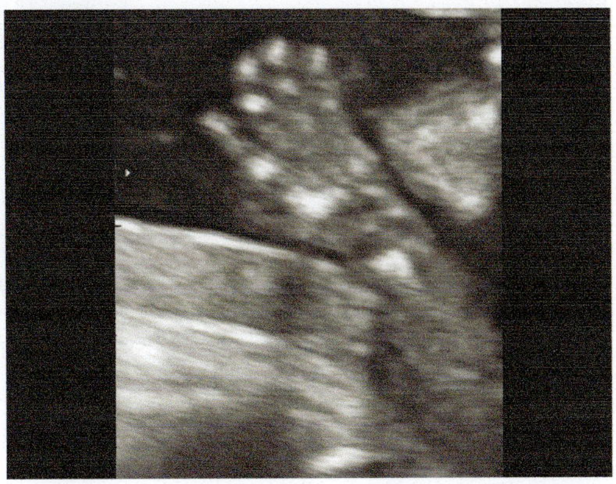

Figure 29: Image shows open hand with fingers and thumb seen individually

Authors prefer to measure femur, humerus and tibia in all fetuses.

Apart from assessment of the fetus, it is preferable to assess the placenta and the umbilical cord insertion in the placenta. Though the placenta and umbilical cord will be discussed more in detail in chapter 11 of this book. Amniotic fluid index is assessed as vertical fluid pouch in all four quadrants. The probe must be always kept vertical during assessment of the amniotic fluid index and the deepest pouch clear of umbilical cord loops or fetal limbs is selected **(Figure 30)**. Though many workers would prefer to assess only

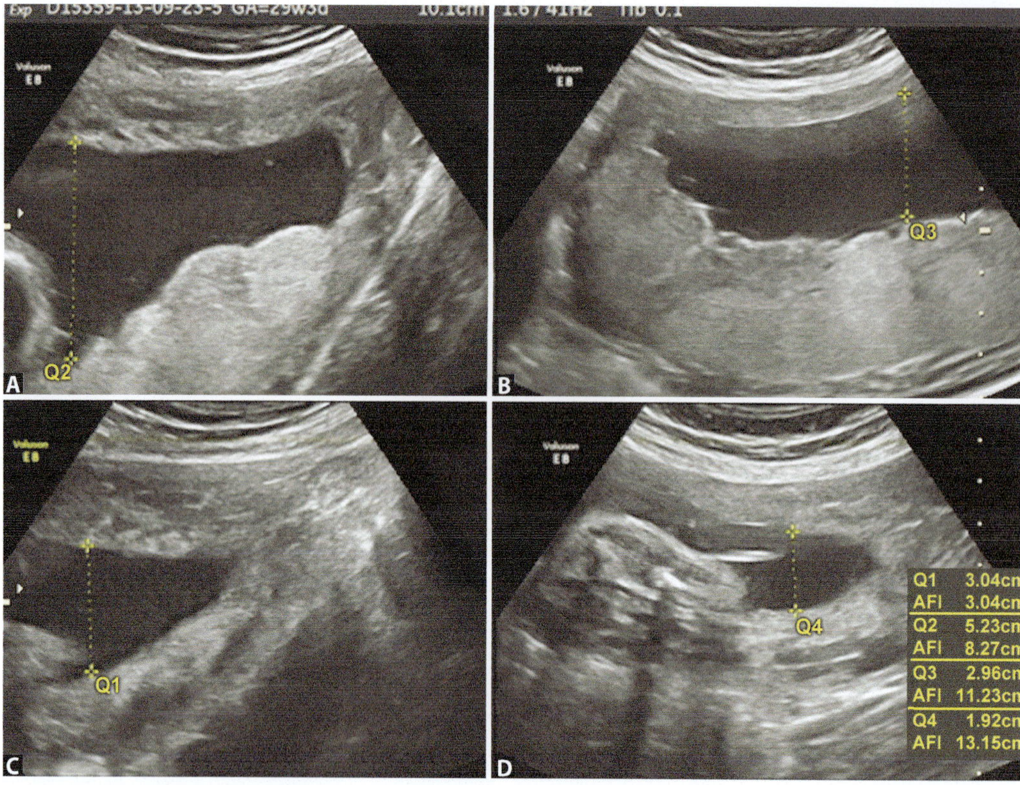

Figure 30: Image shows assessment of the amniotic fluid index in four quadrants

the depth of one largest pocket of amniotic fluid. And a single pocket of 5–8 cms may be considered adequate.

Apart from this the second trimester scan must include assessment of the uterine artery and umbilical artery Doppler. Umbilical artery flow can be assessed in any free loop of umbilical cord but in very mobile fetus, the cord insertion at the placenta may be selected as a site of preference for Doppler assessment of the umbilical artery. Though is thought that the resistance is a little different at the fetal end and the placental end, this difference is not of much clinical significance.

Umbilical artery flow is usually a moderate resistance flow **(Figure 31)** and normally the resistance keeps on decreasing as age advances.

The uterine artery is localized by moving the probe from the symphysis pubis laterally,

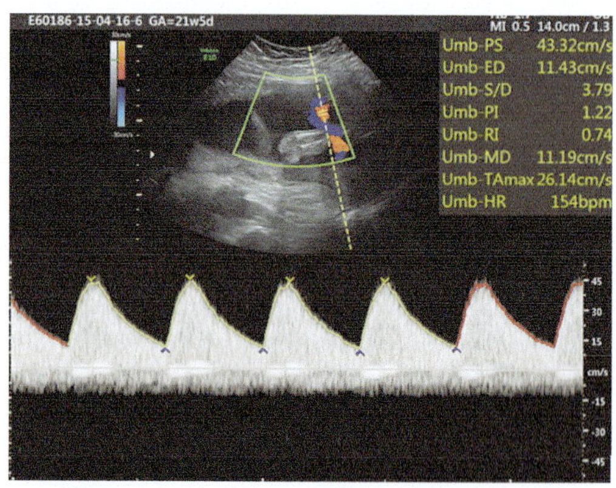

Figure 31: Spectral Doppler of umbilical artery showing its normal waveform

without angulating it. Where the iliac vessels are seen in long axis, a slight medial angulation of the probe shows uterine artery crossing iliac vessels perpendicularly. Uterine arteries are usually high resistance vessels in the early pregnancy but are fairly low resistance vessels in later pregnancy, **(Figure 32)** especially on the side of the placenta if the placenta is not central.

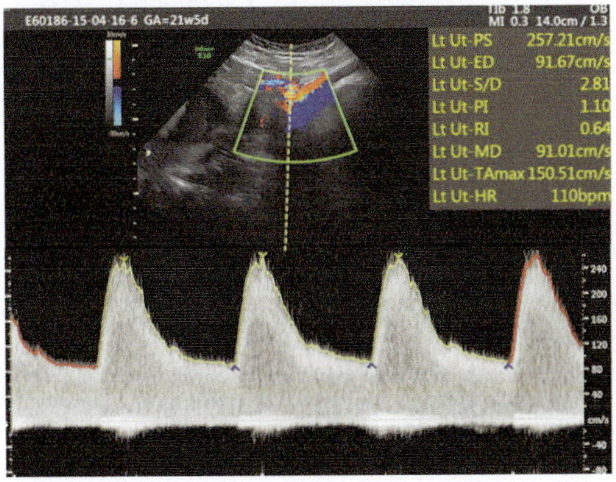

Figure 32: Spectral Doppler of uterine artery normal waveform in 2nd and 3rd trimestera

A systematic scan thus done in the 2nd trimester is capable to excluding almost all major and especially non-progressive abnormalities of the fetus.

REFERENCES

1. Captier G, Faure JM, Bäumler M, Canovas F, et al. Prenatal assessment of the Anteroposterior Jaw relationship in human fetuses: From Anatomical to Ultrasound Cephalometric Analysis. Cleft Palate-Craniofacial Journal. 2011;48(4):465-72.
2. Rotten D, Levaillant JM, Martinez H, Ducou le Pointe H, Vlcaut E. The fetal Mandible: A 2D and 3D sonographic approach to the diagnosis of retrognathia and micrognathia. Ultrasound Obstet Gynecol. 2002;19(2):122-30.

3
CHAPTER

Screening for Down Syndrome: Clinical Perspectives

S Boopathy Vijayaraghavan, Pavithra M Vengetesh

INTRODUCTION

This chapter aims to provide clinicians an insight into the various screening tests for Down syndrome and their performances. It will consider the differences between screening and diagnostic tests with detailed explanation of risk calculation with respect to every screening protocol. The chapter will conclude with the current recommendations put forth by the international bodies, concerning with choosing the appropriate screening approach for the individual pregnant woman.

DOWN SYNDROME

Down syndrome is the commonest chromosomal disorder in clinical practice. It is due to trisomy of chromosome 21. Its incidence is about 1 in 700 live-births.[1] The survival rate for liveborn infants with trisomy 21 is high with 85% of them surviving until their 50s.[2] The extrachromosome disrupts the normal course of development and results in disabilities and morbidities. Children with Down syndrome have characteristic facies and mild to moderate intellectual disability. They reach their developmental milestones later than normal children. Almost half of liveborns have major congenital heart defects and they remain the major cause of early mortality. They have a very high risk to develop leukemia and blood dyscrasia.[3]

Why Should Down Syndrome be Screened?

Prenatal diagnosis of Down syndrome is carried out by karyotyping the fetal tissue obtained by chorionic villus sampling (CVS) or amniocentesis, which are invasive tests. They carry a small risk of miscarriage, which preclude its use on every pregnant woman. Hence, there is a need for screening tests to identify those pregnant women who are at high risk of carrying a fetus with Down syndrome. These women can be offered invasive tests for diagnosis of trisomy 21. The screening also provides an opportunity to reassure most pregnant women that their fetus is unlikely to be affected by the chromosomal disorder. The explicit goal of prenatal screening is to reduce the incidence of disability, social and economic burden in the community. The screening programme for trisomy 21 takes precedence over the screening of other aneuploidies for the following reasons:

- Trisomy 21 is the commonest aneuploidy encountered in clinical practice and therefore there is a greater emphasis for its detection.
- About 80% of fetuses with trisomy 18 and 13, the other two common aneuploidies, miscarry or die in utero between 12 and 40 weeks in contrast to 30% of trisomy 21. So, 70% of trisomy 21 are born alive which is a significant contribution to disability.[4]
- Trisomy 18 and 13 are associated with major structural congenital malformations involving more than one system, which are picked up during prenatal ultrasonography. On the other hand, only 25–30% of trisomy 21 manifests with major anomalies.[5] Hence, if screening for Down syndrome is not emphasized, then there are high chances of trisomy 21 babies to be born.

SCREENING TESTS—CONSIDERATIONS

General Concepts of Screening

Screening is a means of detecting abnormal ones from a healthy population. Screening tests for aneuploidy provide an assessment of the risk of carrying an aneuploid fetus. Every screening test has a defined cut-off risk for its interpretation. Those above the cut-off risk are considered screen positives and they would undergo invasive tests for confirmation. The performances of screening tests are assessed by its sensitivity/detection rate and false positive rate. Detection rate (DR) is defined as the ability of the test to identify the affected fetuses in the population. The false positive rate (FPR) indicates the number of normal fetuses with a screen positive result. This has got important implications in prenatal diagnostics since the normal fetuses in the false positive group would be subjected to unnecessary invasive testing. Thus, a screening test should have a high DR and low FPR. Setting a low cut-off would increase the DR at the expense of a high FPR. A high cut-off would fail to identify some abnormal fetuses but will have a very low FPR. Both these factors have to be taken into consideration while assigning the cut-off for a screening test in order to produce consistent and accurate results. Any screening test should satisfy minimum standards in order to be applicable universally: It should have a DR of atleast 75% with FPR not more than 3–5%. Treatment decisions will not be made upon the results of the screening tests and thus, will require confirmatory tests in succession.

Who Should Be Offered Prenatal Screening Tests?

Until the mid 1980's, testing for aneuploidy was offered to only women above 35 years of age, who constituted just 5% of the pregnant population. It was later observed that such a screening strategy would detect only 30% of pregnancies with trisomy 21 and miss 70%. At present, the recommendation by the American College of Obstetricians and Gynecologists (ACOG) is to offer screening for aneuploidy to all pregnant women presenting for antenatal care before 20 weeks, regardless of their age.[6]

Pretest Counseling

Every screening procedure for aneuploidy should commence with a counseling session. The aim of pretest counseling is to facilitate the couple to make informed choices concerning the pregnancy outcome. It is the prime responsibility of the clinician and his/her team to explain to the couple about the condition to be screened (Down syndrome) and the disabilities and morbidities which the child would face. Information about the screening options relevant to their gestational age and the screening process should be provided. Pregnant women have to be informed that screening tests only target specific chromosomal problems and do not identify all the abnormalities. All women should be counseled regarding the differences between screening and diagnostic tests. Helping them understand the interpretation and perception of risk forms an integral part of counselling. They should be made to understand that when they are screen positive, they should undergo invasive test for confirmation. All of them should be given the option of invasive diagnostic testing.

It is imperative to know their reproductive choices. Termination of pregnancy is not accepted by all couples due to firm religious and social beliefs. If they do not entertain the option of termination in the event of diagnosis of trisomy 21, then the entire screening procedure would become meaningless and unnecessary, adding just expenditure to the couple. The clinician should take into consideration the education status of the couple before presenting the details. The information should be in simple language, balanced and non-directive. The couple should be given every opportunity to discuss with the clinician before they make a final decision.[7] Pre-test counseling is mandatory irrespective of whether the couple accepts or denies the screening test. Due respect have to be paid to their cultural and ethical issues.

Post-test Counseling

The post-test counseling involves explaining the risk (derived from the screening test) and to understand their perception of the concept of risk. If the risk is high enough to warrant an invasive test, they should be provided with all information regarding chorionic villus sampling or amniocentesis (depending on the gestational age). They should be informed about the procedure, the risks associated with them and the cost involved. Their decision to undergo the invasive test should be voluntary. If the risk is borderline, they should be given information about the requirement of further screening tests, available options and guidance for decision.

Understanding and Intrepretation of screening Tests

The results of the screening test are expressed as risk (for example, 1 in 150 means that out of the 150 pregnant women screened, only 1 woman will be carrying a trisomy 21 baby while the rest 149 are normal). Every woman has a risk of carrying a trisomy 21 baby. The risk increases with the maternal age as the chances of meiotic non-disjunction of the ovum and the eventual production of chromosomally abnormal conceptus increases with age. The risk decreases with the gestational age due to spontaneous loss of chromosomally abnormal fetuses. The maternal age and gestation specific risks for trisomy 21 are available.[8]

This background risk which depends upon the maternal age and gestational age is referred to as the 'a priori risk'. For example, the 'a priori risk' for a pregnant woman aged 35 years at 12 weeks of gestation is 1 in 249. If a woman had a previous baby or fetus with trisomy 21, the risk in the current pregnancy is increased by 0.75% than her age-related and gestation age-related risk. For example, 'a priori risk' for a pregnant woman aged 35 years at 12 weeks of gestation, if she had a previous baby or fetus with Down syndrome is increased from 1 in 249 (0.4%) to 1 in 87 (1.15%) by 0.75%. Even before screening every pregnant woman will be assigned 'a priori risk'. After the screening test, 'a priori risk' is multiplied by the likelihood ratio of the test to calculate the new risk. The likelihood ratio (LR) for a given sonographic or biochemical measurement is calculated by dividing the percentage of chromosomally abnormal fetuses by the percentage of normal fetuses with that measurement. This calculated new risk would then become the 'a priori risk' for the next test when sequential screening is performed.[9]

SCREENING TESTS

There are numerous approaches to screening for aneuploidy. They can be employed either in the first or second trimester depending on when the pregnant woman presents for antenatal care. In 1970, screening was restricted to mothers above 35 years. In 1980's, serum analytes were incorporated to the maternal age for screening in the second trimester. This method of screening was found more effective than maternal age alone and the detection improved to 70%. In the 1990's, screening was extended to the first trimester with similar rates of detection.

APPROACH TO SCREENING IN THE FIRST TRIMESTER

The available modalities for aneuploidy screening in the first trimester are ultrasonographic measurement of nuchal translucency (NT) and maternal serum biochemical markers. Screening is performed from 11 weeks to 13 weeks and 6 days. Accurate dating is imperative for risk estimation with NT and serum markers. The lower limit is chosen as 11 weeks for two reasons. Firstly, any screening program should be supported by the availability of a diagnostic test. Chorionic villous sampling is recommended only after 10 weeks since it is associated with transverse limb reduction defects in the fetus, when performed before 10 weeks. Secondly, many major structural fetal defects can be reliably diagnosed after 11 weeks, which if present may make further screening unnecessary. They would be offered CVS for karyotyping. The reasons for assigning 13 weeks and 6 days as the upper limit are to provide women carrying aneuploid fetus, the option of first rather than second trimester termination. Secondly, the presence of abnormal nuchal fluid collection in chromosomally abnormal fetuses is more pronounced before 14 weeks than at 14–18 weeks. The orientation of the fetus is more vertical after 14 weeks, rendering image acquisition and NT measurement difficult.

Nuchal Translucency (NT)

Nuchal translucency (NT) refers to the sonographic appearance of subcutaneous accumulation of fluid behind the fetal neck in the first trimester. The anteroposterior distance is measured in millimeters. Accurate measurement of NT requires adequate training, expertise and adherence to the standard protocols laid by the Fetal Medicine Foundation (FMF), UK. The individual measuring NT should be ideally certified by FMF and his/her performance should be regularly audited. The ultrasound machine should be of high resolution with a video-loop function and callipers that calibrate to one decimal point. NT can be measured accurately by transabdominal route in 95% of cases, while in others transvaginal ultrasonography would be required.

The following protocols are to be followed for precise NT measurement:[4]

- The minimum and maximum CRL should be 45 and 84 mm respectively. The success rate for taking a measurement at 11–13 weeks is 98–100%, which declines to 90% at 14 weeks.
- The magnification should be such that only the fetal head and upper part of the thorax occupy the screen. Each slight movement of caliper produces only a 0.1 mm change in the measurement. Before magnifying the image either pre- or post-freeze, the gain should be turned down to avoid fuzzy margins.
- A perfect sagittal section of the fetus is absolutely essential for measurement. The identification of the following landmarks would assure the correct section—presence of echogenic tip of nose, nasal bone and rectangular shape of palate anteriorly, translucent diencephalon (third ventricle) in the center and nuchal membrane posteriorly. Slight deviations from the midline would result in nonvisualization of the tip of nose and visibility of the zygomatic process of the maxilla.

- The fetal head should be in neutral position (amniotic fluid should be present between the fetal chin and thorax). Hyperextension of the neck will falsely increase NT by 0.6 mm, while hyperflexion will falsely reduce it by 0.4 mm.
- Care must be taken to distinguish between fetal skin and amnion.
- The maximum thickness of the subcutaneous translucency between the skin and the soft tissue overlying the cervical spine should be measured.
- The calipers should be placed on the interface between the tissue (white line) and nuchal fluid that describes the NT—the horizontal line of the crossbar of the caliper should merge with the white line of the margin and not seen in the nuchal fluid.
- It is important to take more than one measurement and record the maximum one.
- In the presence of nuchal cord, the average of two measurements taken on either side of the cord should be recorded.

The intraobserver and interobserver variations in NT are less than 0.5 mm in 95% of cases when the protocols are carefully practised. An ultrasound image in the proper section for measuring NT is shown in **Figure 1**. NT measurements vary with the crown-rump length (CRL). Hence, the gestational age should be taken into consideration for determining whether the NT measurement falls within the normal range (between 5th and 95th centile). The reference ranges of fetal nuchal translucency with respect to CRL is shown in **Figure 2.**[10] NT is a powerful marker of aneuploidy. The numbers of abnormal fetuses increase in direct relation to the NT measurement. When the NT is between 5th and 95th centile, the prevalence of chromosomally abnormal fetus is just 0.2% which increases to 3.5% when NT falls within 95th and 99th centile. The rate of chromosomal abnormality increases exponentially to 65% in fetuses with NT above 6.5 mm. About 75–80% of fetuses with trisomy 21 have NT values above the 95th centile.[4] For the estimation of risk, delta NT (in mm) is obtained by the difference between the measured NT and median NT for that particular CRL. Every delta NT represents a likelihood ratio, which is multiplied by the 'a priori risk' to derive the final risk.[11] Regular auditing of results and continuous assessment of the quality of images are important for successful screening. Increased NT is also associated with increasing number of other fetal defects and genetic syndromes. Early cardiac dysfunction is postulated as the central pathogenesis for increased NT for most of the conditions.

Serum Markers in the First Trimester

Trisomic pregnancies are associated with altered concentrations of fetoplacental

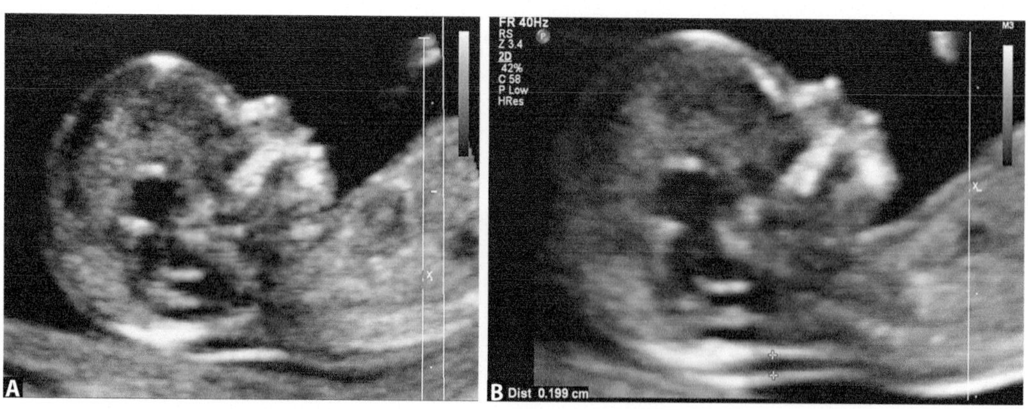

Figure 1: Ultrasound image for the measurement of nuchal translucency (NT)

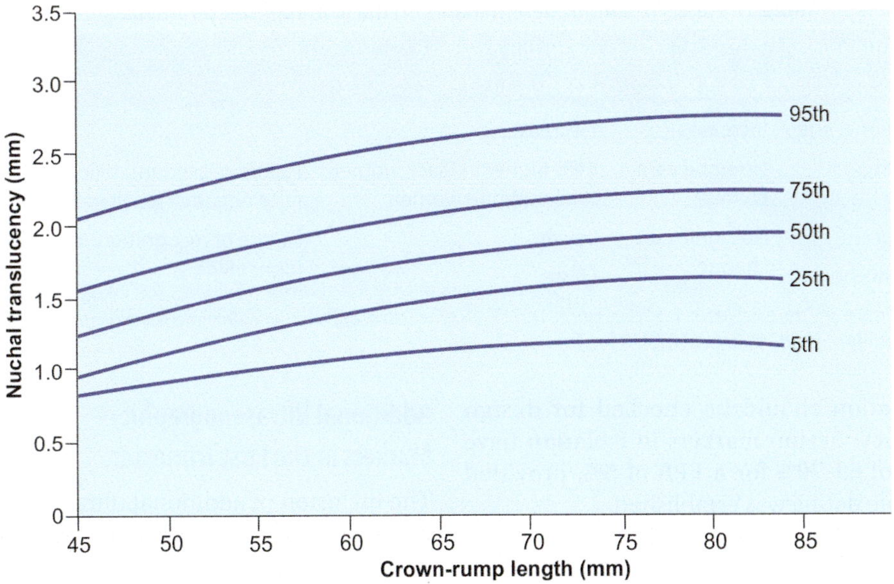

Figure 2: Reference range of fetal nuchal translucency (NT) with crown-rump length (CRL) showing the 5th, 25th, 50th, 75th and 95th centile

Source: Reproduced from Snijders RJM, Noble P, Sebire N, Souka A, Nicolaides KH. UK multicentre project on assessment of risk of trisomy 21 by maternal age and fetal nuchal translucency thickness at 10-14 weeks of gestation. Lancet 1998;351:343-6.

products in the maternal serum. Two such maternal serum analytes have been identified in the first trimester for the purpose of screening: free β-human chorionic gonadotropin (free β-hCG) and pregnancy-associated plasma protein A (PAPP-A). Their serum concentrations are expressed in ng/mL or IU/mL. Their values vary with the gestational age. Free β-hCG and PAPP-A increases and decreases with the gestational age respectively. In order to standardize and eliminate the variation associated with gestational age, they are converted to multiples of median (MoM). The MoM rather than the absolute value is utilized in risk estimation and thus allows comparison between the individual patient and the overall obstetric population for that particular gestational age. In euploid pregnancies the average free β-hCG is 1.0 MoM and PAPP-A is 1.0 MoM. So, PAPP-A value of 1.5 MoM means that a patient has a concentration of PAPP-A that is 1.5 times higher than the median concentration of other pregnant women of the same gestational age. In trisomy 21 at 12 weeks, the maternal serum concentration of free β-hCG is about twice as high (2 MoMs) and PAPP-A is reduced to about half (0.5 MoM) compared to chromosomally normal pregnancies. In trisomy 18 and 13, both the serum markers are reduced. Besides gestational age, the serum markers are influenced by others parameters such as ethnicity etc. Hence, these determinants have to be taken into account and appropriate corrections need to be made to produce accurate patient-specific risks. **Table 1** outlines the various determinants and their effects on the serum markers.[4] The individual risk is derived by the laboratories using software and this risk is compared to the cut-off risk for final interpretation, follow- up and management. The laboratories providing screening services must participate in proficiency testing and monitor their performance through epidemiologic surveillance. Softwares employed for risk

Table 1: Effects of various determinants on the first trimester serum markers

Determinant	Effects on serum markers		Inference
	Free β-hCG	PAPP-A	
Gestational age	Increases	Decreases	
Ethnicity	No significant change	60% higher in Black women than in White women	Failure of accountability will produce false negative result in Blacks
Smoker	No significant change	Lower	Failure of recognition will lead to higher FPR.
IVF conception		Lower	

Source: Data from The Fetal Medicine Foundation. The 11–13+6 weeks scan. http:/www.fetalmedicine.com/synced/fmf/FMF-English.pdf. [Accessed 1 October 2015].

calculation should be checked for design accuracy. Serum markers in isolation have a DR of 60–70% for a FPR of 5%, provided accurate dating was established.

Combined Test

The most effective protocol for the screening of Down syndrome in the first trimester is the "Combined test". It incorporates ultrasonographic measurement of NT and maternal serum markers to estimate the final risk. There is no significant association between fetal NT and maternal serum markers in either trisomic or chromosomally normal pregnancies. Hence, their combination is justified and provides effective screening.[12]

There are two options available:

1. Both the NT measurement and the biochemical markers can be analyzed at the same time at 12 weeks. This option is employed in United Kingdom at OSCAR (One-stop clinic for assessment of risk) clinics, where the results of the combined screen are available in 30 minutes. The DR is 85–90% for a FPR of 5%.
2. Serum biochemical analytes are measured at 10 weeks and NT is done at 12 weeks in two separate visits. It has been estimated that this approach would improve the DR to 93–94%. But, the disadvantage will be an increase in the non-compliance rate that is associated with this method.

The interpretation of risk and further testing are discussed later in this chapter.

Additional Ultrasonographic Markers in the First Trimester

The inclusion of additional ultrasonographic markers to the combined test further improves the DR and reduces the FPR. They can be assessed either in all patients or only those falling under the intermediate risk after combined screening (Contingent I trimester screening). The additional markers assessed are:[4]

Non-ossified or Absent Nasal Bone

For the assessment of nasal bone, the same protocol is followed as for NT. An ideal image should have the same landmarks as mentioned above. When these criteria are met, three distinct lines should be seen at the level of the fetal nose **(Figure 3)**.

- The top line represents the skin
- The underlying line, which is thicker and more echogenic than the overlying skin, represents the nasal bone. These two parallel lines of echogenicity have the shape of an "equal sign".
- A third line in front of the bone and at a higher level than the skin represents the tip of the nose

The nasal bone is considered to be present if it is more echogenic than the overlying skin and absent or non-ossified if it is either not visible or its echogenicity is the same or less than that of the skin. The nasal bone is non-ossified in 60% of fetuses with trisomy 21. In the normal population, the frequency

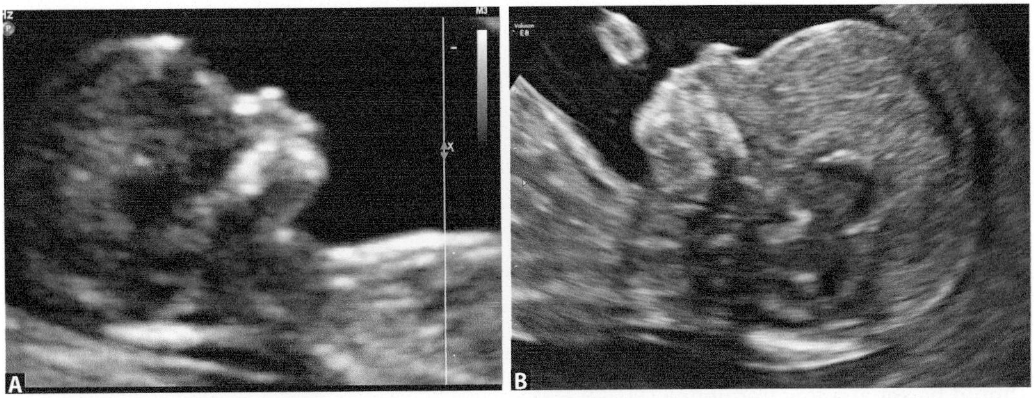

Figure 3: Ultrasound images to illustrate (A) Normal nasal bone and (B) Non-ossified nasal bone

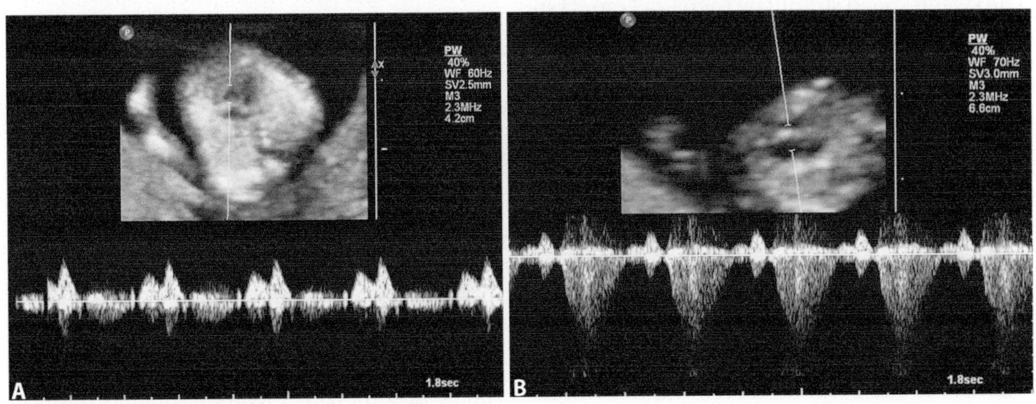

Figure 4: Ultrasound images to show (A) Normal flow across tricuspid valve and (B) Tricuspid regurgitation

of non-ossified nasal bone is related to the ethnicity of the mother. It is 2.2% in Caucasians, 5% in Asians and 9% in the Afro-Caribbeans. This needs to be taken into account while evaluating the individual patient risk.

Tricuspid Regurgitation

For assessment of tricuspid flow, the magnification of the image should be such that the fetal thorax occupies the whole screen. An apical four-chamber view of the fetal heart should be obtained. Color flow mapping should not be used because it is unreliable for the diagnosis of tricuspid regurgitation in the first-trimester. The pulsed Doppler sample should be large (2.0–3.0 mm) and positioned across the tricuspid valve. The insonation angle to the direction of flow should be less than 30 degrees from the direction of the interventricular septum. The sweep speed should be high (2–3 cm/s) so that the waveforms are widely spread for better assessment, as shown in **Figure 4**. The sample volume should be placed across the valve at least three times, in order to interrogate the complete valve.

- Normal flow across tricuspid valve will have no regurgitation during systole.
- Regurgitation during approximately half of systole and with a velocity more than 60 cm/s has been reported in 55% of trisomy 21 fetuses and 1% of euploid fetus.

Abnormal Flow Across Ductus Venosus

The ductus venosus is a short vessel that connects the umbilical vein to the inferior vena cava and preferentially shunts oxygenated blood to the fetal brain. The magnification of the image should be such that the fetal thorax and abdomen occupy the whole screen. A right ventral mid-sagittal view of the fetal trunk should be obtained. Color flow mapping should be used to demonstrate the umbilical vein, ductus venosus and fetal heart. The pulsed Doppler sample should be small (0.5–1.0 mm) to avoid contamination from the adjacent veins and it should be placed in the yellowish aliasing area. The insonation angle should be less than 30 degrees. The filter should be set at a low frequency (50–70 Hz) to allow visualization of the whole waveform. The sweep speed should be high (2–3 cm/s) so that the waveforms are assessed better.

Normally, blood flow in the ductus has a characteristic waveform with:

- High velocity during ventricular systole (S-wave) and diastole (D-wave)
- Forward flow during atrial contraction (a-wave).

The flow is considered abnormal when a-wave is reversed **(Figure 5)** and is observed in 65% of trisomy 21 fetuses and 3% of normal fetuses. With the addition of new sonographic markers to the combined test, the DR would be 93–96% for a FPR of 2.5%.[13]

Advantages of First Trimester Screening

First trimester screening has many advantages:

- The combined test is more effective than second trimester biochemical tests.
- Apart from trisomy 21, trisomy 18 and 13 can also be screened with high sensitivity and specificity.
- NT is raised in many other pathological conditions apart from trisomy 21 which can be evaluated by ultrasonography.
- Other major and lethal congenital malformations can be diagnosed in the first trimester which may modify screening.
- The couple can make their reproductive choice earlier. Abortion procedures in the first trimester are safer than in second trimester.
- The maternal serum analyte PAPP-A is a marker for fetal growth restriction, in which case such pregnancies can be vigilantly monitored.

APPROACH TO SCREENING IN THE SECOND TRIMESTER

Screening in the second trimester for aneuploidy can be accomplished by maternal biochemical analytes or genetic sonogram or both.

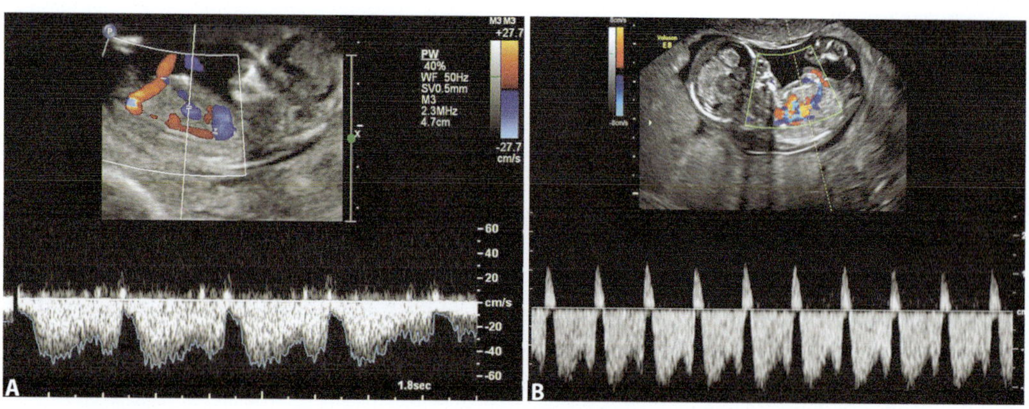

Figure 5: Ultrasound images to depict (A) Normal flow pattern in the ductus venosus (DV) and (B) Reversal of 'a' wave in DV

Maternal Serum Biochemical Analytes: Quadruple Test

The maternal serum concentration of alpha-fetoprotein was routinely measured for the screening of open neural tube defects. It was first reported in 1984 that pregnancies with fetal Down syndrome had lower levels of alpha-fetoprotein during 15–18 weeks.[14] This concept was exploited for screening of aneuploidy from then. With the discovery and inclusion of other biochemical markers, the DR has increased to as high as 70–80%. Triple test involves measuring three biochemical analytes in the maternal serum—Alpha-fetoprotein (AFP), unconjugated estriol (uE3), free β-human chorionic gonadotropin (free β-hCG). Quadruple test includes the fourth marker-Inhibin (Inh A).[15] Screening is preferred between 15 and 19 weeks since this period is optimal for screening open neural tube defects also (AFP). Each of the biochemical analyte is converted to multiples of median (MoM) and final risk is derived, similar to first trimester biochemical screening. The detection rates for triple and quadruple tests are 60–70%, 65–75% respectively, for a false positive rate of 5%.

Genetic Sonogram

With the advances in ultrasound machine, technology and wider accessibility, genetic sonogram is routinely offered to all pregnant women. Genetic sonogram otherwise termed TIFFA (Targeted imaging for fetal anomalies), involves systematic examination of the external and internal anatomy of the fetus. It is performed between 18–22 weeks of gestation. It is essential that genetic sonogram be performed only by those who had received appropriate training and certification of competence. They should subject their results to regular audit for quality assurance. Until the last decade, genetic sonogram was the primary method of risk assessment for aneuploidy. Eventhough the screening paradigm has shifted to first trimester, genetic sonogram still remains the primary modality for the detection of major fetal structural malformations.

Major Structural Malformation

The finding of a major structural anomaly often increases the aneuploidy risk.[16] It needs to be emphasised here that not all aneuploid fetuses will have sonographically detectable major malformations. This is especially true in the case of Trisomy 21 since only 25–30% present with major congenital anomalies.

The identification of a major anomaly obviates the need for further screening tests and calls for diagnostic invasive test because:

- If the abnormalities are either lethal or associated with severe handicap, invasive testing and fetal karyotyping may determine the possible cause and predict the risk of recurrence in future pregnancy.
- If the pregnant woman plans to continue pregnancy in the event of a potentially correctable defect such as diaphragmatic hernia, it is prudent to exclude an abnormal chromosomal defect which will alter the prognosis.

Soft Markers

There are recognized minor sonographic markers referred to as 'soft signs' or 'soft markers' which increase the detection rates of Down syndrome. These markers are employed only for the estimation of risk for aneuploidy. It should be noted that in the absence of major congenital anomalies and normal karyotype of the fetus, they do not carry any significance and do not affect the fetal prognosis as they are not pathological except for ventriculomegaly.

The most widely examined and extensively reported soft markers are:

- Intracardiac hyperechogenic focus
- Ventriculomegaly
- Increased nuchal fold thickness
- Hyperechogenic bowel
- Mild hydronephrosis
- Short humerus
- Short femur
- Aberrant right subclavian artery (ARSA)
- Absent or hypoplastic nasal bone.

Table 2 provides a description of the soft markers. Each marker has positive and

Table 2: Description of second trimester soft markers

S.No	Soft marker	Description
1.	Lateral ventriculomegaly	Diameter of the lateral ventricle ≥ 10 mm, measured at the level of parieto-occipital fissure in the axial section (transventricular plane) of fetal head
2.	Absent or hypoplastic nasal bone	Nasal bone is considered absent when it remains non-ossified. It is considered hypolplastic if its length is < 5th centile for that gestational age of same ethnicity (requires use of normograms)
3.	Increased nuchal fold thickness	Thickness of nuchal fold ≥ 6 mm measured in the transcerebellar plane with posterolateral inclination
4.	Intracardiac echogenic focus	Single or multiple echogenic spots in either or both ventricles of the fetal heart
5.	Aberrant right subclavian artery	Right subclavian artery (RSA) arises directly from the descending aorta at its junction with the ductus arteriosus and courses behind the trachea and the esophagus before turning towards the right shoulder
6.	Hyperechogenic bowel	Echogenicity of the bowel matches with that of the bones
7.	Mild hydronephrosis	Anteroposterior diameter of the renal pelvis ≥ 5 mm, measured in the axial section with the spine positioned anteriorly
8.	Shortened femur or humerus	Femur and humerus are considered shortened if their length is <5th centile for that gestational age (requires use of normograms)

Source: Data from Agathokleous M, Chaveeva P, Poon LCY, Kosinski P, Nicolaides KH. Meta-analysis of second trimester markers for trisomy 21. Ultrasound Obstet Gynecol. 2103;42:247-61.

Table 3: Screening performance of second trimester soft markers

Marker	DR%	FPR%	LR+	LR-	LR isolated marker
Intracardiac echogenic focus	24.4	3.9	5.83	0.80	0.95
Ventriculomegaly	7.5	0.2	27.52	0.94	3.81
Increased nuchal fold	26.0	1.0	23.30	0.80	3.79
Echogenic bowel	16.7	1.1	11.44	0.90	1.65
Mild hydronephrosis	13.9	1.7	7.63	0.92	1.08
Short humerus	30.3	4.6	4.81	0.74	0.78
Short femur	27.7	6.4	3.72	0.80	0.61
ARSA	30.7	1.5	21.48	0.71	3.94
Absent or hypoplastic nasal bone	59.8	2.8	23.27	0.46	6.58

Abbreviations: ARSA, aberrant right subclavian artery; DR, detection rate; FPR, false positive rate; LR+, positive likelihood ratio; LR-, negative likelihood ratio; LR, likelihood ratio

Source: Data from Agathokleous M, Chaveeva P, Poon LCY, Kosinski P, Nicolaides KH. Meta-analysis of second trimester markers for trisomy 21. Ultrasound Obstet Gynecol. 2103;42:247-61.

negative likelihood ratio (LR). Positive LR of a marker is derived by dividing the percentage of confirmed Down syndrome having the marker by the percentage of normal fetus with the same marker. Negative LR results from dividing the number of Trisomy 21 fetuses that do not exhibit the marker by the number of normal fetuses that do not exhibit the marker. The screening performance of each of the markers have been validated in a recent meta-analysis by Agathokleous et al.[17] The pooled estimates of DR, FPR, positive and negative LR for trisomy 21 for each marker are summarized in **Table 3**.

Calculation of the Risk

All the markers are independent of each other except for short femur or humerus. Hence their likelihood ratios can be considered together (with inclusion of LR of either shortened femur or humerus) for the calculation of risk. When any one of the markers is present, the LR for that particular pregnant woman is obtained by multiplying the positive LR of that marker with the negative LR's of the other markers. This is given as isolated LR. When more than one marker is present, the LR will be the product of the positive LR's of the markers identified during the scan and the negative LR's of the other markers not found. When none of the markers are present, the LR would be the product of the negative LR's of all the markers. The LR would be 0.13 if negative LR of shortened femur is considered (excluding that of humerus) and a 7–8 fold decrease in the risk. Finally, the likelihood ratio is multiplied with the 'a priori risk' (in percentage) to derive the post ultrasound risk. The 'a priori risk' would be either the maternal age/gestational age related risk (as in the case of pregnant women who had not undergone any screening procedures previously) or the risk obtained after first or second trimester screening. If the new risk is more than the established cut-off, amniocentesis should be offered for diagnosis. For example: if a 25-year-old pregnant woman undergoes a genetic sonogram and two markers (intracardiac ehogenic focus and ventriculomegaly) are detected, the likelihood ratio would be 27.76 (5.83 × 27.52 × 0.80 × 0.90 × 0.92 × 0.80 × 0.71 × 0.46). Postultrasound risk would be the product of a priori risk 0.087% (1 in 1147) and LR (27.78), which is 2.42%(1 in 41). The presence and absence of sonographic markers increases and decreases the risk for trisomy 21 respectively. Hypoplastic or non-ossified nasal bone is the most powerful marker as it increases the risk by 6–7 folds. The other strong markers of trisomy 21 are ventriculomegaly, nuchal fold thickness and ARSA since each one of them increases the risk by 3–4 times. All the other markers in isolation do not have significant effect on the risk, while the presence of two or more markers will produce significant modification of the risk.

The most recent consensus from the United Kingdom (UK)[18] states that identification of the these soft markers (choroid plexus cyst, dilated cistern magna, 2-vessel cord, echogenic intracardiac foci) in women found to be at low risk through first trimester combined test or second trimester quadruple test, should not be referred for further assessment. Such low risk women would require further assessment only if the following markers are identified:

- Nuchal fold >6 mm
- Ventriculomegaly (Atrium >10 mm)
- Echogenic bowel
- Renal pelvic dilatation >7 mm
- Small measurements <5th centile.

Implications of Genetic Sonogram

In the era of first trimester screening, genetic sonogram has a modest role with a greater impact on FPR rather than on the DR. Nevertheless, it is the only means for detecting structural defects in the fetus. Genetic sonogram has a definite role in case of twin gestation.[19]

NON-INVASIVE PRENATAL SCREENING (NIPS)

Since the discovery of cell free fetal DNA (cffDNA) in the maternal plasma, there has been major progress in the field of prenatal diagnosis. cffDNA is employed in Non-invasive prenatal screening (NIPS). NIPS has been endorsed by the American College of Obstetricians and Gynecologists and the Society for Maternal-Fetal Medicine as screening option for aneuploidy in 2011.[20]

The majority of cell free DNA is maternal in origin, with the fetal origin constituting about 3–13% after 10 weeks of gestation. The fetal DNA are derived from the placental trophoblasts. Testing can be performed at any period of gestation after 10 weeks. Results are generally available within 7–10 days of maternal sampling. NIPS has a sensitivity of 99.3% and a specificity of 99.8% for the detection of trisomy 21.

Condition	*Sensitivity*	*Specificity*
Trisomy 18	97.4%	99.8%
Trisomy 13	91.6%	99.9%
Sex chromosome aneuploidy	91%	99.6%

The reported false-positive rate is 1% and is due to vanishing twin, confined placental mosaicism and maternal malignancy.

Pre-requisites

- Baseline ultrasound is mandatory to determine the viability, number of fetus and gestational age.
- The couple should be counselled about the benefits and limitations of NIPS. A negative test does not assure a chromosomally normal fetus in a very small percentage of patients.

Limitations

- NIPS is expensive and is not applicable for screening general obstetric population. It is not universally available.
- Only trisomy 21, 18 and 13 can be detected. Information about sex chromosomal aneuploidies and other trisomies (trisomy 16 and 22) would be available only if requested for.
- It cannot determine if the trisomy is due to translocation. This information would be important for predicting the risk of recurrence.
- NIPS cannot routinely be offered for the detection of microdeletions. Hence, for the above reasons, NIPS cannot replace conventional karyotype.
- Laboratories require a minimum of 4% fetal fraction for a reportable result, irrespective of the methodology used. Maternal obesity is associated with lesser fetal fraction, leading to 1–8% screen failure.

Recommendations

- NIPS can be offered:
  - As a follow-up test for pregnant women with a high or intermediate risk from a conventional screening test before proceeding for invasive tests. But a normal NIPS result does carry a residual risk of 2% of a chromosomal abnormality in such a situation.
  - To any pregnant woman, provided she understands the benefits and drawbacks of this screening strategy in the context of alternative screening tests. But the use of NIPS to the general obstetric population may produce higher screen false-positives because the positive predictive value is lower in this population due to the lower prevalence of aneuploidy in the general obstetric population.
- NIPS cannot be offered in the following situations:
  - In the event of identification of a structural anomaly by ultrasound which needs a diagnostic test.
  - Multiple pregnancy as it provides only a single composite result for the entire gestation.
  - Couple is unaffordable
  - Non-availability of NIPS.
- Women with a positive test should undergo invasive diagnostic test since NIPS does not replace the accuracy of invasive tests. Knowing the type of trisomy from the karyotype becomes essential for purposes of prediction of recurrence. Management decisions should not be based solely on NIPS results.
- For women, whose NIPS results are not reported or indeterminate should be offered

comprehensive ultrasound evaluation, genetic counselling and invasive diagnostic test for confirmation.

- In addition to NIPS, parallel or simultaneous testing with multiple screening methodologies for aneuploidy is not necessary and should not be performed. But comprehensive anomaly scan should be offered as NIPS does not diagnose structural malformations.

FIRST AND SECOND TRIMESTER SCREENING APPROACHES

Combined first and second trimester screening increases the screening efficacy by improving the DR and reducing the FPR.

This screening paradigm becomes important in the following clinical situations:

- The first trimester combined screen risk is intermediate and further corroborative evidence is desirable for recommending amniocentesis for confirmation.
- The combined test is screen positive (high risk) and the couple requests for further confirmation of the abnormality before proceeding to invasive test.
- The combined screen risk is borderline or high and the couple is unaffordable for NIPS.
- A mere patient request for reassurance after a low risk from first trimester screening.

The combined first and second trimester screening strategies that have been developed are as follows:

- *Integrated screening*: It incorporates the results of the combined test and quadruple test into a single risk. The integrated test has the highest DR and least FPR, thereby reducing unwanted amniocentesis in normal pregnancies. The disadvantage associated with integrated screening strategy lies in ethical issue of not conveying the first trimester result and denying them the option of CVS.
- *Sequential screening*: First trimester combined test is the primary screening modality. The results of the combined test are stratified into low (risk: <1:1000), intermediate (risk ≥ 1:1000 and ≤ 1:51) and high (risk >1:50) risk groups. The results are informed only to women at high risk, thus allowing them to choose the option of CVS. There are two testing strategies in this category:
  - Stepwise sequential screening: Both the low and intermediate risk group would be offered the quadruple test in the second trimester.
  - *Contingent sequential screening*: No further testing would be required for low risk group. For those in the intermediate risk group, quadruple test will be offered. This approach is the most effective for population screening as it obviates the need for second trimester screening in low risk group, who constitute about 85%.

Following the quadruple test, the final risk is calculated after incorporating both the first and second trimester results. When the risk is below the established cut-off, no further screening would be required. When the risk is above the established cut-off, amniocentesis should be offered.

WHAT TO CHOOSE?

The following screening protocol options are recommended by the International Society for Prenatal Diagnosis (ISPD):[21]

For pregnant women presenting in the first trimester (before 14 weeks) for antenatal care:

- Noninvasive prenatal screening (NIPS) which uses cell free fetal DNA (cffDNA) as a primary test in virtue of its high sensitivity and specificity to couples who can afford.
- Combined test (ultrasound nuchal translucency and serum analytes) as a primary test, which is most commonly employed.

Based on the risk, the following steps can be taken.[4]

- Low risk (cut-off: <1 in 1000) group constitutes 83.5% of normal population with euploid foetus and 1% with trisomy 21.
  - No further genetic testing is required. Second trimester anomaly scan can be offered. It is a very useful adjunct to modify the risk and improve detection of anomalies.
- High risk (cut off: ≥1 in 50) group forms 1.5% of normal population and 85% of trisomy 21: They require confirmation by karyotyping.
  - They should be offered chorionic villus sampling if available or amniocentesis at 16 weeks for confirmation.
  - NIPS may also be offered, though not preferable. But a positive result should be followed up by invasive testing for confirmation.
- Intermediate/Borderline risk (cut off: 1 in 51 to 1 in 1000) group constitutes 15% each of pregnancies with euploid and trisomy 21 foetuses. This group of pregnant women can be offered any one of the following options:
  - NIPS can be offered as a secondary test based on the availability and affordability. Positive test should be confirmed by CVS/amniocentesis
  - Contingent first trimester screening with inclusion of additional ultrasound markers (non-ossified nasal bone, tricuspid regurgitation determined by pulse wave Doppler and abnormal blood flow in ductus venosus) can be offered to improve the detection rate.
  - Integrated screening can be offered where CVS is not available.
  - Sequential screening

When the final risk is above the established cut-off, CVS or amniocentesis should be offered for confirmation. No further testing would be required for the low-risk group.

For pregnant women presenting in the second trimester (after 14 weeks) for antenatal care:

Options are few for women seeking antenatal care in the early second trimester. They need to choose screening tests that provide the most accurate results within a short time span since in the event of an aneuploid fetus, the clinician would be faced with issues concerning termination. The clinician should conform to the legal regulations of termination, as in India, termination of pregnancy is not permitted beyond 20 weeks of gestation.

- NIPS as a primary test, when available and affordable by the couple would be the best option with respect to its accuracy.
- Quadruple test
- Genetic sonogram
- Contingent screening (Quadruple test and genetic sonogram).

The following tests are not recommended for screening by the ISPD since they do not meet the minimum requirement criteria:

- Maternal age as a sole criteria
- NT measurement without additional tests (Other ultrasongraphic markers or biochemical analytes)
- Conventional screening tests after an unambiguous NIPS.

A summary of recommended screening options with their performance[21,22] are outlined in **Table 4**.

SCREENING IN SPECIAL CIRCUMSTANCES

Multiple Pregnancy

Multiple pregnancy is on the rise owing to the increased use of assisted reproductive techniques. Determination of chorionicity in the first trimester is mandatory since it has a major impact on the screening process.

Table 4: Performance of different screening protocols for Down syndrome

Screening test	*Detection rate*	*False +ve rate*
First Trimester Tests		
MA+NT	75–80%	5%
MA+first trimester serum markers	60–70%	5%
Combined test (MA+NT+serum markers)	85–90%	5%
Contingent I trimester test (Combined test + NB / TR / DV flow)	93–96%	2.5%
Second Trimester Tests		
Triple test	60–70%	5%
Quadruple test	65–75%	5%
Genetic sonogram	56%	NA
Quadruple test + Genetic sonogram	80%	NA
Combined First and Second Trimester Tests		
Integrated test	90–94%	5%
Stepwise sequential test	90–94%	5%
Contingent sequential test	90–94%	5%
Combined test + Genetic sonogram	88%	NA
Noninvasive prenatal screening (NIPS)	99%	NA

Abbreviations: MA, maternal age; NT, nuchal translucency; NB, nasal bone; DV, ductus venosus; TR, tricuspid regurgitation; NA, not available

Source: Data from Benn P, Borrell A, Chiu RW, Cuckle H, Dugofff L, Faas B, et al. Position statement from the Chromosome Abnormality Screening Committee on behalf of the Board of the International Society for Prenatal Diagnosis. Prenat Diagn.2015 Aug;35(8):725-34. Nicolaides KH. Screening for fetal aneuploidies at 11 – 13 weeks. Prenat Diagn 2011; 31: 7-15.

First Trimester

Maternal Age and Nuchal Translucency

Screening with maternal age and nuchal translucency is the method of choice for aneuploidy screening of twins in the first trimester.[23] Monochorionic twins are always monozygotic and each fetus has the same risk of being affected. The NT measurements of the twins are averaged to derive a single pregnancy—specific risk. Such an approach was estimated to have a sensitivity of 100% for a FPR of 4.2%. This method is currently preferred since increased NT in one of the twins could be an early manifestation of twin-to-twin transfusion syndrome. If this aspect is not taken into consideration, then there would be an increase in the false positives and unnecessary invasive testing.[24] In dichorionic pregnancies, a fetus-specific risk is calculated since each fetus has an independent risk of having aneuploidy. The detection rates are similar to singleton pregnancy approaching 75% for a FPR of 6.8%.[25] Although about 10% of dichorionic pregnancies are monozygotic, the same approach for dichorionic twins is employed as it does not seem to affect the screening accuracy in this population.

Combined Test

Aneuploidy screening in twins with maternal serum markers requires adjustment of the calculated multiples of the median to account for the presence of two fetuses. For adjustment of β-hCG, the observed MoM is divided by 2.023. For PAPP-A, the correction factors are 2.192 and 1.788 for dichorionic and monochorionic twins respectively. For a FPR of 5%, this method has a detection rate of 70% in dichorionic twins and 84% in monochorionic twins.[26] Its performance is better in monochorionic twins. Combined test may be considered due to its better performance by decreasing the FPR. Combined test has been criticized because abnormal levels will be brought closer to the mean by the normal cotwin.

Second trimester

Serum Screening

Second trimester screening with serum markers is feasible and preferable to screening by maternal age alone for those pregnant women with twin gestation presenting in the second trimester. It has a DR of 50–70% and a high FPR (10%). This may lead to higher rates of invasive tests. This testing strategy should be restricted only when NT has been missed.

Genetic Sonogram

The current recommendation does not support for or against the use of ultrasound soft markers for aneuploidy screening in twins.[27]

Integrated screening has not been prospectively validated in twin pregnancies.

CONCLUSION

Screening for Down syndrome is the most emphasised screening procedure in the field of obstetrics and fetal medicine for more than a decade globally. Pre-test and post-test counseling are imperative to allow the couple to make an informed choice. At present, the ideal screening module for India is the "Combined test" in the first trimester-nuchal translucency and dual serum markers. The protocols for measurement of NT with regular audit of NT and serum markers by the laboratory should be practised diligently in order to achieve the DR and FPR obtained by the proponents. If this is not adhered to, the DR and FPR will be much below the standards resulting in under diagnosis on one hand. On the other hand, with higher false positive diagnosis, there would be an increased risk of losing more number of normal fetuses due to invasive test and phenomenal increase in the expenditure to the society in general. Other screening paradigms can be chosen to increase the performance depending on the availability of the facility and expertise. In future, when the cost becomes affordable, the NIPS would be the much preferred and ideal screening method.

REFERENCES

1. Parker SE, Mai CT, Canfield MA, et al. Updated national birth prevalence estimates for selected birth defects in the Unites States, 2004-2006. Birth defects. Res A Clin Mol Teratol. 2010;88:1008-16.
2. Kingston HM. ABC of clinical genetics. Chapter 5; Common chromosomal disorders. BMJ books. 2002;3:pp 18-24.
3. CDC. (2011). Facts about Down syndrome. Retrieved October 10, 2015 from http://www.cdc.gov/ncbddd/birth defects/DownSyndrome.html
4. The Fetal Medicine Foundation. The 11 – 13+6 weeks scan. http://www.fetalmedicine.com/synced/fmf/FMF-English.pdf. [Accessed 1 October 2015].
5. Vintzileos AJ, Egan AJ. Adjusting the risk for trisomy 21 on the basis of second- trimester ultrasonography. Am J Obstet Gynecol. 1995;172(3):837-44.
6. American College of Obstetricians and Gynecologists. ACOG Practice Bulletin No. 77. Screening for fetal chromosomal abnormalities. Obstet Gynecol. 2007;109: 217-27.
7. Rodeck CH, Whittle MJ. Fetal Medicine: Basic science and clinical practice. Chapter 17. Conveying information about screening. Churchill Livingstone Elsevier. 2009;2:p.225-33.
8. Snijders RJM, Sundberg K, Holzgreve W, Henry G, Nicolaides KH. Maternal age and gestation-

specific risk for trisomy 21. Ultrasound Obstet Gynecol. 1999;13:167-70.
9. Snijders RJM, Nicolaides KH. Sequential screening. In:Ultrasound markers for fetal chromosomal defects. Parthenon Publishing, Canforth, UK. 1996;p109-13.
10. Snijders RJM, Noble P, Sebire N, Souka A, Nicolaides KH. UK multicentre project on assessment of risk of trisomy 21 by maternal age and fetal nuchal translucency thickness at 10-14 weeks of gestation. Lancet. 1998;351: 343-6.
11. Spencer K, Bindra R, Nix ABJ, Health V, Nicolaides KH. Delta NT or NT MoM: which is the most appropriate method for calculating accurate patient-specific risks for trisomy 21 in the first trimester? Ultrasound Obstet Gynecol. 2003a;22:142-8.
12. Spencer K, Souter V, Tul N, Snijders R, Nicolaides KH. A screening program for trisomy 21 at 10-14 weeks using fetal nuchal translucency, maternal serum free b-human chorionic gonadotropin and pregnancy associated plasma protein A. Ultrasound Obstet Gynecol. 1999;13:231-7.
13. Nicolaides KH. Nuchal translucency and other first-trimester sonographic markers of chromosomal abnormalities. Am J Obstet Gynecol. 2004;191:45-7.
14. Merkatz IR, Nitowsky HM, Macri Jn, et al. An association between maternal serum alpha fetoprotein and fetal chromosomal abnormalities. Am J Obstet Gynecol. 1984;148:886.
15. Arias F, Daftary SN, Bhide AG. Practical guide to high risk pregnancy and delivery. A South Asian perspective. Chapter 2, Prenatal Diagnosis of chromosomal abnormalities. Reed Elsevier India Pvt. Ltd. 2008;3:p.32-61.
16. Cunningham FG, Levono KJ, Bloom SL, Hauth JC, Rouse DJ, Spong CY. Williams Obstetrics. Chapter 13, Prenatal Diagnosis and fetal therapy. McGraw Hill Companies Inc, New York. 2010;3:p.287-311.
17. Agathokleous M, Chaveeva P, Poon LCY, Kosinski P, Nicolaides KH. Meta-analysis of second trimester markers for trisomy 21. Ultrasound Obstet Gynecol. 2013;42:247-61.
18. http://www.gov.uk/government/publications/fetal-anomaly-screening-programme-handbook.
19. Odibo AO, Ghidini A. Role of second trimester genetic sonogram for Down syndrome screen in the era of first-trimester screening and noninvasive prenatal testing. Prenat Diagn. 2014;34(6):511-17.
20. Cell-free DNA screening for fetal aneuploidy. ACOG Committee Opinion No. 640. Committee on Genetics Society for Maternal-Fetal Medicine. American College of Obstetricians and Gynecologists. Obstet Gynecol. 2015;126(3):e31-e7.
21. Benn P, Borrell A, Chiu RW, Cuckle H, Dugofff L, Faas B, et al. Position statement from the Chromosome Abnormality Screening Committee on behalf of the Board of the International Society for Prenatal Diagnosis. Prenat Diagn. 2015;35(8):725-34.
22. Nicolaides KH. Screening for fetal aneuploidies at 11-13 weeks. Prenat Diagn. 2011; 31:7-15.
23. Francois Audibert, Alain Gagnon. SOGC Genetics Committee: CCMG Committee on Prenatal Diagnosis. Prenatal screening for and diagnosis of a Aneuploidy in twin pregnancies. SOGC Clinical Practice Guideline No. 262. J Obstet Gynaecol Can. 2011;33(7):754-67.
24. Snijders RJ, Thom EA, Zachary JM, Platt LD, Greene N, Jackson LG et al. First trimester trisomy screening: nuchal translucency measurement training and quality assurance to correct and unify technique. Ultrasound Obstet Gynecol. 2002;19:353-9.
25. Spencer K, Nicolaides KH. Screening for trisomy 21 in twins using first trimester ultrasound and maternal serum biochemistry in a one-stop clinic: a review of three years-experience. BJOG. 2003;110:276-80.
26. Wald NJ, Rish S, Hackshaw AK. Combining nuchal translucency and serum markers in prenatal screening for Down syndrome in twin pregnancies. Prenat Diagn. 2003;23:588-92.
27. Morin L, Lim K. SOGC Diagnostic Imaging Committee; SOGC Genetics Committee; SOGC Maternal Fetal Medicine Committee. Ultrasound for twin pregnancies. SOGC Clinical Practice Guideline No.260. J Obstet Gynaecol Can. 2011;33:643-56.

4
CHAPTER

Abnormalities of Central Nervous System

KV Sridevi, Binodini Mahendra Chauhan

INTRODUCTION

Fetal cerebral abnormalities are one of the common congenital abnormalities detected during the prenatal period. CNS malformations amount to about 1–2 per 1000 births.[1] Advanced high-resolution ultrasound machines, use of transvaginal ultrasound and 3D ultrasound have improved the detection of these abnormalities as early as first trimester. The brain continues to develop in the second half of gestation and into the neonatal period thus limiting the detection of anomalies of neuroproliferation, migration and some acquired lesions, such as hemorrhage and tumors, which can occur at any gestational age and therefore, a second trimester ultrasound may not detect these late-onset pathologies. However, screening for fetal brain malformations is commonly performed at 19–21 weeks gestation. Sensitivity of detection of CNS abnormalities by transabdominal ultrasound in low-risk patients undergoing basic examination is 80%.[2-4]

The fetal head is commonly evaluated using transverse scanning planes. Coronal and sagittal views are done when necessary.

Transabdominal sonography is the technique of choice to investigate the fetal CNS during first, second and third trimesters of gestation in low-risk pregnancies. Cerebral structures are visualized in the transventricular, transthalamic and transcerebellar planes.

Brain anomalies, which can be identified by the axial scanning planes, are discussed first followed by other cerebral anomalies.

VENTRICULOMEGALY AND HYDROCEPHALUS

Hydrocephalus and ventriculomegaly both are the terms used to describe dilatation of the lateral ventricles. However, these two should be distinguished from each other. Hydrocephalus signifies dilated lateral ventricles that resulted from increased amount of CSF inside the ventricles and increased intracranial pressure, while ventriculomegaly is dilatation of lateral ventricles without an increased intracranial pressure, due to cerebral hypoplasia or CNS anomaly.[5,6] Ventriculomegaly can sometimes change into hydrocephalic state. Obliterated subarachnoid space and dangling choroid plexus are observed in hydrocephalus, in contrast to ventriculomegaly in which both these are well preserved. Subarachnoid space is difficult to evaluate in the axial plane; therefore it is suggested that the evaluation of enlarged ventricles should be done in the parasagittal and coronal views by transvaginal approach or by 3D analysis. Atrial width of cerebral lateral ventricles of 10.0–15 mm—mild ventriculomegaly, >15 mm—severe ventriculomegaly.[7]

Mild ventriculomegaly is defined as isolated if there is no sonographic evidence of associated malformation or markers of aneuploidy at the time of the initial presentation.[7,8] Isolated mild ventriculomegaly represents a considerable diagnostic dilemma as it can be an apparently benign finding, but can also be associated with abnormalities like congenital infection, vascular abnormalities and hemorrhagic causes. Several studies have reported an incidence of associated anomalies (neural and extraneural), as high as 50%. For women with pregnancies in which mild ventriculomegaly is suspected, detailed neurosonographic evaluation should be performed by an expert.[7] Congenital infections can cause mild ventriculomegaly and possible pathogens include *Toxoplasma*, rubella, and CMV.[8-10] CMV infection is of particular concern because of the poor prognosis. Incidence of CMV as a cause of mild ventriculomegaly varies from 0 to 5%.[11,12] On the other hand, cerebral CMV is one of the common prenatal ultrasound abnormalities in fetuses with proven intrauterine transmission of CMV present in around 18% of cases. Poor prognosis in affected children, the potential for treatment, and the simplicity of the screening test should prompt maternal serum studies to be considered. Isolated ventriculomegaly has been associated with chromosomal abnormalities, mainly 1.4% in trisomy 21 fetuses providing a likelihood ratio of 9 for the risk of aneuploidy. Investigation for aneuploidy in the presence of the finding therefore is appropriate.[13] Follow-up USG examination should be performed, suggested time interval being 2 weeks.[14] The risks of progression of ventricular dilatation is about 11% (increase in the ventricular measurement of more than 3 mm is considered as progression). Abnormalities not seen at the initial scan can also be identified later; therefore one additional detailed ultrasound examination of the fetus should be performed between 28 and 34 weeks in order to search for cerebral and extra cerebral abnormalities. There is no solid data to suggest an increased frequency of neurological/neuropsychiatric disorders in infants with prenatal diagnosis of isolated mild ventriculomegaly.[4] Fetal MRI may add important information in 6–10% cases.

The factors that influence the prognosis of fetus with isolated mild ventriculomegaly are:

1. Fetal sex (there is a male preponderance)
2. Gestational age at diagnosis
3. Bilateral vs. unilateral
4. Symmetrical vs. asymmetric
5. Finally, the progression (cases with progression seem to be worse than those with no progression)

Moderate-to-Severe Ventriculomegaly

(Atrial width of more than 15 mm)

The term "hydrocephalus" does not signify a specific disease but is a pathological condition, because of abnormal circulation of cerebrospinal fluid (CSF). Congenital hydrocephalus is classified into three categories based on the causes which disturb the CSF circulation pathway: (a) simple hydrocephalus, (b) dysgenetic hydrocephalus (c) secondary hydrocephalus.[6]

a. *Simple hydrocephalus:* simple hydrocephalus, caused by developmental abnormality, which is localized within CSF circulation pathway, includes aqueductal stenosis, atresia of foramen of Monro, and maldevelopment of arachnoid granulations type of hydrocephalus, due to various sites of obstruction to CSF flow.

b. *Dysgenetic hydrocephalus:* Dysgenetic hydrocephalus indicates hydrocephalus as a result of cerebral developmental disorder and includes hydranencephaly, holoprosencephaly, porencephaly, shizencephaly, Dandy-Walker malformation, dysraphism, and Chiari malformation.
c. *Secondary hydrocephalus:* Hydrocephalus caused by intracranial pathologic condition, such as brain tumor, intracranial infection and intracranial hemorrhage.

In cases with progressive hydrocephalus, there may be seven stages of progression;

1. Increased fluid collection of lateral ventricles
2. Increased intracranial pressure
3. Dangling choroid plexus **(Figure 1)**
4. Disappearance of subarachnoid space
5. Excessive extension of the dura and superior sagittal sinus
6. Disappearance of venous pulsation
7. Enlarged skull.[6]

To evaluate enlarged ventricles, examiners should carefully observe the structure below and specify the cause of hydrocephalus:

- Choroids plexus, dangling or not
- Subarachnoid space, obliterated or not
- Ventricles , symmetry or asymmetry
- Visibility of third ventricle
- Pulsation of dural sinuses
- Ventricular size (3D volume calculation if possible)

ABSENT SEPTUM PELLUCIDUM

Absence of the septum pellucidum is either primary, as part of ventricular induction disorder or secondary to a disruptive process,[15-17] with or without associated anomalies. Isolated absent septum pellucidum is rare but can occur. A combination of transvaginal and transabdominal ultrasound approach is needed to image the place and extent of ventricular communication, cleavage or non cleavage of hemispheres, callosal anomalies, position of the choroid plexus and presence of CNS and other anomalies.[18] Absent CSP may be associated with various congenital brain malformations such as Holoprosencephaly, septo-optic dysplasia, agenesis of corpus callosum and schizencephaly.

Ultrasound features for differentiation between hydrocephalus and holoprosencephaly are seen in the table.

Flowchart used in differential diagnosis of fetuses with absent septum pellucidum **(Flowchart 1)**

- **Incidence:** Extremely Rare 2–3:100000
- **Etiology:** Maternal drug abuse, such as valproic acid and cocaine. Autosomal recessive, HESX 1 homeodomain gene mutation.[19]
- **Differential diagnosis:** Dysgenesis of the corpus callosum, lobar holoprosencephaly.

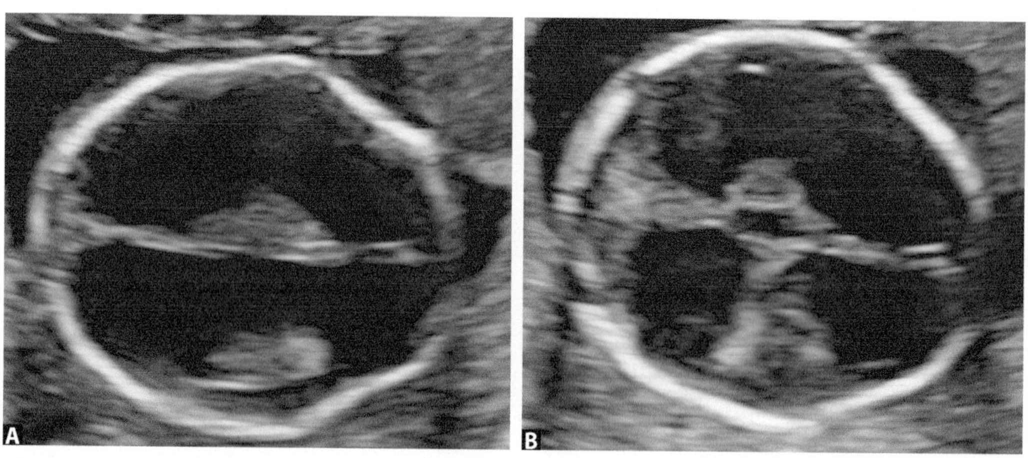

Figure 1: (A) Bilateral dialted lateral ventricles and dangling choroid plexus; (B) Dilatation of the third ventricle

Flowchart 1: How to proceed for absent septum pellucidum[20]

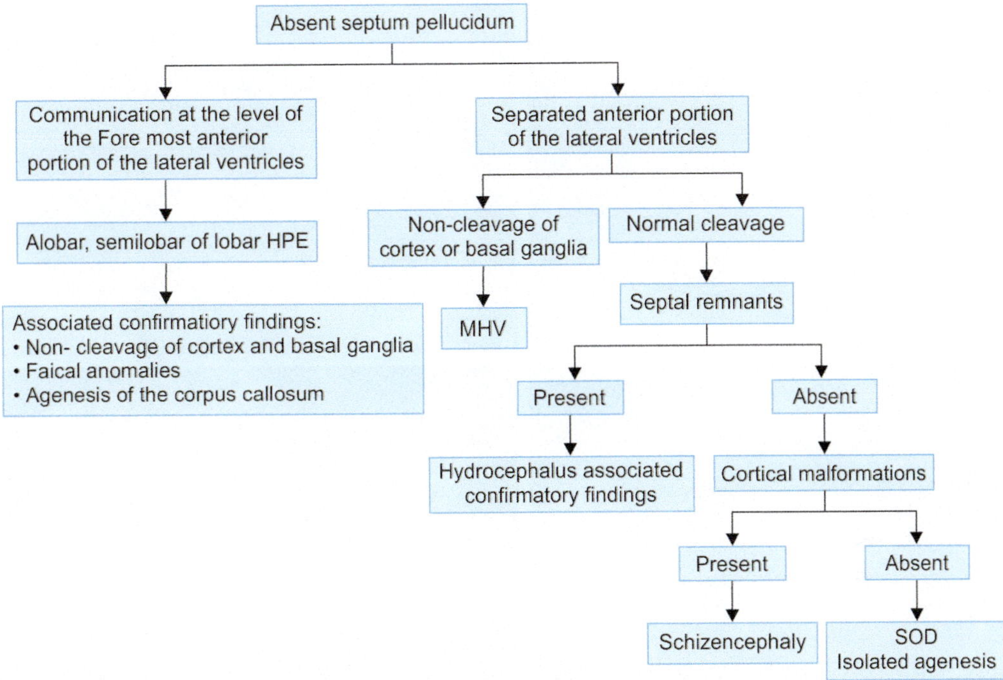

- **Prenatal diagnosis:** Transventricular, transthalamic and transcerebellar views show absent CSP.[21]
- **Prognosis:** Depends upon the associated anomalies, degree of mental deficit, presence of multiple endocrine dysfunction. Absence of septum pellucidum in most of the cases is associated with developmental abnormalities. If isolated, the prognosis may be good.
- **Recurrence risk:** Unknown
- **Management:** Endocrine dysfunction should be investigated and corrected. Shunt procedure is advised in cases of progressive ventriculomegaly and genetic counseling.

Agenesis of the Corpus Callosum

- Complete agenesis: complete absence of corpus callosum.
- Partial agenesis: absence of splenium of posterior portion in various degrees
- Incidence—0.3-0.7—1000.

Etiology: variable environmental factors, such as alcohol abuse, infections, ischemia and maternal phenylketonuria and genetic factors.

Prenatal diagnosis: Corpus callosum is detected by ultrasound after 18 weeks of gestation. Diagnosis is difficult prior to 18 weeks of gestation, even in expert hands.

Complete agenesis: absence of corpus callosum-cavum septum pellucidum complex in sagittal and coronal planes. Axial planes usually do not allow diagnosis with certainty but reveal important clues, such as:

1. Absent CSP **(Figure 2A)**
2. Ventriculomegaly (tear drop configuration of the lateral ventricles—colpocephaly) **(Figure 2B)**
3. Upward displacement of third ventricle and formation of radial sulcus **(Figure 2C).**
4. Abnormal midline lesions, cysts and lipomas.

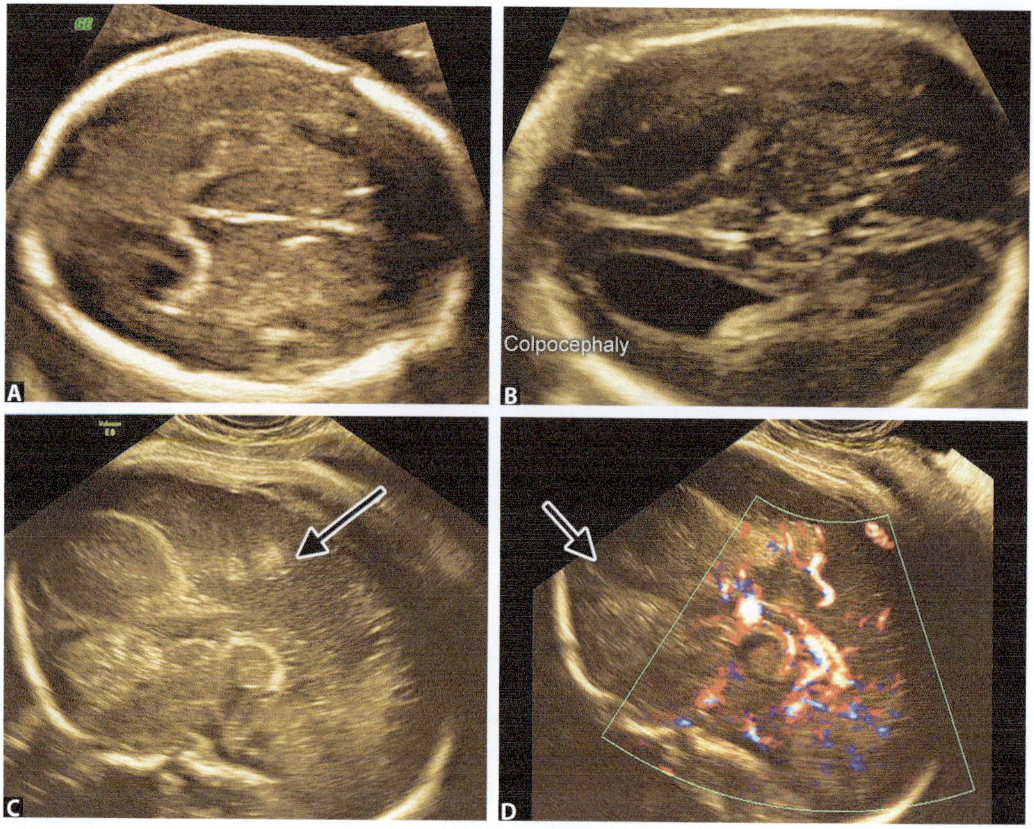

Figure 2: Transventricular scan of the fetal brain showing: (A) Absent CSP; (B) mild dilatation of lateral ventricle (colpocephaly) while the anterior part is normal; (C) sagittal view: Typical radial sulcus formation; (D) 3D power Doppler normal callosomarginal artery does not exist

Partial agenesis—affects the most posterior portion and is usually associated with less degree of distortion.

Color Doppler examination—in complete agenesis, semicircular loop of the pericallosal artery is lost. With partial agenesis, it is much shortened **(Figure 2D)**.

3D ultrasound is useful. MRI may be more informative.

Associated anomalies—Chromosomal anomalies (Trisomes 18, 13 and 8) are seen in 20% of cases. Neural anomalies are seen in 85% of cases and extraneural anomalies in 62% of cases.

Prognosis: It depends upon associated anomalies. Cases of isolated ACC are asymptomatic and neurological prognosis is good. Complete ACC has a worse prognosis than partial agenesis. Epilepsy, intellectual impairment and psychiatric disorders are noted.

Recurrence risk: It depends upon etiology.

Management: Chromosomal evaluation is offered and standard obstetric care is recommended.

HOLOPROSENCEPHALY

- **Classification:** Holoprosencephaly is classified into three varieties:
  - **Alobar type**: A single cerebral structure with a single common ventricle, **(Figure 3)** posterior large cyst of third ventricle

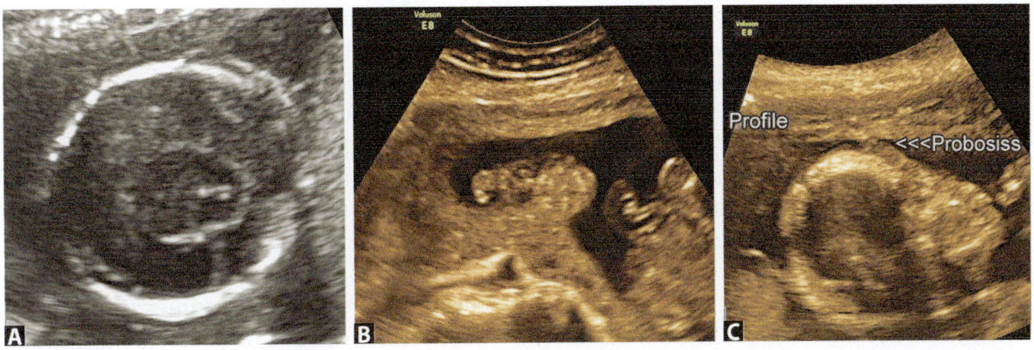

Figure 3: Alobar holoprosencephaly: Axial scan at the level of the thalamus showing the single ventricle, absence of midline structures, and fused thalamus; (B) face-proboscis

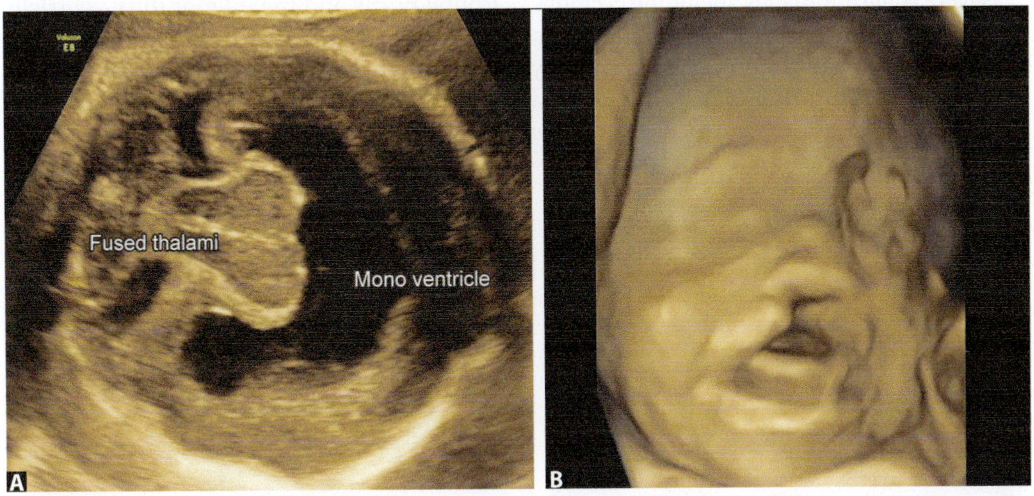

Figure 4: Alobar holoprosencephaly: Axial scan at the level of the thalamus showing (A) the single ventricle, absence of midline structures, and fused thalamus; (B) median cleft lip palate; semilobar holoprosencephaly

(dorsal sac), absence of olfactory bulbs and tracts and a single optic nerve.
 - **Semilobar type**: With formation of a posterior portion of the interhemispheric fissure.
 - **Lobar type**: With formation of interhemispheric fissure anteriorly and posteriorly but not in the mid hemispheric region. The fusion of the fornices is seen.
- **Incidence:** 1 in 15,000–20,000 live births
- **Etiology:** Heterogeneous. Genetic causes are identified in 15–50% of cases. Chromosomes 2,3,7,13,18 and 21 have been implicated in holoprosencephaly.[22] Particularly, trisomies 13 and 18 have most commonly been observed. An association with several teratogens has been suggested, including maternal diabetes, alcohol and retinoic acid consumption.
- **Pathogenesis:** Failure of the prechordal mesenchyme to induce cleavage of the forebrain and midfacial development is thought to result in a combination of cerebral and facial defects.
- **Associated anomalies:** Facial abnormalities, such as cyclopia, cebocephaly, flat nose, cleft lip and palate **(Figure 4)** are invariably associated with holoprosencephaly. Extra

cerebral abnormalities are also invariably associated due to a very early derangement of embryogenesis, such as renal and cardiac anomalies, omphalocele, etc.

- **Prenatal diagnosis:** In typical cases of alobar holoprosencephaly, sonographic diagnosis is straightforward and has been reported as early as 9 weeks of gestation. There are no midline structures in the anterior part of the brain. The boomerang-shaped ventricle is outlined anteriorly by a rim of cortex and posteriorly by the bulb shaped thalami **(Figures 4 and 5)**. Severe facial anomalies, including cyclopia, hypotelorism, proboscis and median cleft lip are seen commonly.[23,24] Many anatomical variations result in different sonographic appearances, such as the pancake, the cup and the ball types.[25]

Alobar and semilobar varieties have similar appearances and are difficult to differentiate. Sonographic clue is visualization of the hippocampal fornix. In alobar type, hippocampal fornix and rudimentary gyrus are separated from the brain stem. In semilobar type the hippocampus is seen close to the thalami forming the echogenic ambient cistern.

Specific diagnosis of lobar holoprosencephaly is difficult at times. Sonography will show some degree of enlargement of lateral ventricles, absence of the septum pellucidum and a wide communication between the frontal horns and the inferior third ventricle. Differentiation of disruption of the septum pellucidum and lobar holoprosencephaly and hydrocephalus are sometimes difficult. Some of the differences between hydrocephalus and holoprosencephaly are given below **(Table 1)**.

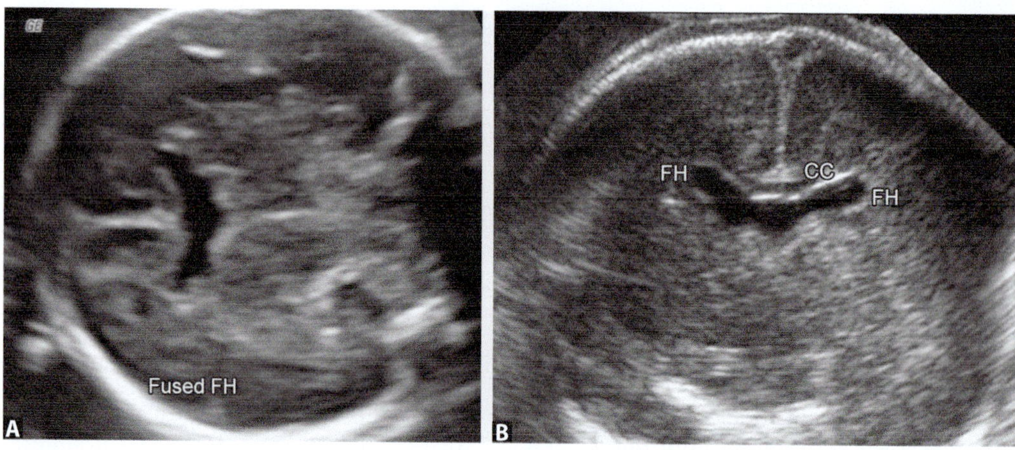

Figure 5: Lobar holoprosencephaly: Ultrasound image showing the interhemispheric fissure anteriorly with fussion of the frontal horns

Table 1: Differential diagnosis of severe hydrocephalus and holoprosencephalus[20]

	Hydrocephalus	*Holoprosencephaly*
1	Anterior portion of the lateral ventricles separated by the falx	The communication begins at the anterior portion of the lateral ventricles
2	The communication between the ventricles is only in the medial portion	The communication between the ventricles is always anteroposterior
3	Normal cleavage of the hemispheres	Non-cleavage of the hemispheres
4	Separated thalami	Non-cleavage of the thalamus
5	Normal corpus callosum	Agenesis of the corpus callosum
6	Both choroid plexus in the same side	No choroid plexus
7	Normal face	Extreme hypotelorism

Differential Diagnosis

Hydrocephalus, hydranencephaly

Prognosis

Alobar holoprosencephaly is considered a lethal condition. Semilobar is associated with extremely severe neurologic compromise.[26]

Recurrence Risk

6% but much lower in sporadic or trisomy cases and much higher in genetic cases.

Management

Chromosomal evaluation and genetic consultation are to be offered. Severe forms are almost always associated with poor prognosis; therefore termination of pregnancy should be discussed with the couple (according to the law of the particular country).

Posterior Fossa Anomaly

The algorithm for the main abnormalities of the posterior fossa that can be depicted on routine ultrasound (Axial plane) is seen below.

Diagnostic Ultrasound Criteria (Figure 6)

1. Increased cisterna magna: Increased fluid filled space of the posterior fossa.
2. Abnormal transcerebellar diameter
3. Abnormal cerebellar anatomy

Increased fluid-filled space of the posterior fossa: The main anatomic land mark is the position of the cerebellar tentorium and torcular. In the case of ascent of the torcular, the increased fluid-filled retro-or pericerebellar space is related to an expansion of the fourth ventricle, and this is characteristic of Dandy-Walker malformation. In case of normal positioning of the torcular the main criterion on which to base the diagnosis is anatomy and biometry of cerebellum. If the cerebellum is biometrically and anatomically normal, the increased fluid, filled space is related either to a rotation of normal vermis with or without blake's pouch cyst, or to an arachnoid cyst or a megacisterna magna.

Abnormal transcerebellar diameter: Decreased cerebellar biometry can be associated with either normal or abnormal cerebellar anatomy. Decreased cerebellar biometry with normal anatomy can be either focal or global. Global decrease needs focus on brain stem to differentiate cerebellar hypoplasia from ponto cerebellar hypoplasia. Decreased cerebellar biometry can also be focal.

Abnormal cerebellar anatomy: Abnormal cerebellar anatomy (banana sign) and the non identification of obliterated cisterna magna are seen in Chari II malformation. Analysis of

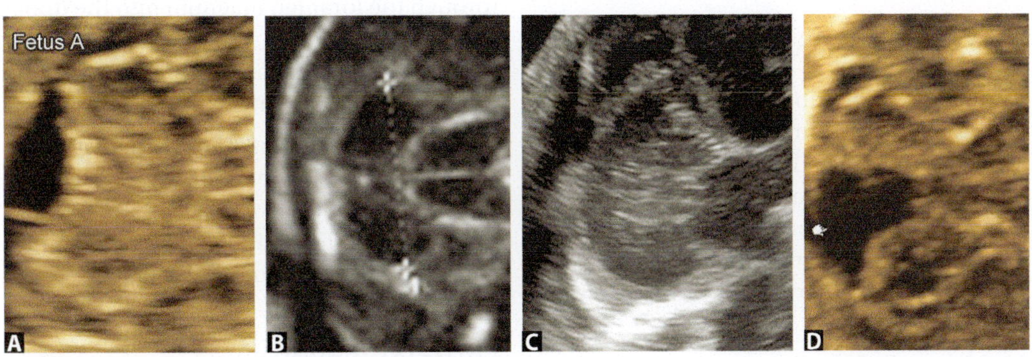

Figure 6: (A) normal dumbell shaped cerebellum and cisternamegna; (B) disappearance of cisterna magna and banana-shaped cerebellum-chiari malformation; (C) fussed cerebellum with absent vermis—rhombencephalosynapsis; (D) abnormal dilatation of fourth ventricle cyst communication with cisterna magna—Dandy-walker malformation

Flowchart 2: Following the posterior cranial fossa lesions

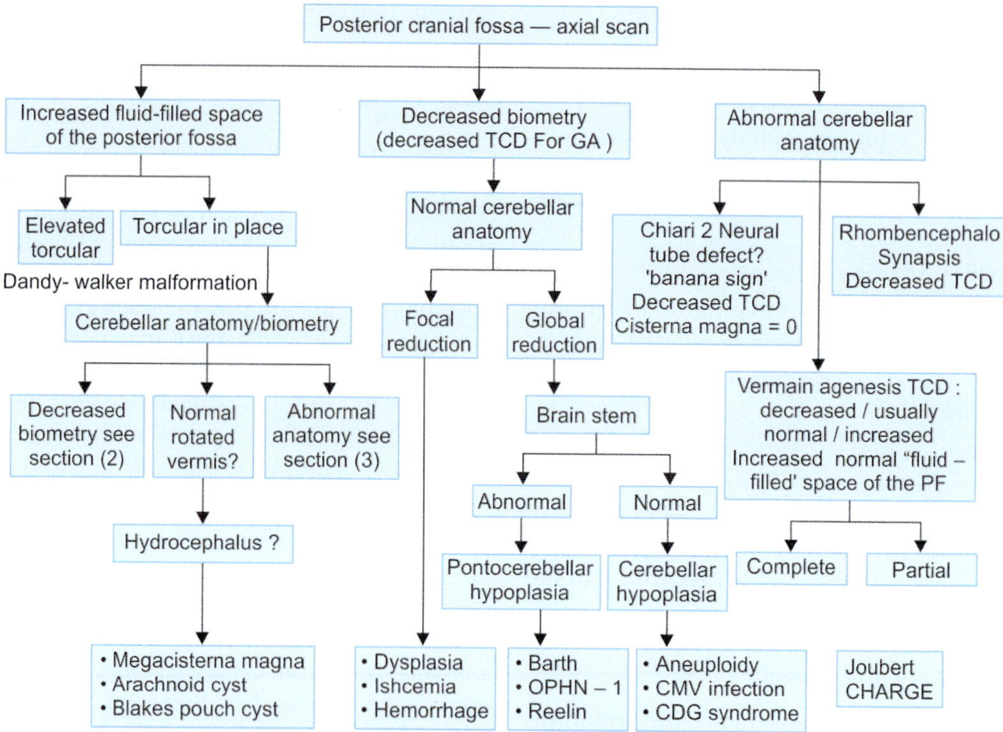

vermian fissures, cerebellar hemispheres and identification of fourth ventricle are important to differentiate rhombencephalosynapsis from partial and complete agenesis[27-29] of vermis **(Flowchart 2)**. In this chapter Chiari malformation and Dandy-Walker malformation are discussed in detail.

CHIARI MALFORMATION

Cerebellar herniation into the spinal canal is classified into three types based on the contents of herniated tissue.

- Type 1—lip of cerebellum
- Type 2—part of cerebellum, fourth ventricle and medulla oblongata and pons
- Type 3—large herniation of the posterior fossa.

Incidence: 1:1000

Synonyms: Arnold Chiari malformation

Etiology: Depends on the types.

Pathogenesis: Chiari malformation occurs due to (i) inferior displacement of the medulla and the fourth ventricle into the upper cervical canal, (ii) elongation and thinning of the upper medulla and lower pons and persistence of the embryonic flexure of these structures, (iii) inferior displacement of the lower cerebellum through the foramen magnum into the upper cervical region, and (iv) a variety of bony defects of the foramen magnum, occiput, and upper cervical vertebrae.

Associated anomalie: 88% of fetuses with open spina bifida develop ventriculomegaly, and the majority do so by 21 weeks of gestation. Other CNS abnormalities, foot and other system anomalies may be associated with it.

PRENATAL DIAGNOSIS

Lemon and banana signs are[30,31] evidences of Chiari malformation **(Figure 7)** which are

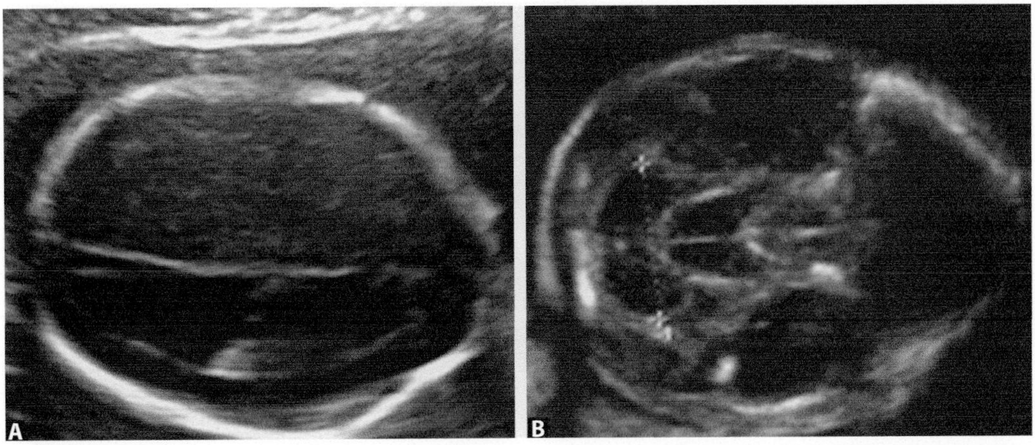

Figure 7: (A) Dilatation of the lateral cerebral ventricles and "lemon sign" are clearly seen; (B) Disappearance of cistern megna and banana-shaped cerebellum

easily demonstrated in the second trimester. Lemon sign indicates deformity of the frontal bone; banana sign indicates abnormal shape of cerebellum without cisterna magna space.

Prognosis: Feeding distrurbances, laryngeal stridor or apnoeic episodes, are found in approximately 9–30% of cases. Prognosis is often poor.

Recurrence risk depends on the type of malformation.

Dandy-Walker malformation, Dandy-Walker variant, megacisterna magna.

The term Dandy-Walker complex is used to indicate a spectrum of anomalies of the posterior fossa. Dandy - Walker malformation, Dandy-walker variant, and megacisterna magna seem to represent a continuum of developmental anomalies of the posterior fossa.[32]

CLASSIFICATION

Dandy-Walker malformation (classic): Cystic dilation of fourth ventricle, enlarged posterior fossa, elevated tentorium and complete or partial agenesis of the cerebellar vermis **(Figure 8)**.

Dandy-Walker variant: Variable hypoplasia of the cerebellar vermis with or without enlargement of the posterior fossa.

Megacisterna magna: Enlarged cisterna magna with integrity of both cerebellar vermis and fourth ventricle.

Incidence of Dandy-Walker malformation (classic): about 1:30,000 births.

Incidence of Dandy-Walker variant and megacisterna magna is unknown.

Etiology: Chromosomal aberrations, such as partial monosomy/trisomy, viral infections and diabetes.

Pathogenesis: During development of roof of the fourth ventricle, there is a delay or total failure of the foramen of Magendie to open, allowing a build up of CSF and development of the cystic dilation of the fourth ventricle. Despite the subsequent opening of the foramina of Luschka, cystic dilation of the fourth ventricle persists and CSF flow is impaired.

Associated anomalies of Dandy-Walker malformation: Cranial abnormalities, such as hydrocephalus, agenesis of corpus callosum, holoprosencephaly and occipital encephalocele. Extracranial abnormalities,

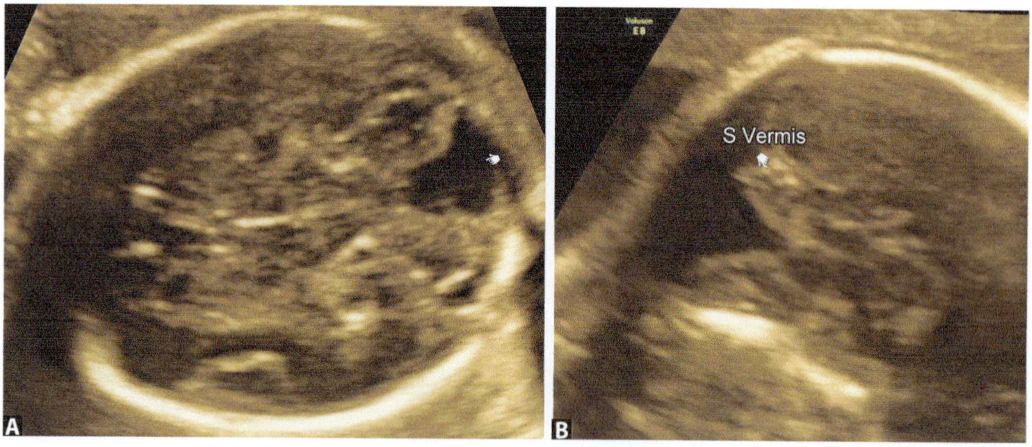

Figure 8: (A) Vermian hypoplasia with posterior fossa cyst; (B) Ascent of the torcular, the increased fluid filled retro or pericerebellar space is related to an expansion of the fourth ventricle, and this is characteristic of Dandy–Walker malformation

such as congenital heart diseases, neural tube defects and cleft lip/palate.

Prenatal diagnosis: *Increased fluid-filled space of the posterior fossa, an ascent of the torcular, the increased fluid-filled retro-or pericerebellar space is related to an expansion of the fourth ventricle, and this is characteristic of Dandy-Walker malformation* (perhaps this should be simplified).

Differential diagnosis: Infratentorial arachnoid cyst, other intracranial cystic tumors, hydrocephalus, cerebellar dysplasia.

Prognosis: Outcome is generally poor. Nearly 40% of affected fetuses die, and 75% of survivors exhibit cognitive deficits.

Recurrence risk: Depends on etiology. Generally 1–5% (Dandy-Walker malformation)
Management: Standard obstetric care and shunting procedures after birth.

NEURONAL MIGRATION DISORDERS

Neuronal migration disorders are caused by the abnormal migration of neurons in the developing brain and nervous system. Neurons must migrate from the area where they are born to the surface of the brain. The process of neuromigration results in an increase in the surface of the cortex, leading to formation of sulci and gyri. Neuronal migration disorders can result in incomplete formation of the cortical layers leading to structurally abnormal or missing areas of the brain in the cerebral hemispheres, cerebellum, brainstem or hippocampus, leading to, schizencephaly, porencephaly, lissencephaly, agyria, macrogyria, pachygyria, microgyria, micropolygyria, neuronal heterotopias (including band heterotopia), agenesis of the corpus callosum, and agenesis of the cranial nerves.[33]

LISSENCEPHALY

Lissencephaly is characterized by a lack of gyral development. The surface of the brain appears smooth. There are several types of lissencephaly. Classification is based on the associated malformations and etiology. On this basis, five major groups of lissencephaly can be recognized.[34]

1. Classical lissencephaly (previously known as type 1 lissencephaly):
   - Lissencephaly due to LIS 1 gene mutation, which is subdivided into
     - Type 1 isolated lissencephaly

   - Miller - Dieker syndrome
     - ♦ Lissencephaly due to double cortin (DCX) gene mutation
     - ♦ Lissencephaly, type 1, isolated, without other known genetic defects.
2. Lissencephaly X-linked with agenesis of the corpus callosum (ARX gene)
3. Lissencephaly with cerebellar hypoplasia, including
   - Norman - Roberts syndrome (mutation of reelin gene)
4. Microlissencephaly (Lissencephaly and microcephaly).
5. Cobblestone lissencephaly, including
   - Waker - Warburg syndrome, HARD (E) syndrome
   - Fukuyama syndrome
   - Muscle-Eye-Brain (MEB) disease.

Incidence: Rare.

Pathogenesis: Failure of migration of the neurons results in a reduction or absence of cerebral convolutions (smooth brain surface) and four rather than six, layers in the cortex.

Associated anomalies: Polyhydramnios, decreased fetal movement, colpocephaly, agenesis of the corpus callosum, Dandy - Walker malformation, micrognathia, flat nose, high forehead, low - set ears and cardiac anomalies are noted.

Prenatal diagnosis: Incomplete opercularization of the insula, abnormal/delayed formation of sulci and gyri, borderline ventriculomegaly, increased subarachnoid space. Some cases are also associated with microcephaly during third trimester.

Prognosis: Prognosis is poor. Severe seizures, mental disorders and death in the first year of life are common.

Recurrence Risk: Depends upon etiology.

Management: Conservative, as the diagnosis is made during the third trimester. Genetic workup is recommended.

SCHIZENCEPHALY

Incidence: Rare

Definition: A disorder characterized by congenital clefts in the cerebral mantle, lined by pia - ependyma. These clefts communicate with the subarachnoid space laterally and the ventricular system medially. 63% of cases are unilateral and 37% are bilateral.

Etiology: Etiology is uncertain. In certain familial cases, a point mutation in the homeobox gene, EMX 2 was found. Cytomegalovirus infection was also related in some cases.[35]

Pathogenesis: Neuronal migration disorder

Associated anomalies: Ventriculomegaly, polymicrogyria, gray matter heterotopias, dysgenesis of the corpus callosum, absence of the septum pellucidum are frequently found.

Prenatal diagnosis: Cleft in the cortex in the area of the Sylvian fissures communicating with enlarged lateral ventricles and subarachnoid space laterally.

Differential diagnosis: Porencephaly, arachnoid cyst or other intracranial cystic masses. MR imaging is useful in diagnosis of schizencephaly.

Prognosis: Variable. Patients generally suffer from mental retardation, seizures and developmental delay.

Recurrence risk: Unknown.

MICROCEPHALY

Microcephaly is defined as a head circumference that is more than 2 standard deviations below the normal mean for age, sex, race, and gestation.

Incidence: 1.6 per 1000

Etiopathogenesis: Microcephaly usually results from either primary (congenital) or secondary (acquired) brain dysgenesis.

Primary dysgenesis results from a developmental field defect or genetic abnormality.

Secondary brain dysgenesis occurs from an insult to a well formed brain (vascular accident, infections etc)

Differential diagnosis: Craniosynostosis.

Prenatal diagnosis: Head circumference less than 2SD below the mean for gestational age, abnormal shape of the head, sloping forehead, ventriculomegaly, abnormal sylvian fissure, lissencephaly, periventricular echogenic halo, corpus callosal abnormalities **(Figure 9)**. Diagnosis by ultrasound is limited. In severe cases, intracranial contents may not be visible as a result of narrowing of the sutures.

Prognosis: Prognosis depends upon associated anomalies. Hyperactivity and moderate to severe mental retardation are common occurrences. Convulsions may also occur. Motor ability varies, ranging from clumsiness in some to spastic quadriplegia in others.

Recurrence risk: Unknown.

Treatment: No specific treatment exists for microcephaly. Treatment is symptomatic and supportive.

INTRACRANIAL TUMORS

Incidence: Extremely rare. 34 per million live births.

Pathology: Teratomas are most commonly reported tumors and nonteratomatous tumors include neuroepithelial tumor, such as medulloblastoma, astrocytoma, choroid plexus papilloma, choroid plexus carcinoma,

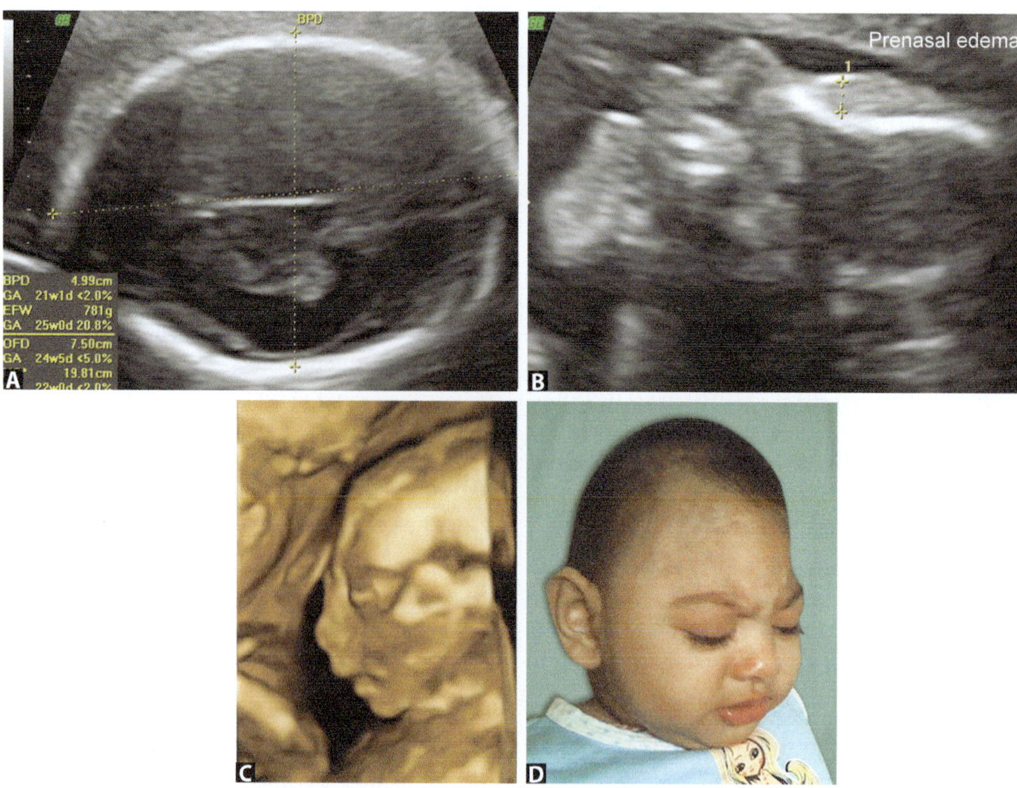

Figure 9: Microcephaly (A) Cephalobiometry less than 2 SD; (B) Face sagittal view—flat face with frontal bone and nasal bone on a single line 2D US picture; (C) 3D sagittal view; (D) postnatal picture of the child

hemangioma and meningioma and others are lipoma of the corpus callosum, subependymal giant-cell astrocytoma associated with tuberous sclerosis.[36,37]

LOCATION OF TUMOR

Most lesions are supratentorial whereas infratentorial predominance is seen in older children. Choroid plexus papilloma is located within the lateral ventricles.

Associated abnormalities: Macrocrania or local skull swelling, secondary hydrocephalus, intracranial hemorrhage, intraventricular hemorrhage, polyhydramnios, heart failure by high cardiac output and hydrops.

Prenatal diagnosis: Intracranial masses with solid, cystic or mixed pattern with or without visualization by ultrasound and fetal MRI. Brain tumor should be considered in cases with unexplained intracranial hemorrhage.

Differential diagnosis: Arachnoid cyst, vein of Galen aneurysm, porencephaly, schizencephaly, periventricular leukomalacia, subdural hemorrhage.

Prognosis: Prognosis in neonates is generally poor, but depends on timing of diagnosis and the type of tumor.

Recurrence risk: Unknown.

Management: Cesarean section may be considered. Neurosurgical tumor resection and chemotherapy are possible treatments for neonatal tumors.

INTRACRANIAL CYSTS: ARACHNOID CYST, INTERHEMISPHERIC CYST

Congenital or acquired cysts are filled with fluid collection which is of the same character as the cerebrospinal fluid. The number of cysts is mostly single, but two or more cysts can occasionally be observed.

Location of arachnoid cyst is varied; approximately 50% of cysts arise from the Sylvian fissure, 20% from the posterior fossa, and 10–20% each from the convexity, suprasellar, inter hemispheric, and quadrigeminal cistern in the pediatric population.[38]

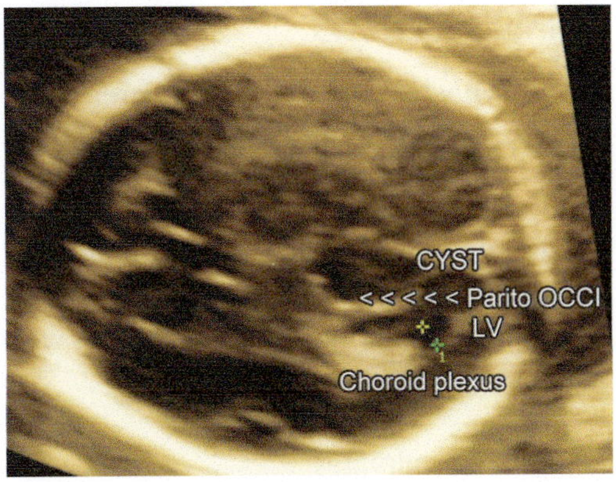

Figure 10: Arachnoid cyst: Well-defined anechoic cyst seen medial to occipital horn of the lateral ventricle

Prevalence: 1% of intracranial masses in newborns.

Etiology: Unknown.

Pathogenesis: Congenital arachnoid cyst is formed by maldevelopment of the arachnoid membrane. CSF accumulation is (seen in) the subarachnoid space or intra-arachnoid layers.

Associated anomalies: Unilateral or bilateral hydrocephalus, macrocrania.

Prenatal diagnosis: Well-defined anechoic lesion with adjacent mass effect occasionally associated with hydrocephalus **(Figure 10)**.

Differential diagnosis: Porencephaly, schizencephaly, third vein of Galen, aneurysm.

Prognosis: Generally good. Postnatally, many cysts are asymptomatic and remain quiescent for years, although others expand. Neurological symptoms are caused by compression of adjacent brain.

Recurrence risk: Unknown.

Obstetrical management: Arachnoid cysts may increase or decrease in size. Therefore, expectant management of antenatally diagnosed cases is suggested.

CRANIOSYNOSTOSIS

Craniosynostosis is defined as premature closure of cranial suture, which may affect one or more cranial sutures. Simple sagittal synostosis is most common. Various cranial shapes are seen depending on the affected suture **(Figure 11)**.

Incidence: Unknown and associated with many syndromes.

Associated Syndromes

Crouzon syndrome: Acrocephaly, synostosis of coronal, sagittal and lambdoid sutures with ocular proptosis, maxillary hypoplasia.

Apert syndrome: Brachycephaly, synostosis of coronal and/or sagittal sutures with hypertelorism, broad thumbs and toes, partial syndactyly.

Antley-Bixler syndrome: Brachycephaly, multiple synostosis, especially of coronal suture with maxillary hypoplasia, radio humeral synostosis, choanal atresia, arthrogryposis.

Etiology: Genetic—mutation in FGFR genes.[40]

Pathogenesis

1. Cranial vault bones with decreased growth potential
2. Asymmetrical bone deposition at perimeter sutures

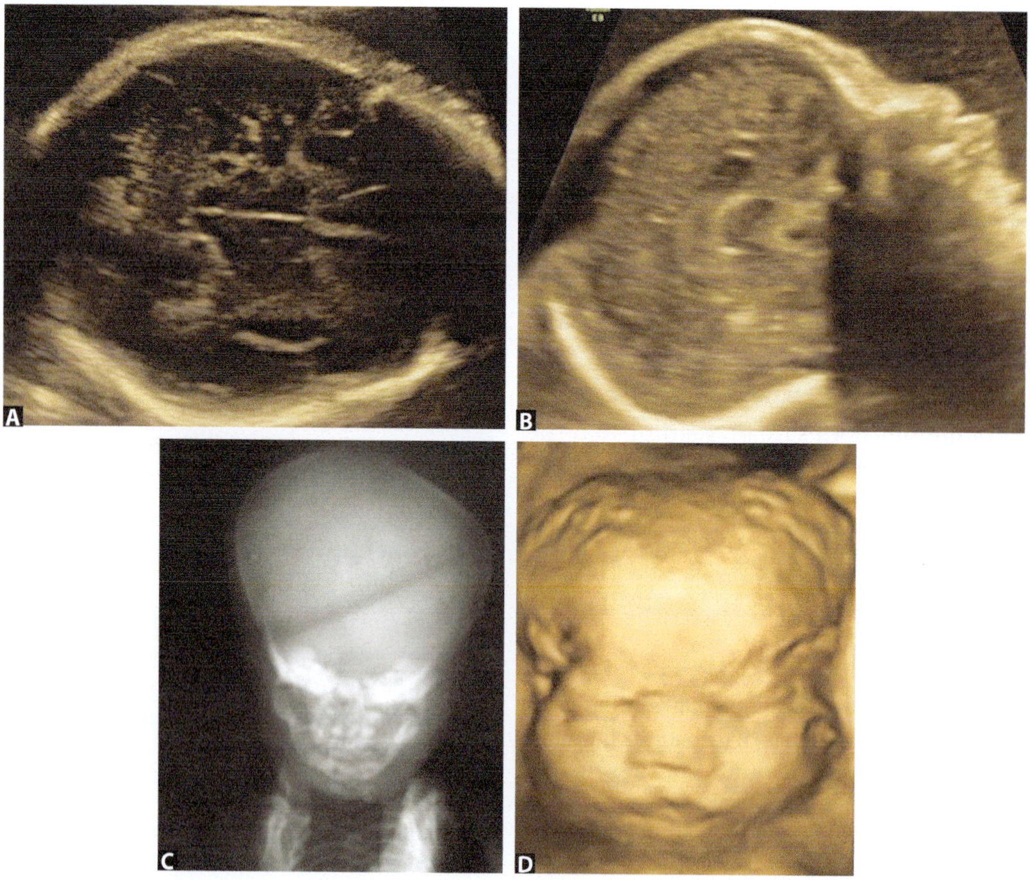

Figure 11: Craniosynostosis: (A) Clover leaf skull with craniosynostosis in a case of thanatophoric type 2; (B) Abnormal profile view; (C) Postnatal X-ray; (D) 3D image of the same fetus inutero

3. Sutures adjacent to the prematurely fused sutures not contiguous with the closed sutures
4. Enhanced symmetrical bone deposition occurs along both sides of a non-perimeter suture continuing prematurely closed suture **(Figure 11C)**.

Associated anomalies: Hypertelorism, syndactyly, polydactyly, exophthalmos, frontal bossing, and low nasal bridge.

Prenatal diagnosis: Abnormal craniofacial appearance can be detected by 2D/3D ultrasound.

Prognosis: Varies. In some cases of trigonocephaly and syndromic types, prognosis is poor.

Recurrence risk: Depends on etiology.

Management: Operative aim of cranioplasty is improvement.

ACQUIRED BRAIN ABNORMALITIES IN UTERO

Intracranial Hemorrhage

Intracranial hemorrhage includes subdural hemorrhage, intraventricular hemorrhage and intraparenchymal hemorrhage and intracerebellar hemorrhage.[41]

Incidence: Unknown.

Etiology: Trauma, alloimmune and idiopathic thrombocytopenia, von willebrand's disease, illicit drug abuse, seizures, fetal conditions including congenital factor-10 and factor-5 deficiencies, intracranial tumor, twin-twin transfusion, demise of a co-twin, vascular diseases, feto maternal hemorrhage and extracorporeal membrane oxygenation (ECMO).[41]

On prenatal ultrasound, it is diagnosed as hyperechoic lesions inside the ventricles, distorting the normal smooth ventricular margins **(Figure 12)**.

Associated anomalies: Hydrocephalus, hydranencephaly, porencephaly, or microcephaly.

Differential diagnosis: Intracranial tumor.

Prognosis: Uncertain. It depends upon the cause of hemorrhage. Some cases of local cerebral hemorrhage/intraventricular hemorrhage have good prognosis. Poor prognosis is seen in premature infants, apnea, seizures, and other neurological symptoms.

Recurrence risk: Depends upon etiology.

Management: Ventriculo-peritoneal shunt if hydrocephalus progresses.

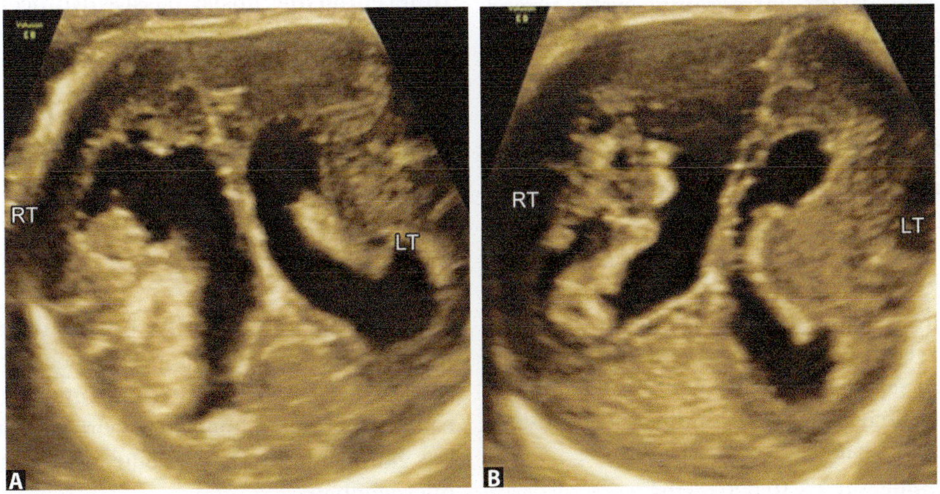

Figure 12: Intracerebral hemorrhage

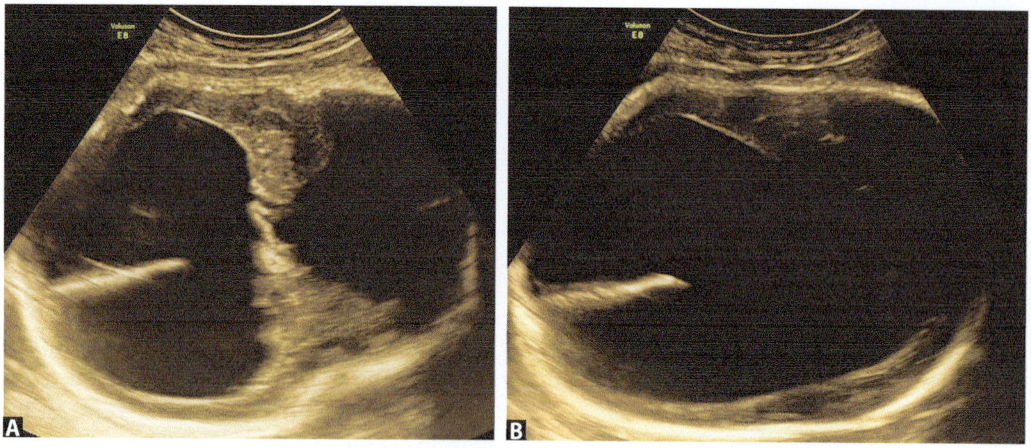

Figure 13: Hydrancephaly: Large cystic mass filling the entire cranial cavity with absence or discontinuity of the cerebral cortex and the midline echo

Porencephaly

Porencephaly is defined as fluid-filled spaces replacing normal brain parenchyma, which may or may not communicate with lateral ventricles or subarachnoid space.

Incidence: Unknown.

Etiopathology: Ischemic injury is strongly related to porencephaly, trauma, demise of one twin, intracerebral hemorrhage, cytomegalo virus infection.[42,43]

Differential diagnosis: Schizencephaly, arachnoid cyst, intracranial cystic tumor, other cysts.

Prognosis: Varies, depending upon the timing of occureence and size of the lesion.

Recurrence risk: Unknown.

Management: Ventriculoperitoneal shunt if hydrocephalus progresses.

Hydranencephaly

Hydranencephaly is a condition in which there is absence of the cerebral hemispheres and a sac-like structure containing cerebral spinal fluid is seen surrounding the brainstem and basal ganglia.

Incidence: 1–2.5:10,000 births.

Etiopathology: Ischemic injury is strongly related to porencephaly and hydranencephaly.[44]

Ischemic episode, trauma, demise of one twin, intracerebral hemorrhage, occlusion of the supraclinoid segment of the internal carotid arteries or the middle cerebral arteries are some of the causes.

Prenatal diagnosis: Large cystic mass filling the entire cranial cavity with absence or discontinuity of the cerebral cortex and the midline echo **(Figure 13)**.

Differential diagnosis: Massive hydrocephalus, alobar holoprosencephaly, porencephaly.

Prognosis: Extremely poor.

Recurrence risk: Unknown.

Management: No active treatment. Termination of pregnancy can be offered.

CONGENITAL INFECTIONS

Maternal infection during pregnancy may result in congenital infection. Cytomegalovirus (CMV) infection and toxoplasmosis may cause fetal brain damage. Zika virus infection has gained importance recently as a cause of microcephaly.

Prenatal diagnosis:[49] Fetal CMV infection remains undetected with routine sonography in most cases. Intracranial abnormalities include multiple calcification, abnormal periventricular echogenicity in association with diffuse lissencephaly or cerebellar hypoplasia.

Zika virus infection: Ultrasound features are periventricular and cerebral parenchymal calcifications, progressive pattern of posterior fossa lesions with mega cistern magna, cerebellar hypoplasia and vermis destruction, mild to severe ventriculomegaly, growth restriction, and arthrogryposis.

(NORMAL VARIANTS) CHOROID PLEXUS CYSTS

Cysts with fluid collection within the choroid plexus which may be unilateral or bilateral. They are detected in the second trimester and usually resolve by the 24th week of gestation **(Figure 14)**.

Incidence: 0.61–2.89% of all fetuses scanned.[46-48]

Pathogenesis: Choroid plexus is located within the ventricular system and produces cerebrospinal fluid. Choroid plexus cyst exists, within the choroidal villi, surrounded by the loose stroma of the choroid plexus. They probably result from entrapment of cerebrospinal fluid within tangled villi of the fetal ventricular system.

Associated anomalies: In cases of trisomy 18, the associated anomalies include growth retardation, congenital heart disease, overlapping fingers, facial anomaly and cerebellar dysplasia.

Prenatal diagnosis: Sonolucent area in the choroid plexus of the lateral ventricles with a diameter of greater than 2 mm.

Differential diagnosis: Intraventricular hemorrhage.

Management: An isolated choroid plexus cyst is an indication to perform a detailed and accurate examination of other markers of aneuploidy. If the choroid plexus cyst is an isolated finding by detailed scan, there is no reason to perform amniocenesis.

VASCULAR ANOMALIES

Vein of Galen Aneurysm

These are vascular anomalies, which are a congenital malformation of blood vessels of the brain. The incidence is rare and the etiology and recurrence risk are unknown. The main structure is direct arteriovenous fistula in which blood shunts from choroidal and/ or quadrigeminal arteries into an overlying

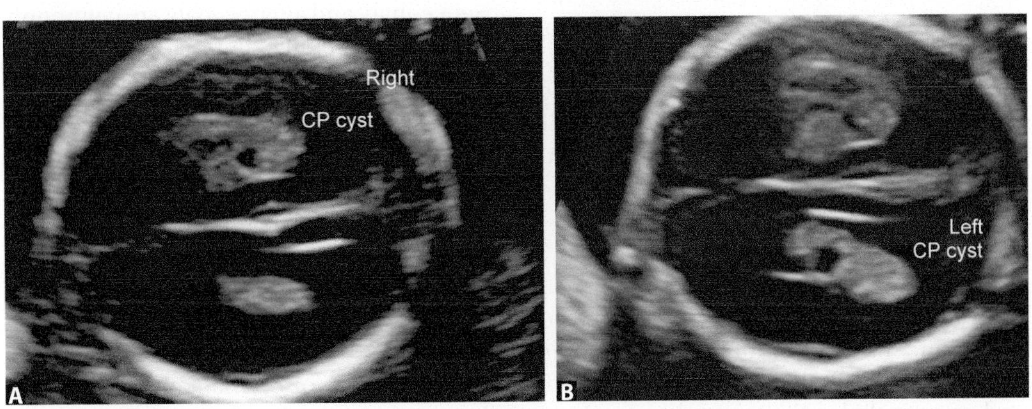

Figure 14: Isolated bilateral choroid plexus cyst–hypoechoeic areas in the choroid plexus

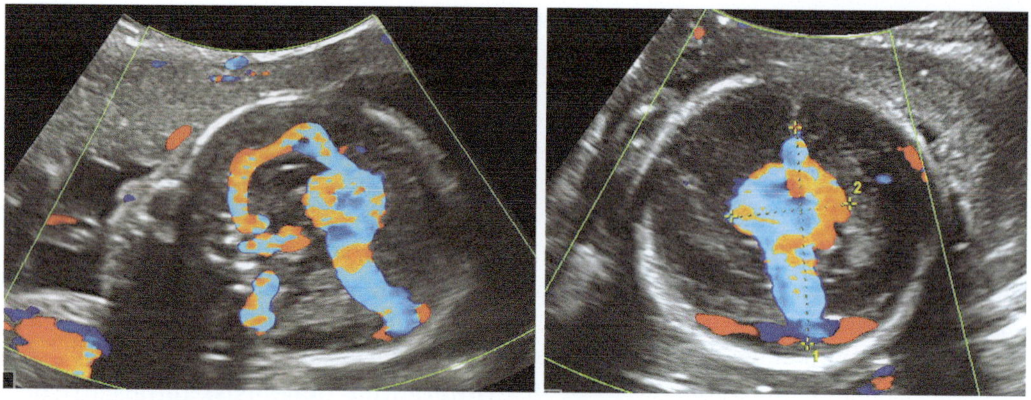

Figure 15: Vein of Galen aneurysm. Anterior cerebral artery and the pericallosal artery feeder into the VOG aneurysm. Drainage via the dilated straight sinus and the transverse sinuses is seen

single median venous sac. This leads to progressive aneurysmal dilatation of the vein, whose wall becomes thick and tough. Vein of Galen aneurysm is not a real aneurysm' but an arteriovenous malformation.[49,50]

Prenatal diagnosis: Elongated anechoic area at the level of the cistern of the vein of Galen. Color Doppler helps in identifying the origin of the vessels feeding the lesion. Cerebral architecture may be intact or distorted **(Figure 15)**.

Differential diagnosis: Arachnoid cyst, porencephalic cyst, and intracranial teratoma.

Prognosis: Outcome did not differ between treated and non-treated cases and over 80% of cases died. However, recent advances in treatment have improved outcome, such that 60 to 100% survive and over 60% have a good neurological outcome. Therefore referral to paediatric tertiary care unit is required. Percutaneous embolization by micro coils is recent main postnatal treatment with remarkably improved outcome.

NEURAL TUBE DEFECTS

Neural tube defects are birth defects of the brain, spine, or spinal cord. The most common neural tube defects are spina bifida and anencephaly. NTDs can be classified, based on embryological considerations and the presence or absence of exposed neural tissue, as open or closed types.[51]

Open NTDs result from failure of primary neurulation,neural tube is exposed with CSF leakage.

Closed NTS result from a defect in secondary neurulation,neural tissue is not exposed (skin closed dysraphism).

Cranium bifidum is classified into four types[6]

Encephaloschisis (including anencephaly and exencephaly), meningocele, encephalo-meningocele, encephalocystocele, and cranium bifidum occultum. Encephalocele occurs in the occipital region in 70-80% of cases. Acrania (absent skull valult- **Figure 17**), exencephaly and anencephaly are commonly used as synonyms. It is considered that dysraphia (absent cranial vault) occurs in very early stage and disintegration of the exposed brain (exencephaly) during the fetal period results in anencephaly.[52]

Prenatal diagnosis: Acrania is absence of calvaria above the bony orbits Prenatal ultrasound exencephaly has abnormal head shape with sonolucent spaces with in the exposed and disintegrating brain due to the absence of cranial vault. The outer shape of the exposed two hemispheres

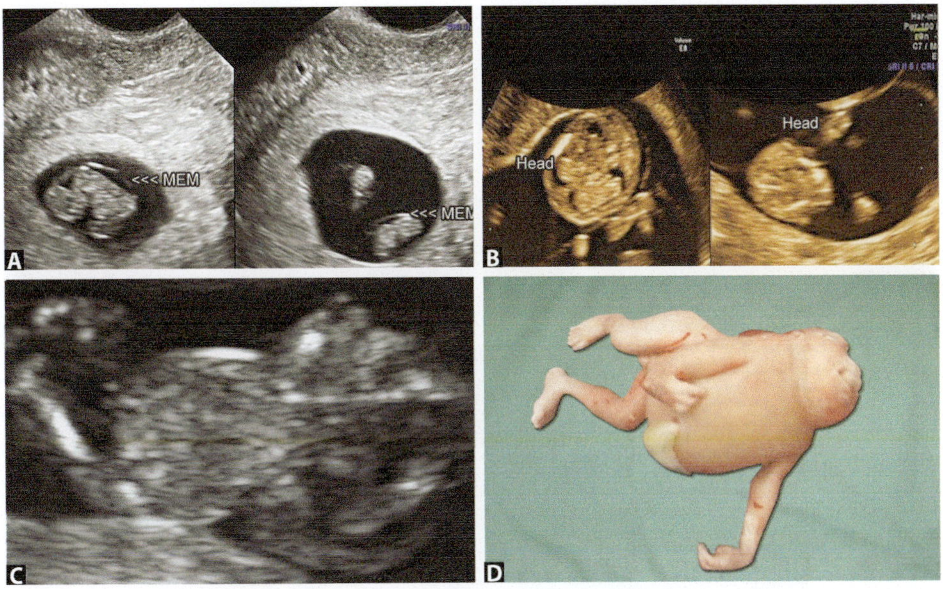

Figure 16: (A) Monochorionic diamniotic twins at 8 weeks discrepency in the CRL noted; (B) cranial vault absent in one twin at 10 weeks; (C) absent cranial vault,retroflexion of the neck and the spinal defect noted; (D) post abortal picture (fetus had multiple anomalies)

fall to the side giving Mickey mouse head appearance. Exencephaly observed during first trimester typically evolves into anencephaly.[53]

Anencephalic fetus **(Figure 16)** can be diagnosed as early as 9 to 10 weeks, definitively by 12 weeks. Dystrophic exposed brain tissue with no skull above the orbits anteriorly and above the cervical spine posteriorly. Polyhydramnios develops in upto 50% of cases during second and third trimester.

Cephalocele are cranial defects through which the brain and/or meninges have herniated outside of the skull. The occipital, frontal,parietal,orbital,nasal or nasopharyngeal region of the head can be involved,but most occur posteriorly.

Sonographic appearance of cephalocele is a defect of the bony skull with protruding sac like structure which may contain anechoic cerebrospinal fliud (meningocele), brain tissue (encephalocele) or a combination of both[54] **(Figures 18 and 19).** Cephaloceles are usually isolated but may be part of a syndromes such as Meckel-Gruber or Walker -Warburg syndrome.

Inencephaly is a rare,lethal anomaly with a defect in the occiput ,retroflexion of the entire spine (occiput is directed towards lumbar spine and the fetus look upwards),open spinal defects of variable degrees.[55] This is typically described as star gazing fetus **(Figure 20)**.

Spinal Dysraphism

Protrusion of spinal contents through a bony defect in the spine. Myelocele is a midline plaque of neural tissue (neural placode that is flush with the fetal surface and not covered by skin. The bony defect is identified as asymmetry and non-parallelism of the ossification centres of the vertebral column. The overlying skin may or may not show a breech. With discontinuity of the overlying skin, it is an open spinal canal defect, where as with the intact skin it is an occult defect. These abnormalities may be seen as early as end of

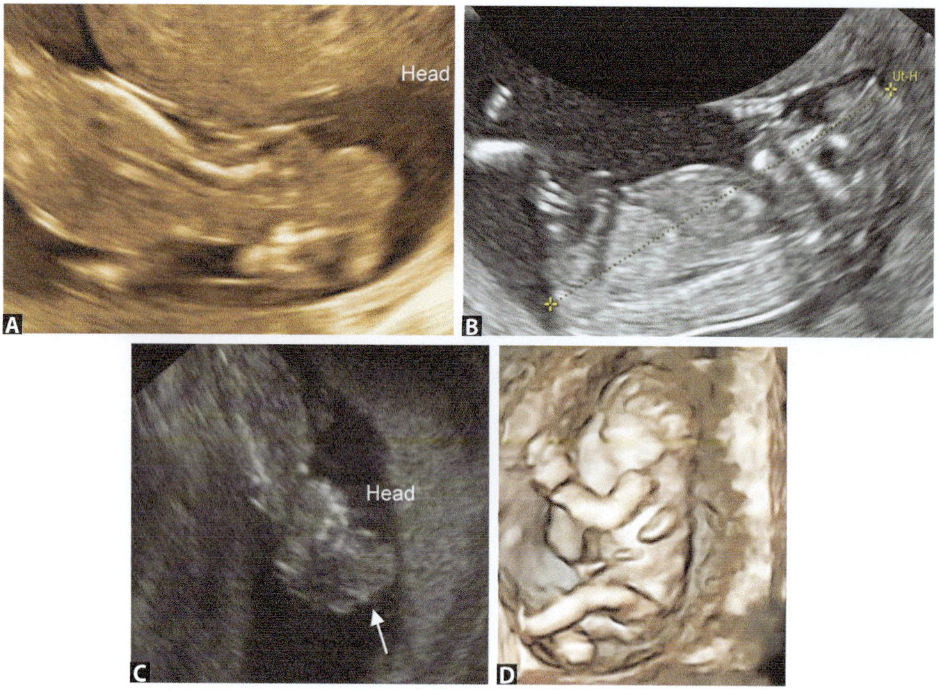

Figure 17: (A, B and C)cranial vault absent with dystrophic intracranial structures of 14 weeks fetus (D) 3d picture of acrania fetus at 14 weeks

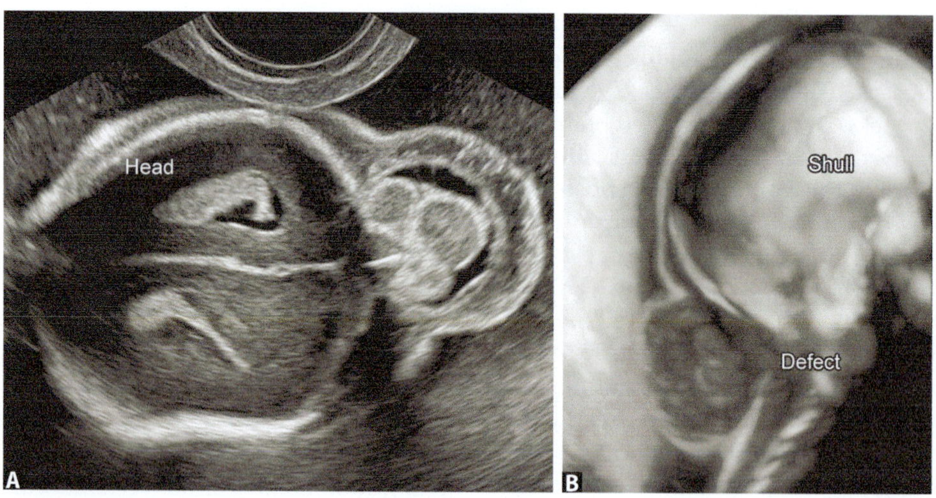

Figure 18: (A) axial view occipital encepholocele is seen (B) 3D picture of the same fetus with the defect at the occipital region

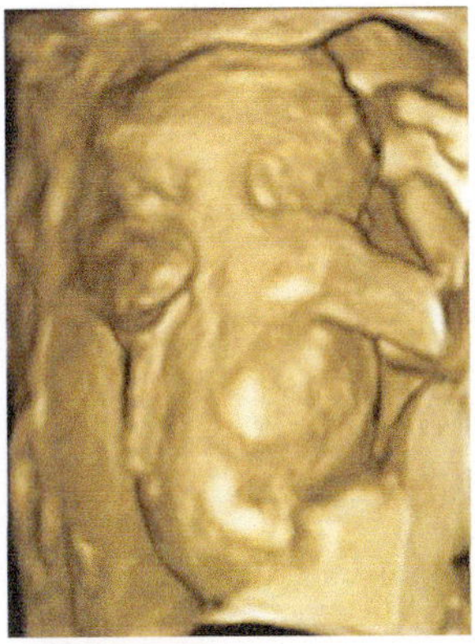

Figure 19: Defect in the occiput ,open spinal defects seen from occipital region to the lumbosacral region

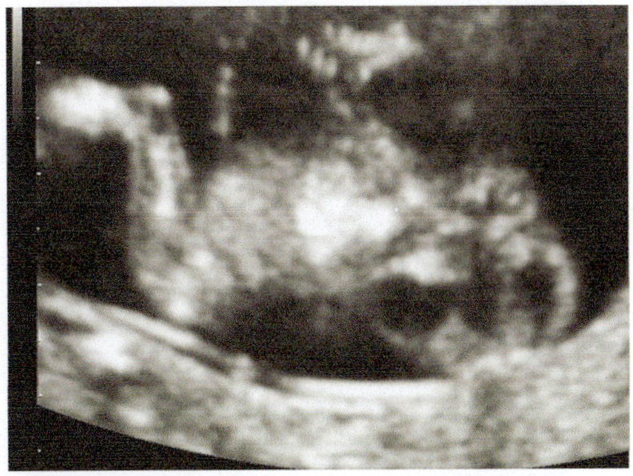

Figure 20: Iniencephaly on B mode ultrasound

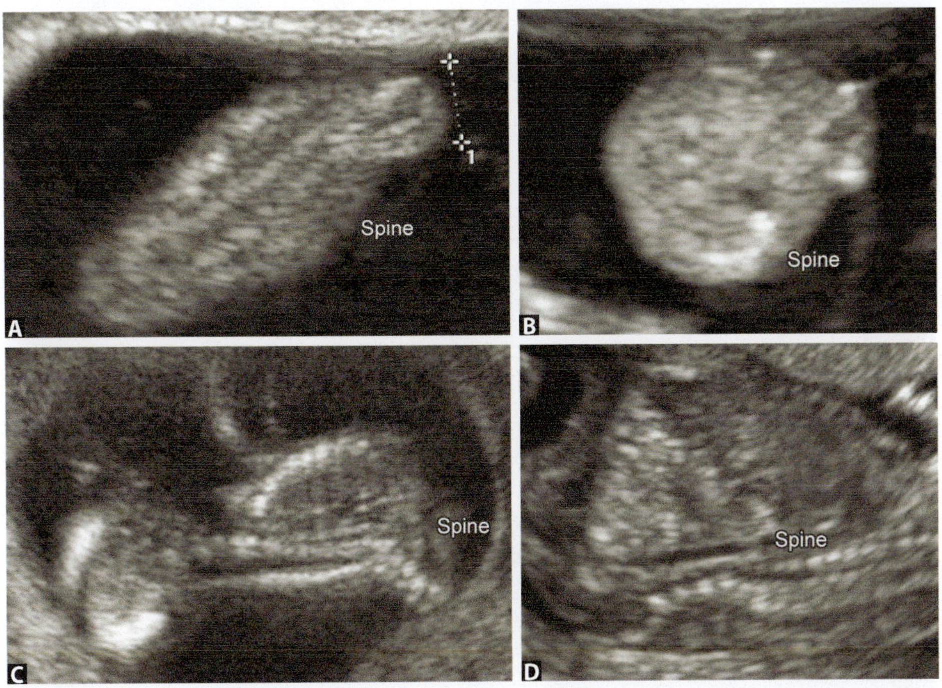

Figure 21: (A) Irregularity of spine at 9 weeks in the coronal view (B) transverse view skin defect (C and D) same fetus at 11 weeks open spinal defect at the lumbar region

the first trimester, but become more evident later in the pregnancy (**Figure 21**).

Through the bony defect, the meninges alone or along with the spinal cord may herniate. Myelomeningocele is a buldging defect in which the elevated neural plate and meninges are contiguous laterally with the subcutaneous tissue[56] **(Figures 22 to 25)**.

This herniation leads to caudal pull on the posterior brain structures leading to the typical lemon skull (collapsed frontal bones)

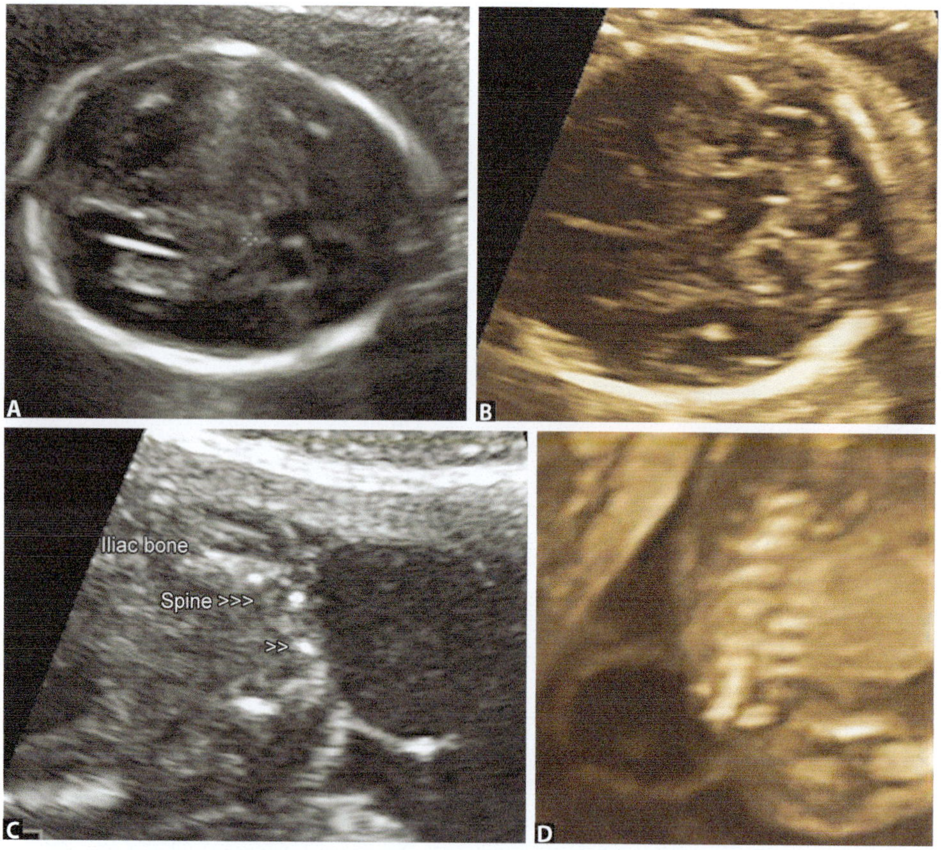

Figure 22: (A) normal ventricular measurement (B) normal posterior cranial fossea (C and D) sacral open spinal defect with protrusion of meninges and CSF – sacral meningocele

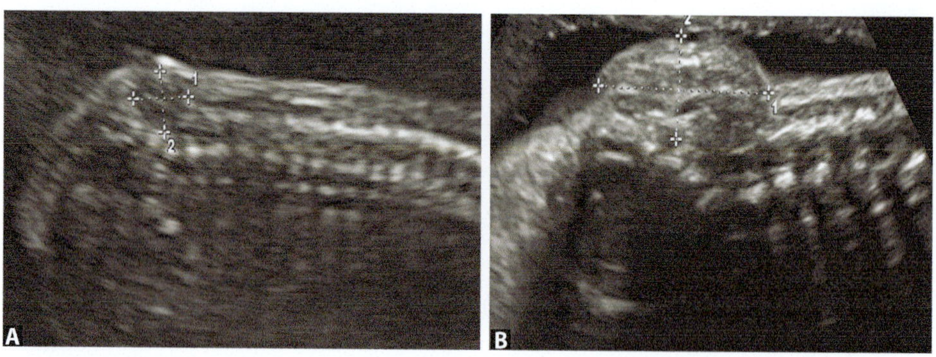

Figure 23: (A) 5 × 7 mm closed spinal defect in the sacral region of a dichorionic diamniotic twin at 16 weeks (B)Repeat scan at 28 weeks gibbus was formed

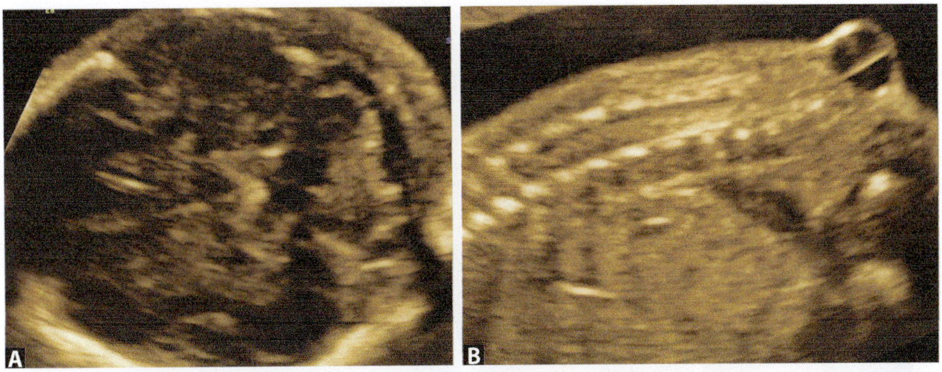

Figure 24: (A) Normal intra cranial anatomy (b) small sacral meningolcele

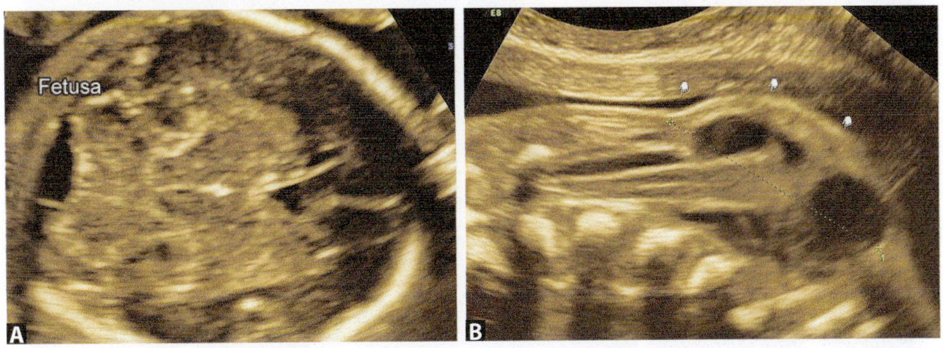

Figure 25: (A)Normal intracranial anatomy (B) skin closed spinal defect

and banana shaped cerebellum (obliteration of the vermian notch due to downward pull) **(Figure 26)**. This leads to constriction of the aqueduct and results in ventricular dilatation and hydrocephalus in the course.

As consequences of herniation of the spinal cord, due to injury and inflammation, there may be abnormal control of the sphincters as well as lower limb muscles. This may result into abnormalities like talipes equino varus **(Figure 27)**.

Prevalence: Neural tube defect (NTD) is 0.58-1.17 / 1000 births.[57]

Etiology: Multifactorial inheritance, single mutant genes, specific teratogens (valproic acid), maternal diabetes, environmental factors.

Pathogenesis: Failure of anterior neural tube closure or a restricted disorder of neurulation.[6]

Associated anomalies: Open spinal bifida (iniencephaly), Chiari type 3 malformation, bilateral renal cystic dysplasia and postaxial polydactyly with occipital cephalocele (Meckel - Gruber syndrome), hydrocephalus and polyhydramnios.[6]

Prognosis: Anencephaly is a uniformly lethal anomaly. Other types of cranium bifidum, various neurological deficits may occur. Spinal defects prognosis depends on the lesion level,thoracic lesions or myeloschisis children are nonambulatory,higher lesion levels are associated with dysphagia,absence of covering membrane was associated with scoliosis and bladder dysfunction.[52]

Recurrence Risk: 5-13%

Obstetrical management: Termination of pregnancy can be offered in cases with anencephaly .

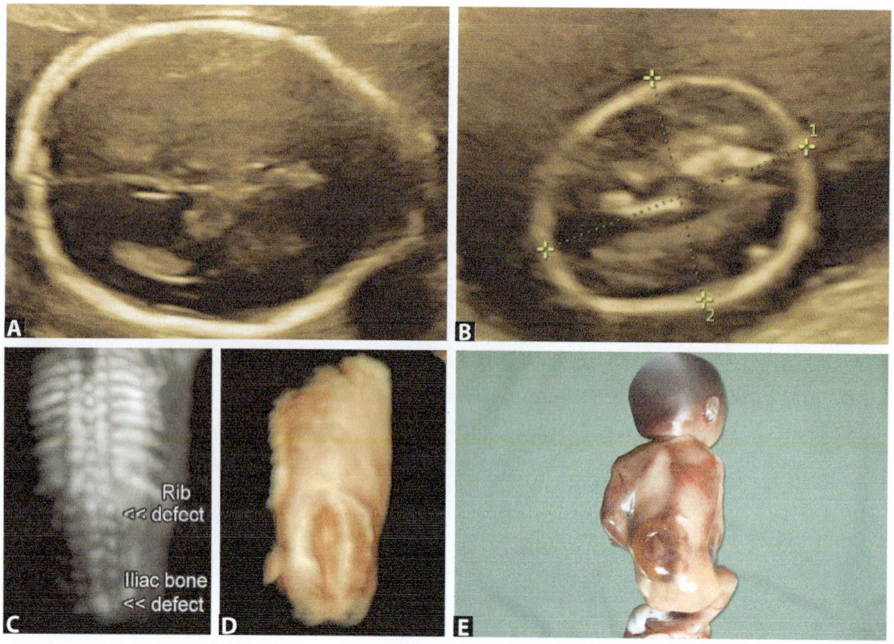

Figure 26: (A) lemon shaped skull (B)meningomylocele (C and D) 3d spinal defect (E)postabortal picture

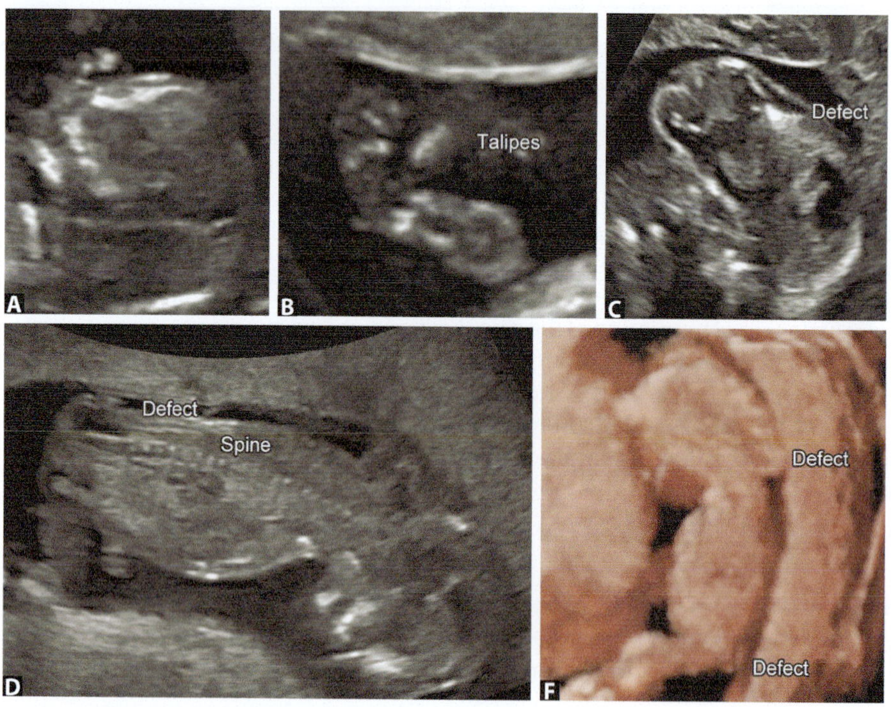

Figure 27: (A) sloping forehead (B) talipes deformity of the leg (C) occipital encephalocele (D) spinal defect with protrusion of meninges at the sacral region in a fetus with 13 weeks gestational age (E) 3d image of the same fetus showing both occipital and spinal defect

REFERENCES

1. McIntosh R, Merrit K, Richards M. The incidence of congenital anomalies. A study of 5,964 pregnancies. Paediatrics. 1954;14:505.
2. Crane JP, LeFevre ML, Winborn RC, Evans JK, Ewigman BG, Bain RP, et al. A randomized trial of prenatal ultrasonographic screening: Impact on the detection, management and outcome of anomalies fetuses. The RADIUS Study Group. Am J Obset Gynecol. 1994;171:392-9.
3. Ewigman BG, Crane JO, Frigoletto FD, Lefevre ML, Brain RP, McNellis D. Effect of prenatal ultrasound screening on prenatal outcome. The RADIUS Study Group. N Engl J Med. 1993;329:821-7.
4. Sonographic examination of the fetal central nervous system: guidelines for performing the 'basic examination' and the 'fetal neurosonogram'. Ultrasound obstet gynecol. 2007;29:109-16.
5. Pooh RK, Maeda K, Pooh KH, Kurjak A. Sonographic assessment of the fetal brain morphology. Prenatal Neonat Med. 1999;4: 18-38.
6. Pooh RK, Maeda K, Pooh KH. An atlas of fetal central nervous system disease. Diagnosis and management. Parthenon CRC Press, London, New York. 2003.
7. Vergani P , Locatelli A, Strobelt N, Cavallone M, Ceruti P, Paterlini G, et al. Clinical outcome of mild fetal ventriculomegaly. Am J Obstet Gynecol. 1998;178:218-22.
8. Pilu G, Falco P, Gabrielli S, Perolo A, Sandri F, Bovicelli L. The clinical significance of fetal isolated review cerebral borderline ventriculomegaly: report of 31 cases and review of the literature. Ultrasound Obstet Gynecol. 1999;14:320-6.
9. Senat MV, Bernard JP , Schwarzler P, Britten J, Ville Y. Prenatal diagnosis and follow-up of 14 cases of unilateral ventriculomegaly. Ultrasound Obset Gynecol. 1999;14:327-32.
10. Beke A , Csabay L, Rigo J , Harmath A, Papp Z. Follow-up studies of newborn-babies with congenital ventriculomegaly. J Perinant Med. 1999;27:495-505.
11. Greco P, Vimercati A, De Cosmo L, Laforgia N , Mautone A , Selvaggi L. Mild ventriculomegaly as a counseling challenge. Fetal Diagn Ther. 2001;16:398-401.
12. Graham E, Duhl A, Ural S, Allen M, Blkaemore K, Witter F. The degree of antenatal ventriculomegaly is related to paediatric neurological morbidity. J Matern Fetal Med. 2001;10:258-63.
13. Van DenHof MC, Wilson RD. Diagnostic Imaging Committee, Society of Obstetricians and Gynaecologists of Canada; Genetics committee, Society of Obstetricians ultrasound. J Obstet Gynaecol Can. 2005;27:592-636.
14. French recommendation of the High Authority of Health regarding the management of fetal cerebral ventriculomegaly.
15. Rakic P. Yakovlev PI. Development of the corpus callosum and cavum septi in man. J Comp Neurol. 1968;132:45-72.
16. Jou HJ , Shyu MK , Wu SC, Chen SM , Su CH, Hsieh FJ. Ultrasound measurement of the cavum septi pellucid. Ultrasound obstet Gynecol. 1998;12:419-21.
17. Barkovich AJ, Norman D. Absence of the septum pellucidum: a useful sign in the diagnosis of congenital brain malformations. Am J Roentgenol. 1989;152:353-60.
18. Aicardi J. Malformations of the central nervous system. In: Disease of the nervous system in childhood. Mac Keith Press: London, UK. 1998;87-9.
19. Dattani MT, Martinez-Barbera JP, Thomas PQ, Brickman JM, Gupta R, Martensson IL, et al. Mutations in the homeobox gene HESX1/Hesx1 associated with septo-optic dysplasia in human and mouse. Nat Genet. 1998;19:125-33.
20. Differential diagnosis in foetuses with absent septum pellucidum. Ultrasound Obstet Gynecol. 2005;25:42-9.
21. Sonography of fetal agenesis of the corpus callosum: a survey of 35 cases. Ultrasound obstet gynecol. 1993;3:318-29.
22. Cohen MM. An update on the holoprosencephalic disorders. J Pediatr. 1981;101:865-9.
23. Blaas HG, Eriksson AG, Salvesen KA, Isaksen CV, Christensen B, Mollerlokken G, et al. Brains and faces in holoprosencephaly: pre- and post-natal description of 30 cases. Ultrasound Obset Gynecol. 2002;19(1):24-38.
24. Blass HG, Eik- NEs SH, Vainio T, Isakesen CV. Alobar holoprosencephaly at 9 weeks gestational age visualized by two- and three-dimensional ultrasound. Ultrasound Obset Gynccol. 2000;15(1):62-5.

25. Cohen MM Jr. Holoprosencephaly: clinical, anatomic, and molecular dimensions. Birth defects. Res A clin Mol Teratol. 2006;76(9): 658-73.
26. Pilu G, Sandri F, Perolo A, Giangaspero F, Giangaspero F, Cocchi G, Salvioli GP, et al. Prenatal diagnosis of lobar holoprosencephaly. Ultrasound Obset Gynecol. 1992; 2(2):88-94.
27. Plea for an anatomical approach to abnormalities of the posterior fossa in prenatal diagnosis. Ultrasound obset Gynecol. 2006;27: 477-81.
28. Laing F, Frates M, Brown DL, Benson CB, Di Salvo DN , Doubilet PM. Sonography of the fetal posterior fossa: false appearance of megacisterna magna and Dandy-Walker variant. Radiology. 1994;192:247-51.
29. Chong BW, Babcook CJ, Pang d, Ellis WG. A magnetic resonance template for normal cerebellar development in the fetus. Neurosurgery. 1997;41:924-8.
30. Volpe JJ. Neural tube formation and prosencephalic development. Neurology of the Newborn. WB Saunders; Philadelphia. 2001;4:pp3-44.
31. Nicolaides KH, Campbell S, Gabbe SG, Guidetti R. Ultrasound screening for spina bifida : cranial and cerebellar signs . Lancet. 1986;12;2 (8498):72-4.
32. Barkovich AJ, Kjos BO, Normal D, et al. Revised classification of the posterior fossa cysts and cyst like malformations based on the results of multiplanar MR imaging. AJNR. 1989;10:977-88.
33. Ritsuko K Pooh. Fetal Neurology Neuroscan of congenital Brain Abnormality. Chapter-4.
34. Dobyns WB, Leventer RJ. Lissencephaly: the clinical and molecular genetic basis of diffuse malformations of neuronal migration. In: Disorder of neuronal migration. PG Bath, (ed). International Review of Child Neurology Series. Mac Keith Press, London. 2003;24-57.
35. Innaetti P, Nigro G, Spalice A , Faiella A, Boncelli E. Cytomegalovirus infection and schizenchephaly: case reports. Ann Neurol. 198;43:123-7.
36. Wakai S, Arai T, Nagai M. Congenital brain tumours. Surg Neurol. 1984;21:597-609.
37. Volpe JJ. Brain tumors and vein of Galen malformation. Neurology of the Newborn. WB Saunders, Philadelphia. 2001;4:41-56.
38. Barkovich AJ, Simon EM, Walsh CA. Callosal agenesis with cyst: a better understanding and new classification. Neurology. 2001;56(2):2207
39. Elbers SE, Furness ME. Resolution of presumed arachnoid cyst in utero. Ultrasound Obset Gynecol. 1999; 14:353-5.
40. Delashaw GE, Suthers GK, Hann EA, Thompson E, David DJ, Gecz J, et al. Mutation detection in FGFR 2 craniosynostosis syndromes. Hum Genet. 1997;99:251-5.
41. Sherer DM, Anyaegbunam A, Onyeiji C. Antepartum fetal intracranial hemorrhage, predisposing factors and prenatal sonography: A review. Am J Perinatol. 1998;15:431-41.
42. Moinuddin A, McKinstry Rc, Martin KA, Neil JJ. Intracranial hemorrhage progressing to porencephaly as a result of congenitally acquired cytomegalovirus infection—an illustrative report. Prenat Diagn. 2006;23: 797-800.
43 . Volpe JJ. Hypoxic—Ischemic encephalopathy: Neuropathology and pathogenesis. Neurology of the newborn. WB Saunders, Philadelphia. 2001;4:296-330.
44. Stevenson DA, Hart BL, Clericuzo CL. Hydranencephaly in an infant with vascular malformations. Am J Med Genet. 2001;15:104:295-8.
45 . Nigro G, Adler SP, La Torre R, Best AM. Congenital cytomegalovirus collaborating group. Passive immunization during pregnancy for congenital cytomegalovirus infection. New Eng J Medicine. 2005;353:1350-62.
46. Kupferminc Mj, Tamura RK, Sabbagha RE, Parilla BV, Cohen LS, Pergament E. Isolated choroid plexus cyst (s): An indication for amniocentesis. Am J Obset Gynecol. 1994; 171:1068-71.
47. Reinsch R. Choroid plexus cysts - association with trisomy: prospective review of 16,059 patients. Am J Obset Gynecol. 1997;176:1381-3.
48. Snijders RJ, Shawa L, Nicolaides KH. Fetal choroid plexus cysts and trisomy 18: assessment of risk in the second - trimester fetus: Is amniocentesis really indicated ? Radiology. 1992;185:545-8.
49. Pooh RK , Kurjak A, Tikvica. Fetal neurology normal and abnormal brain vascularity. Chapter -3.
50. Wakai S, Arai T, Nagai M, et al. Congenital brain tumors. Surg Neurol. 1984;21:597-609.

51. Tortori-Donati P,Rossi A, Cama A. Spinal dysraphism. A review of neuroradiological features with embryological correlations and proposal for a new classification - Neuroradiology. 2000;42;471-91.
52. Monteaogudo A, Timor-Tritsch IE. Fetal neurosonography of congenital brain anomalies. Ultrasonography of the prenatal and neonatal brain.2nd ed. McGraw-Hill, Newyork 2201,p151-258.
53. China-U.S. Collaborative Project for Neural Tube Defect Prevention. N Engl J Med. 1999; 341:1485.
54. Copp AJ, Stanier P, Greene ND. Neural tube defects: recent advances, unsolved questions, and controversies. Lancet Neurol. 2013; 12:799.
55. Mitchell LE. Epidemiology of neural tube defects. Am J Med Genet C Semin Med Genet 2005;135C:88.
56. Up to date. Authors: Monteagudo A, Timor-Tritsch IE. Literature review current through: Jan 2017. This topic last updated: Nov 30, 2016.
57. Mathews TJ, Honein MA, Erickson JD. Spina bifida and anencephaly prevalence—United States, 1991-2001. MMWR Recomm Rep. 2002;51-911.

5 CHAPTER

Ultrasound of the Fetal Face

Ashok Khurana

The fetal face with its irregular non-geometric shape is one of the most difficult areas to image in ultrasound scans. And yet, evaluation is important not only because of psychosocial aspects of a facial anomaly but because the face is an important component of chromosomal and syndromic anomalies. The impact of isolated anomalies, such as microphthalmia, anophthalmia, hypertelorism and micrognathia can also not be ignored. This treatise presents evaluation protocols for assessing the fetal face, the increasing role of 3D and 4D imaging, specific isolated anomalies, an approach to evaluation of the abnormal midface, nose, cleft lip and palate and gross facial anomalies. The approach to facial anomalies followed in this treatise is largely based on the practical and systematic approach recommended in a recent release on the subject by Paladini and Volpe in their textbook entitled *Ultrasound of Congenital Anomalies: Differential Diagnosis and Prognostic Indicators (CRC Press)*. The reader is referred to the extensive bibliography of this text for further insights into the complex subject of fetal facial anomalies.

It must be emphasized at the outset that the human phenotype has a huge number of variants and facial diagnosis may, therefore, be frequently missed or overdiagnosed.

TECHNICAL CONSIDERATIONS IN FACIAL ULTRASOUND

This section takes the reader through information on the optimal time for facial evaluation, standard scanning planes and additional views, malformations that can be assessed in each of these views and 3D/4D applications that enhance fetal diagnosis.

Timing of Examination

The fetal face evolves through gestation **(Figure 1)** just as it continues to do through childhood, puberty, adulthood and senescence. This includes some bone remodeling, cartilaginous ossification and accumulation of facial fat. Fat accumulation is most marked in the cheek, chin and neck. The fetal face, therefore, often appears thin and pinched if scans are performed prior to 23–24 weeks of gestation. Consequently, even though the face is assessed as part of the protocol of the midtrimester anomalies scan, it is wise to evaluate it again after 24 weeks

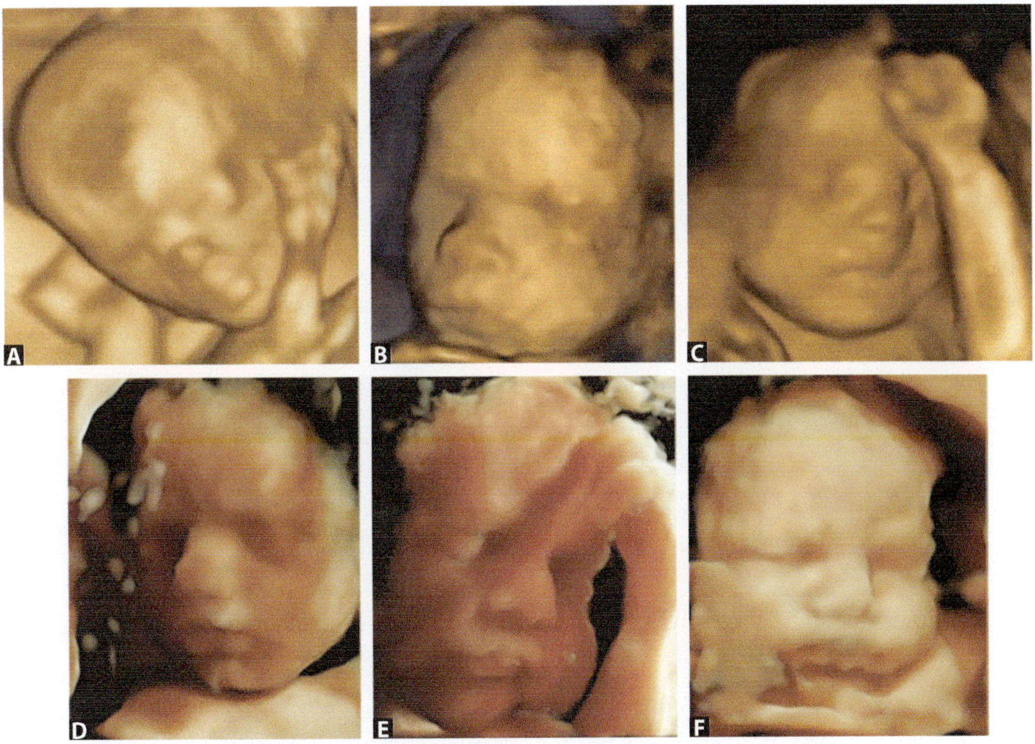

Figure 1: Normal 3D facial appearance at 12, 19, 15, 29, 32 and 37 weeks of gestation. Note the gradual change from a pinched appearance to a filled out face. Fat accumulation is most marked in the cheek and chin with advancing gestation and is the largest contributor to this change

in those clinical situations where there is a previous or family history, and in all fetuses with an anomaly in any system detected at 18–22 weeks where the parents have opted to continue the pregnancy. This later evaluation may not be useful for the option of termination, but can have tremendous bearing on referral to the type of neonatal care unit that would be able to give the anomalous fetus an optimal outcome.

Standard Ultrasound Scanning Planes in the Midtrimester Anomalies Scan

Most guidelines suggest the inclusion of three 2D facial scan planes **(Figure 2)**:

1. Anterior (Ventral) axial/Lateral view of the orbit,
2. Tangential view of the nostril and upper lip, and,
3. Midsagittal view.

Additional 2D views recommended for a detailed evaluation include **(Figure 3)**:

1. Clear delineation of the lens in an anterior view.
2. Anterior axial view for the maxilla and lips.
3. Anterior axial or lateral view for the tongue.
4. Anterior view for the mandible.
5. Lateral or posterior coronal views for the ears.

The recommended 2D view for the face in the 11-14 weeks scan **(Figure 4)** include:

1. The NT Plane with nasal bone and hard palate.
2. Anterior view of orbits and premaxillary area.

Appropriate combinations of these views permits a detailed evaluation of the slope of the forehead, orbital presence, size and contents including cataract, the configuration of the nose, upper lip, alveolar ridge of the maxilla and mandible, palate, mandible and

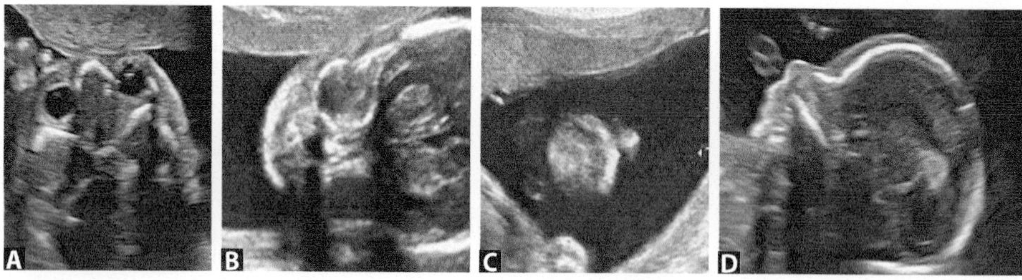

Figure 2: Standard views of the face: These include an anterior axial view of the orbits (A) or a lateral view (B), a tangential view displaying the nostrils and the upper lip (C), and a midsagittal view delineating the nasal bone (D)

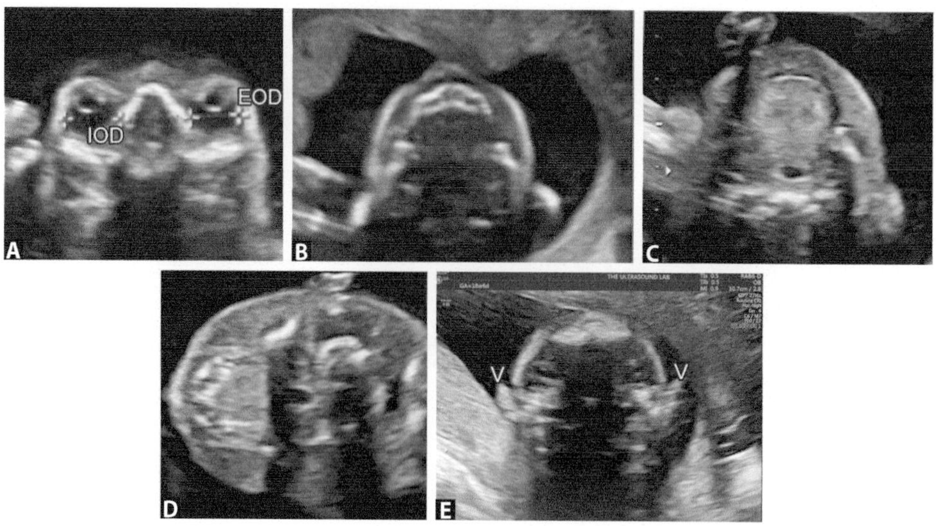

Figure 3: Additional views of the face need to be assessed only in special situations such as a history of a previous malformation or teratogenic exposure. These are tailored views which are largely axial and are used to delineate the lenses (A), anterior axial projections for the alveolar ridge of the maxilla (B), axial views to show the tongue (C), anterior axial views of the mandible (D), and posterior coronal views to demonstrate the ears (E)

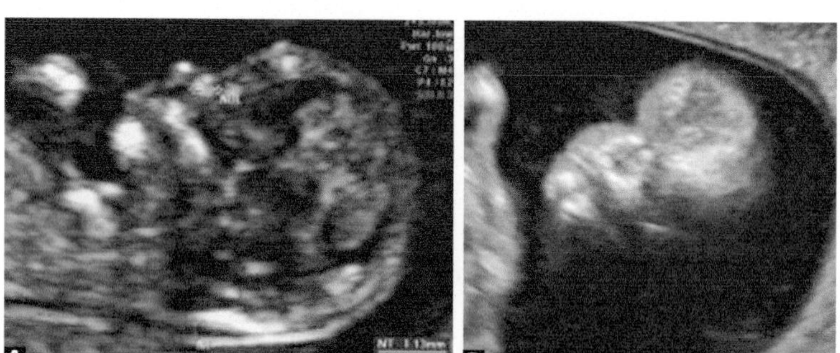

Figure 4: Components of the fetal face are well seen in the standard midsagittal view obtained routinely for the nuchal translucency. This view when correctly taken always delineates the nasal bone and the hard palate (A). Anterior views show the zygoma and the anterior hard palate (B)

chin and the cheeks. The ears can be assessed when indicated, such as in the scenario of a family history, other facial anomalies and extra facial anomalies.

Quantification of facial anomalies is not part of standard guidelines. However, routine assessment of the binocular distance, ocular diameter and interocular distance enhances diagnosis of several facial abnormalities and numerous fetal syndromes. Facial angles have been suggested and used and may be useful to confirm a qualitative suspicion. Their routine use is cumbersome for most workers but should not be rejected altogether. It is wide to "practice" such measurements at regular intervals so that the operator remains in touch with normal patterns and how to obtain these. Using them after a long gap for confirming a suspicion is fraught with inaccuracy. Extensive charts for orbital measurements, facial angles and 3D facial measurements can be found as free download on a Google search. One can access these and even use them for user programming of ultrasound scanners with the assistance of brand specific applications personnel.

The information that can be obtained from the more commonly employed views is as follows:

1. The tangential view of the front of the face displays clefts of the lips and oropharyngeal masses. If the fetus yawns at the time of examination, the entire palate can be seen through the mouth.
2. The sagittal view will delineate micrognathia, retrognathia, premaxillary protrusion, proboscis, frontal bossing, flattened nasal bridge, nasal anomalies and masses (neck, oral).
3. The anterior view of the orbits will reveal hypotelorism, hypertelorism, microphthalmia, anophthalmia, aphakia, cataract and other intraocular abnormalities.
4. Anterior axial view of the alveolar ridges is an excellent view for assessing the lips, facial and palatal clefts and the uvula.

3D/4D Evaluation

Surface rendering of the face with three dimensional (3D) and real time four dimensional ultrasound truly made these new technologies "famous" and surface rendering remains one of the most superior methods of imaging the fetal face **(Figure 5)**. The availability of rotation in X,Y and Z planes enabled visualization from any possible perspective. This was rapidly followed by the availability of adjustable curves (curved ROI) and automated ROI settings **(Figure 6)** as the window to 3D/4D reconstruction and further enhanced the information available. 3D/4D evaluation has for many years moved beyond surface rendering to yield additional information. This includes navigating the data in orthogonal planes, multislice views and slice "any which way" planes **(Figure 7)**. These have vendor specific brand names and, although bewildering initially, emerge as great tools for analysis for further information. Fortunately, learning these techniques has a short learning curve. Surface rendering can also be enhanced using newer rendering engines **(Figure 8)** and light/shadow effects to increase the information that can be extracted from a volume dataset.

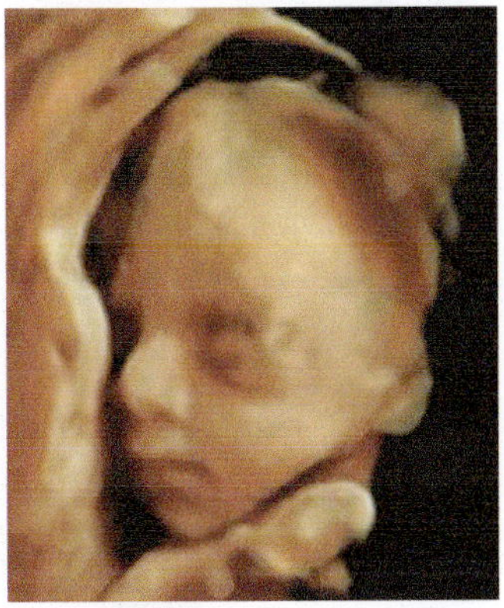

Figure 5: Surface rendering with 3D and real time 3D (4D) is now routine practice to delineate the face in many clinical situations

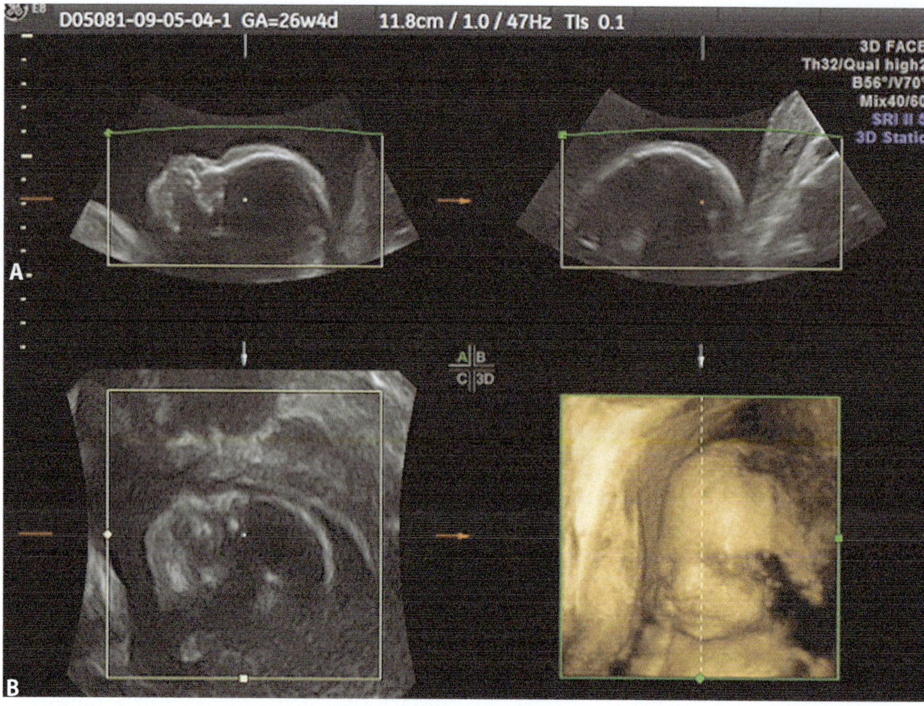

Figure 6: Older 3D software acquires information along a linear plane (A). Newer software uses a curved or customised rendering line (B). This has revolutionized depiction of details of the fetal face

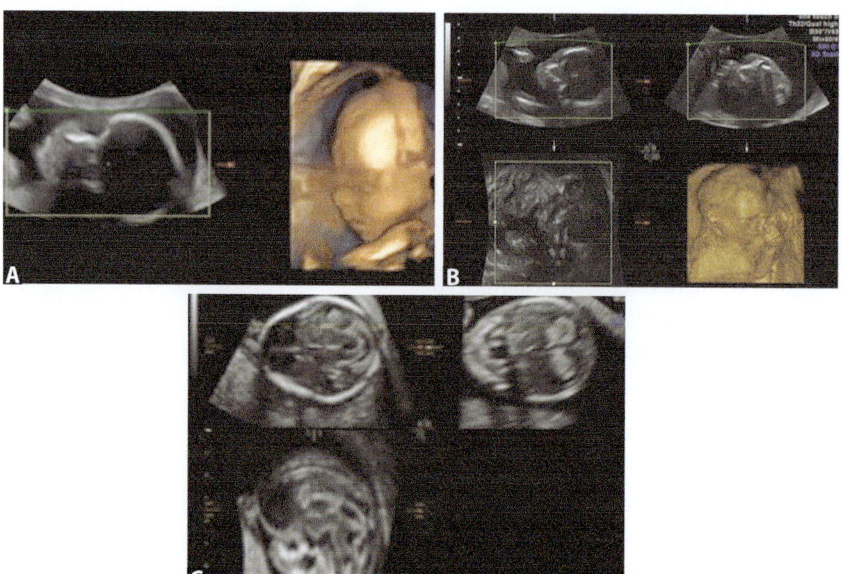

Figure 7: After a volume of the face has been acquired it is possible to navigate through it with parallel slices in any geometric plan (A), random non-geometric slice planes (B) or in orthogonal planes (C). This software goes by several proprietary names

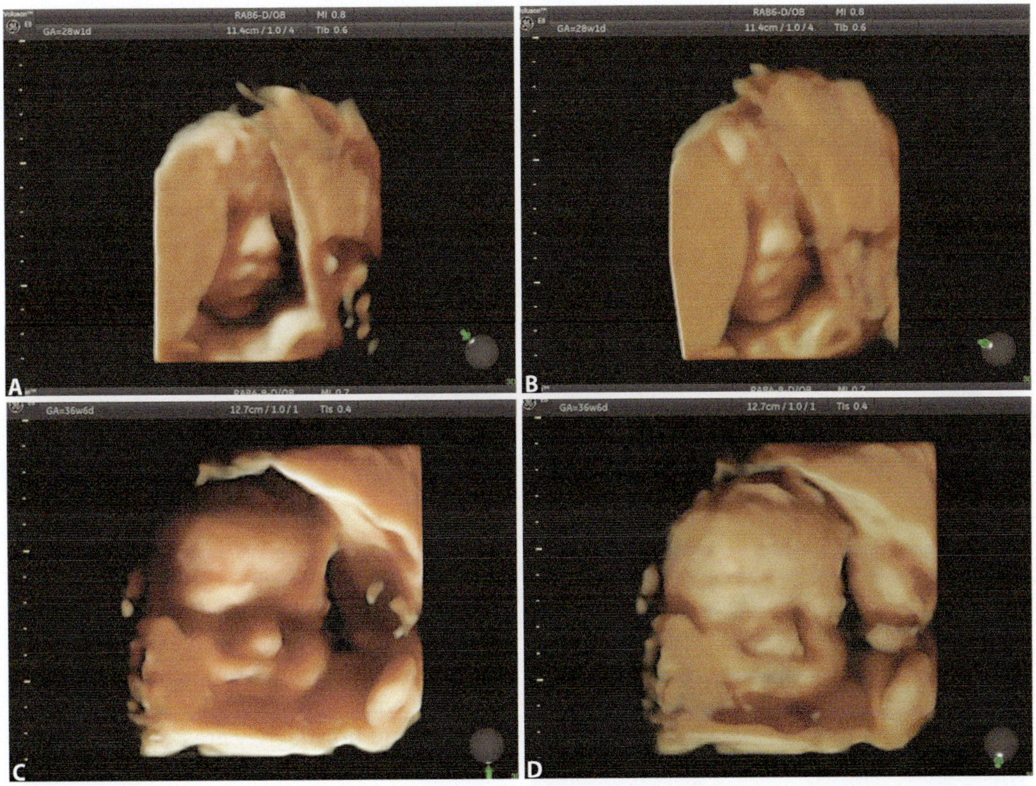

Figure 8: There are two sets of two images seen showing fetal face. In both sets in both images the light source is from different direction. The direction of the light source is demonstrated as a green arrow on the gray colored circular shadow in right lower corner in each image. Change in the direction of the light source, high lights different parts of the fetal face

Preset modes for skeletal rendering are now widely available and are used in conjunction with surface rendering to demonstrate palatal, facial and cranial skeletal anomalies in order to yield a more "complete" diagnosis **(Figure 9)**. It must be remembered that 3D and 4D methods acquire volumes and not just two-dimensional planes and, therefore, the entire volume included during the acquisition can be analysed online, offline and in retrospect. Although resolution is best in the plane of acquisition, newer equipment yields excellent detail in rendered planes as well.

3D measurements have been reported by a few groups, but these are very elaborate and, in their current form, cumbersome and time-consuming for routine use. They do, however, hold promise for refinement and automation in the future.

From a futuristic perspective, 4D surface rendering holds promise for fetal neurodevelopmental evaluation by assessing changesx in the face, such as a grimace, a smile, yawning, etc.

SPECIFIC FACIAL FINDINGS IN PERSPECTIVE

Anophthalmia/Microphthalmia

Anophthalmia and microphthalmia refer to absence or hypoplasia of the eyeball **(Figure 10)**. The lens may be absent or there may be a cataract. The condition may be unilateral or bilateral and each eye may be

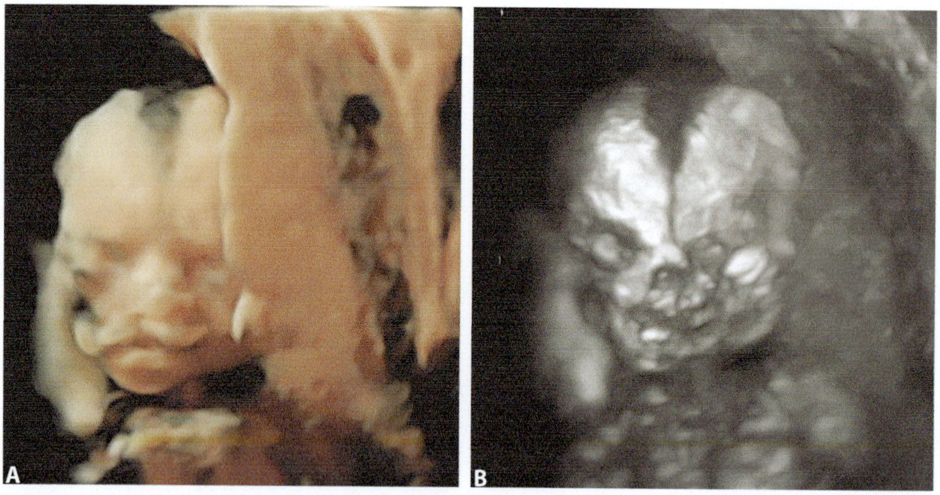

Figure 9: A set of two 3D ultrasound rendered images of fetal face with unilateral cleft lip and palate, derived from the same acquired volume where the first one is rendered on surface mode and the second one on the bony texture mode

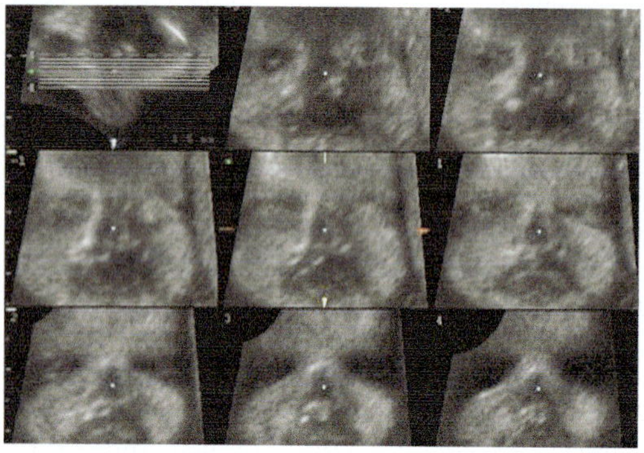

Figure 10: Multislice coronal imaging in a diabetic mother with a previous blind child. Images reveal one very small orbit and one small orbit with a misshapen lens

affected to a varying degree. The associated morbidity may vary from a cosmetic deformity to complete blindness. The diagnosis is made by a subjective evaluation and/or measurements in an anterior or lateral view of the orbits and several nomograms exist that may be referred to.

The incidence of chromosomal anomalies and syndromic associations is high and include trisomy 13, del(13q). Associated holoprosencephaly is a major pointer for trisomy 13. In Goldenhahr syndrome, there is an associated cleft lip and palate, hemifacial hypoplasia and vertebral anomalies. In Meckel Gruber syndrome cephalocele, polycystic kidneys and polydactyly are pointers. Walker Warburg syndrome shows microphthalmia, Dandy-Walker malformation, cataract and ventriculomegaly. Fraser syndrome shows associated ear anomlies, cleft lip and palate, congenital heart disease and renal agenesis. Arthrogryposis and micrognathia are markers for cerebro-oculo-facial-skeletal (COFS) syndrome. Consequently, the presence of an abnormally small orbit should prompt a detailed anatomical evaluation of the fetus.

Cataract

Cataract denotes partial or complete opacity of the lens **(Figure 11)**. It may be partial or complete and unilateral or bilateral. Bilateral cataracts are usually syndromic and have a poor prognosis.

Catarcts may be consequent to intrauterine infection especially rubella and cytomegalovirus, or, even cosequent to nonspecific maternal fever in the first trimester. Chromosomal anomalies are rare. Syndromic anomalies are common and

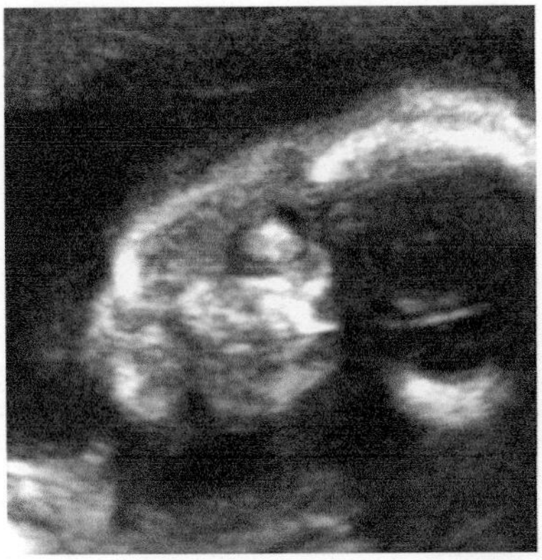

Figure 11: Congenital cataract. Note the echogenic lens seen here compared to the echo free lens shown in Figure 3A

include cerebro-oculo-facial-skeletal (COFS) with arthrogryposis and micrognathia, Walker Warburg syndrome with ventriculomegaly and Dandy Walker malformation, chondrodysplasia punctata with rhizomelic dwarfism and stippled epiphyses and Neu Laxova syndrome with joint contractures, growth restriction, polyamnios, agenesis of the corpus calllosum, cerebellar hypoplasia, hypertelorism, micrognathia, short limbs and syndactyly.

The diagnosis is made in an anterior view of the orbits. It is important to note that an echogenic lens is always associated with a cataract but that the absence of hyperechogenecity in a lens does not exclude a cataract.

Hypertelorism

Hypertelorism refers to an increased interocular distance. Technically this distance should be greater than the 95th centile **(Figure 12)**. It is not always associated with an increased binocular distance. It is a rare anomaly and even rarer in the fetus. It can be consequential to arrest of the medial migration process or the result of an anterior cephalocele that mechanically limits the migration process. It may also be consequent to anomalous cranial bones. The diagnosis is made on an axial view of the orbits with a lateral or anterior approach. The risk of chromosomal anomalies is rare, although a few associations have been reported. The risk of nonchromosomal syndromes is high. In Neu-Laxova syndrome there are joint contractures, early onset growth restriction, polyhydramnios, microcephaly, agenesis of the corpus callosum, severe cerebellar hypoplasia, cataract, micrognathia, short limbs and syndactyly. In Median Facial Cleft syndrome there is an associated facial clefting and an anomalous nose. In Apert's syndrome there is macroglossia, syndactyly, fusion of cervical vertebrae, hypertelorism, renal anomalies and congenital heart disease. In frontonasal dysplasia there is often an anterior cephalocele, median cleft lip and bifid nose.

Hypotelorism

Hypotelorism refers to reduced interocular and binocular distances **(Figure 13)**. These are less than the 5th centile. Holoprosencephaly is a common association. Variations in the phenotype are abundant and range from severe hypotelorism to cyclopia (fusion of the orbits). The diagnosis is usually subjective and can be confirmed by measuring the interocular and binocular distances. Trisomy 13 is the most frequent association.

Anomalies of the Nose

Nasal anomalies include congenital absence, single nostril, proboscis and the non-specific abnormal morphology of the nose **(Figure 14)**. There is a high association with holoprosencephaly and trisomy 13. These are best evaluated in a sagittal plane and with 3D.

Proboscis refers to a single midline appendage of soft tissues arising from the nasal route area. The single nostril is also referred to as cebocephaly and presents as a single nasal opening. Complete absence of the nasal bones and the nares is referred to an ethmocephaly or arhinia.

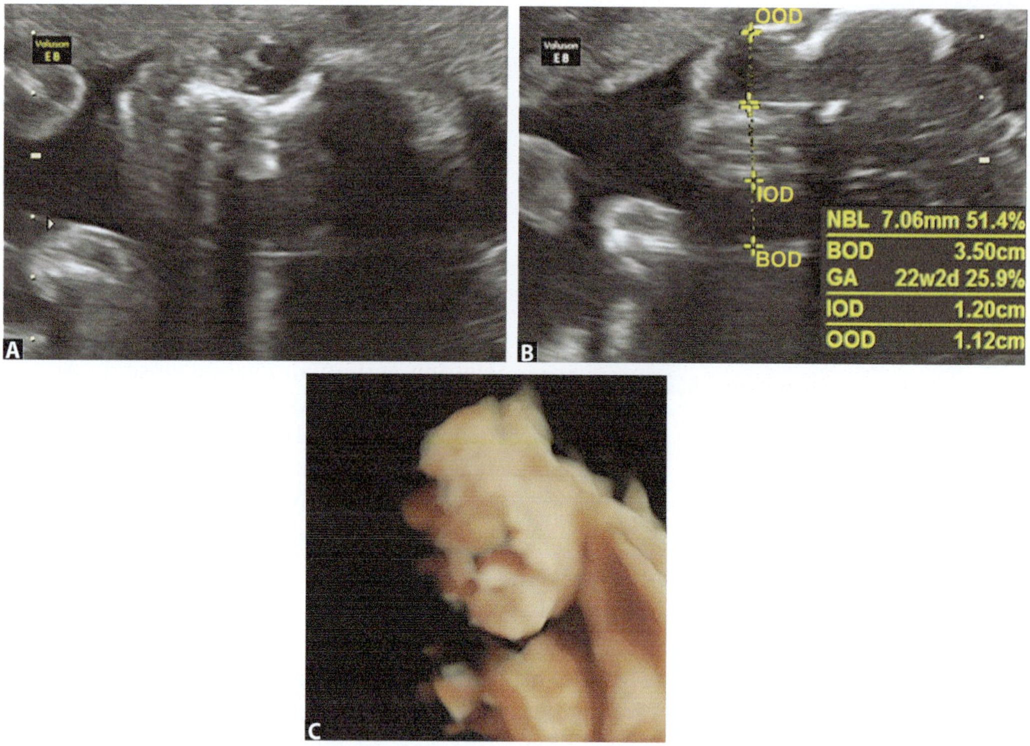

Figure 12: B mode ultrasound and 3D ultrasound image of the fetal face showing increased distance between the two orbits—hypertelorism. The 3D ultrasound image also shows central cleft lip and palate

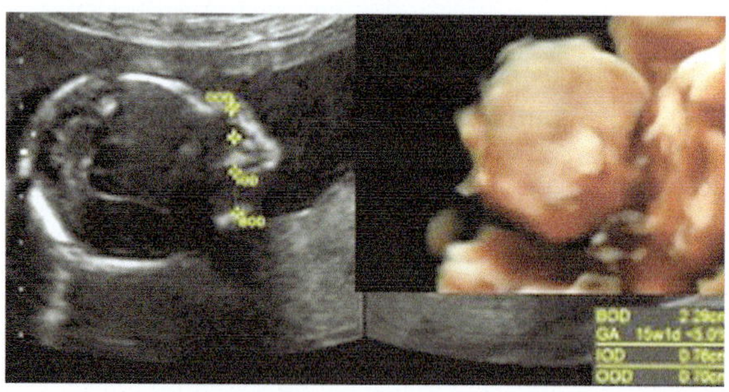

Figure 13: Measurements of the orbits and face are useful to confirm a subjective suspicion of hypotelorism. Measurements shown at the bottom left show a decreased interocular distance. Norms for these are extensively available on the internet

2D sagittal views and 3D/4D surface rendering have revolutionized the evaluation of the nose and enhanced the correlation of findings described in treatises of dysmorphology. This works in two ways. Firstly, in a scenario where a group of fetal findings need further information for syndrome diagnosis and, the other, where a group of findings need specific midfacial evaluation for a differential diagnosis.

Clefts of the Lip, Alveolus and Palate

Clefts may be confined only to the lip or variably extend into the alveolar ridge of the maxilla, into the hard palate and soft palate.

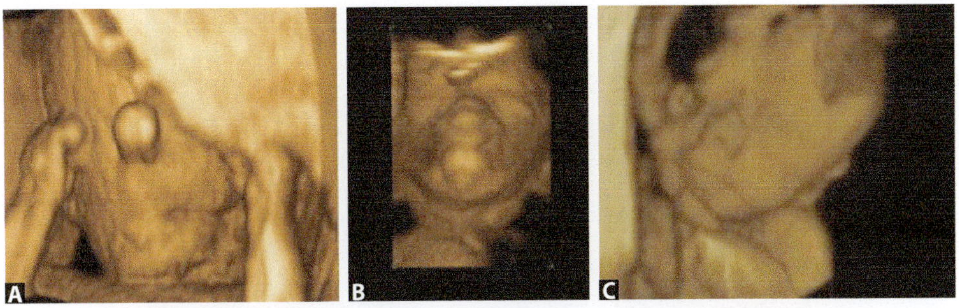

Figure 14: Midline fetal face anomalies: Proboscis (A), Arhinia (B), and a single nostril (C)

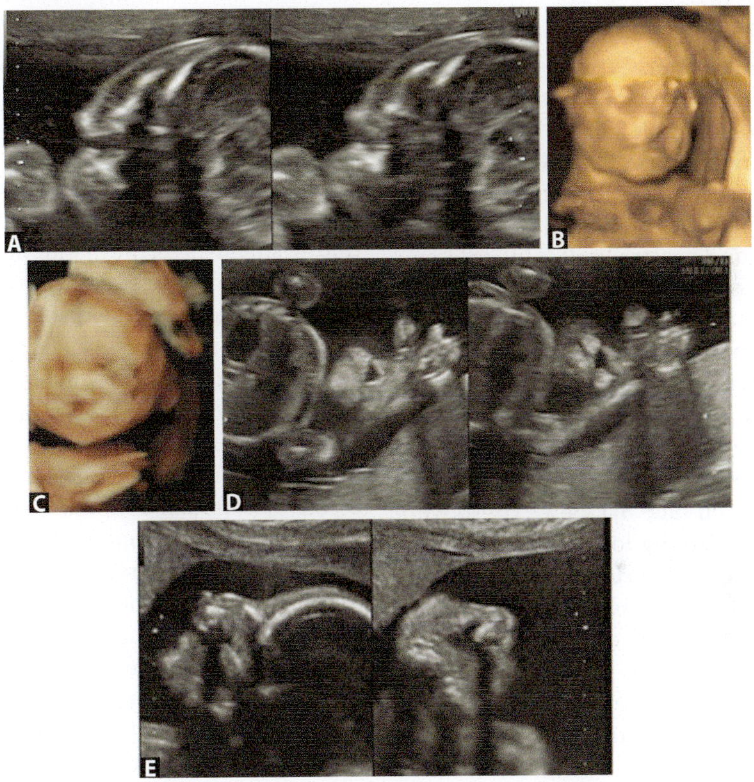

Figure 15: A combination of frontal 3D rendering and 2D coronal and axial views is the method of choice for delineating clefts of the lips, alveolus and palate. Images show a unilateral cleft lip (A), unilateral cleft palate (B), bilateral cleft lip (C), bilateral cleft palate (D) and a median cleft lip and palate (E)

Clefts may be unilateral, bilateral or median **(Figure 15)**. It must be remembered that there may be isolated hard and soft palatal defects without clefts of the lip. These often go undetected. Their detection rate and the general detection rate of soft palatal clefts can be enhanced by visualization of the uvula. When fluid is present in the pharynx, the margins of the uvula get enhanced and appear as an "=" sign **(Figure 16)**. This excludes most clefts of the soft palate. Very occasionally, isolated defects of the soft palate may occur without a cleft of the uvula.

Even though facial clefts have been described in the 11–14 weeks window, these are difficult to detect and it must be

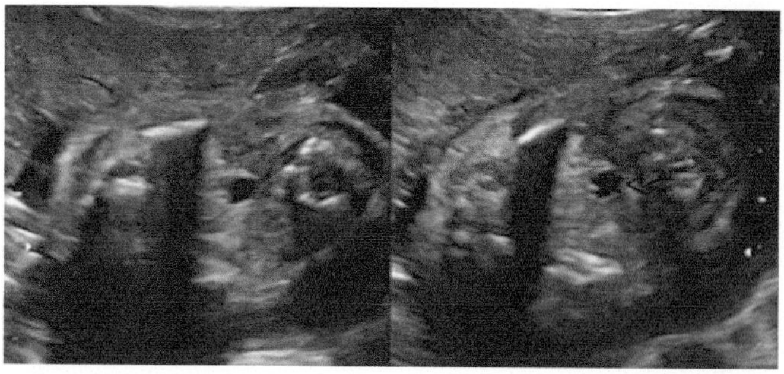

Figure 16: The uvula can be seen as an = sign in an axial plane if the pharynx contains swallowed fluid

emphasized that the detection rate at this early gestation is poor.

A tangential or anterior (ventral) axial view is ideal for assessing cleft lip.

The anterior (ventral) axial view of the maxilla is best for assessing the presence, depth and width of palatal defects. Beam penetration and scatter limit a lateral view. Cut any-plane views are ideal for a rapid and more complete assessment. Surface rendering improves appreciation of the cosmetic and functional aspects of facial clefts by clinicians and families of patients. From a historical viewpoint, authors have from time to time suggested views, such as a reverse face 3D view and flipped face 3D view. These were largely limited by shadowing from osseous elements in the field of view.

Congenital heart disease is frequently associated with facial clefts and must be carefully looked for.

Median clefts have an association with holoprosencephaly and chromosomal anomalies. The risk for chromosomal anomalies is also high for unilateral cleft lip and palate. The association of CLP with trisomy 13 is also high.

Syndromes that are more frequently associated with facial clefts include Goldenhar (unilateral microphthalmia and hemifacial microsomia), Fraser (laryngeal atresia, congenital heart disease, microphthalmia, renal agenesis), Fryn's (diaphragmatic hernia, CNS anomalies), Frontonasal dysplasia (median cleft lip and palate, anterior cephalocele, hypertelorism) and ectrodactyly-ectodermal dysplasia (maxillary hypoplasia, lobster claw anomaly of hands and feet).

Retrognathia and Micrognathia

A reduced anteroposterior extent of the mandible is referred to as retrognathia and a diffuse smallness of the mandible is referred to as micrognathia. Very often, the two conditions coexist **(Figure 17)**. These conditions are relatively more common facial anomalies and are often syndromic. The incidence of trisomy 13 and 18 is also high when this finding is evaluated further. Although, a fair number of measurements have been described to assess mandibular abnomalities, a subjective evaluation is the usual method of diagnosis. It must be remembered that smallness of the mandible may not be evident until after 24 weeks of gestation and may, therefore, not be diagnosed in the routine midtrimester anomalies scan. In the scenario of a previously affected child, therefore, it may be useful to resort to measurements of the mandible in the anomalies scan window for a diagnosis. Interestingly, some of these conditions can be diagnosed at the 11–14 weeks evaluation window as well.

More frequent conditions where the mandible is abnormal include Pierre-Robin anomaly, Treacher-Collins syndrome, Neu Laxova and Pena-Shokier syndrome and multiple pterygium syndrome. It must be noted that the condition may be a primary disorder of skeletal formation or consequent to neuromuscular disorder.

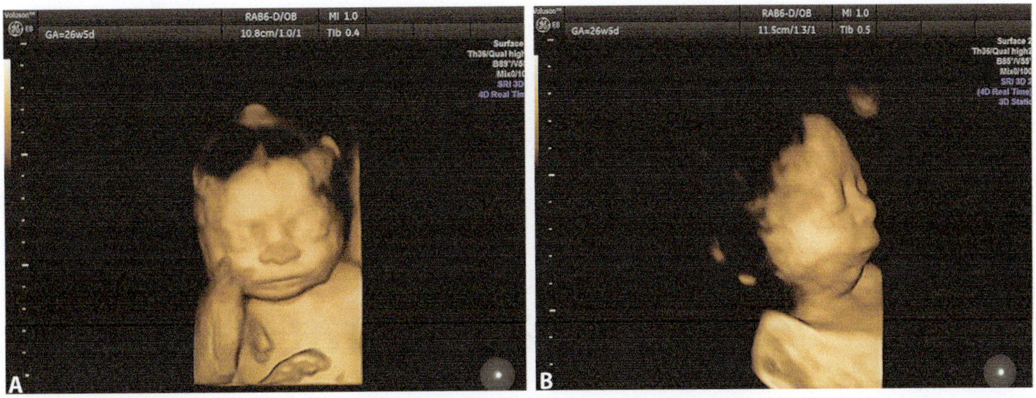

Figure 17: Retrognathia and micrognathia. Note that 3D views give greater diagnostic confidence and that lateral projections are necessary to assess the anomaly

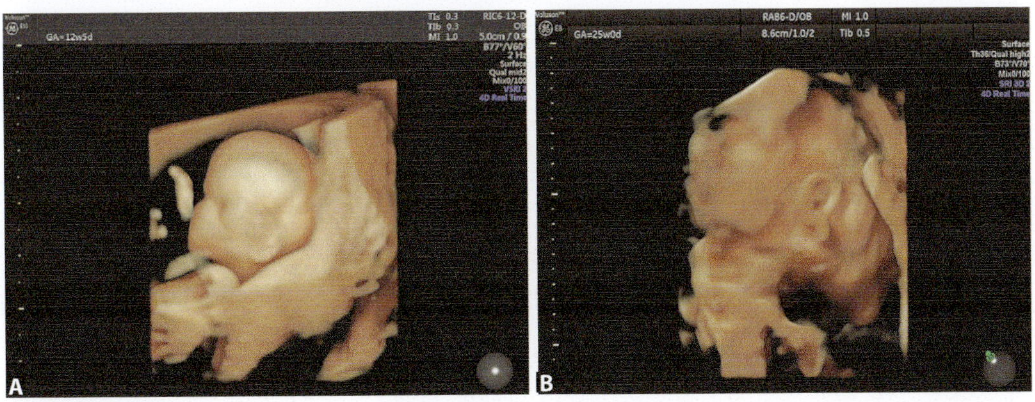

Figure 18: (A) Pinna of the ear, seen on 3D ultrasound image at 12.5 weeks; (B) pinna of the ear, seen on 3D ultrasound image at 25 weeks

External Ear Anomalies

These are common anomalies but seldom detected on antenatal ultrasound because evaluation of the pinna is not part of standard protocol **(Figure 18)**. It is, however, recommended to assess the ears if there is a relevant family history or any other anomaly. There is an unusually high incidence of autosomal trisomies and a very high incidence of Goldenhar, Fraser, Nager and Treacher—Collins Syndromes.

CONCLUSION

The array of facial anomalies and associated syndromes and sequences is truly bewildering. This should not put off the focus of the ultrasound operator and treating practitioner. An incomplete evaluation and a hasty referral to a tertiary center is not the way to approach these anomalies. An ideal approach is one that tackles the problem from two systematic perspectives. The first is where a facial anomaly is identified. In this situation, a thorough fetal evaluation is warranted to assess for associated abnormalities and a final. The second clinical scenario is when an extrafacial fetal anomaly is delineated. For a complete diagnosis a facial anomaly must be looked for. Syndromes and chromosomal anomalies are a largely neglected group compared to isolated anomalies. Prognosis is based on the extent of the anomalies and the opportunity to offer a charted prognosis should not be missed.

6

CHAPTER

Fetal Thoracic Lesions

BS Ramamurthy

The thoracic contents include the cardia, great vessels, lungs and thymus. Superiorly, it is limited by the clavicles and inferiorly by the diaphragm. The fetal spine, ribs and sternum and the overlying soft tissues form the circumferential limits.

The fetal thorax can be studied in the axial, parasagittal, midsagittal and coronal planes. The axial four-chamber view is the standard view used to assess the thorax. Any abnormality in this view should prompt assessment with additional planes of section. In the four-chamber view, the Lungs are faintly hyperechoic and homogeneous. The right lung is larger than the left lung as the cardia is more to the left. The three-vessel view is the other axial plane to display the thymus and the great vessels. The thymus is relatively hypoechoic compared to the lungs and is seen between the great vessels and the sternum in the superior mediastinum. The mid and parasagittal planes demonstrate the diaphragm as a hypoechoic line between the lungs and the liver and stomach. High frequency transducers demonstrate the lung thymus echogenicity difference well. There is no pleural fluid seen normally. A thin film of pericardial fluid may be seen with high frequency transducers. These findings are well seen in the mid trimester anomaly scan (18–23 weeks). With advancing gestational age rib shadowing limits direct sagittal and coronal view. Thoracic anomalies may evolve (progress or regress) with time and hence evaluation in the third trimester is necessary. Sagittal or coronal planes reconstructed from an axially acquired thoracic 3D volume yields better images with less rib shadowing.

The thoracic lesions discussed in this chapter include congenital diaphragmatic hernia, congenital pulmonary airway malformation, pulmonary sequestration, congenital high airway obstruction sequence and pulmonary agenesis.

CONGENITAL DIAPHRAGMATIC HERNIA

Congenital defect in the diaphragm results in the migration of abdominal contents into the thorax. Congenital diaphragmatic hernia (CDH) may be left posterior (Bochdalek) in 85–90%, right sided in 10–15% and bilateral very rarely. The defect itself is not the problem. Herniation of abdominal organs through the defect into the thorax may cause long-standing compression of the lungs during the pseudoglandular, canalicular, saccular and alveolar phases resulting in pulmonary hypoplasia (of ipsilateral and contralateral lungs). This may be compounded by postnatal pulmonary hypertension. Prognostication is centered around prediction of these complications. The factors that decide the presence of pulmonary hypoplasia include the time of onset of herniation, the volume of herniation, duration of herniation and whether the herniation is sliding or not.[1] Herniation may occur as early as 12 weeks or as late as postnatal with the first few breaths of the neonate. Associated structural or chromosomal abnormalities occur in more than half of the cases.[2] 10% of cases of CDH are associated with chromosomal abnormalities. Polyhydramnios is seen in about 75% of cases of CDH.[3]

Sonographic Features of Left CDH

a. Inability to find the stomach in the abdomen.
b. Presence of stomach (90%) and intestines in the left hemithorax as seen in the four-chamber view. The presence of paracardiac liver between the cardia and the stomach is the liver up sign **(Figure 1A)**. The stomach intimately in contact with the cardia without intervening liver echoes is the liver-down sign. Liver-up or liver-down signs help prognostication. Color Doppler landmarking of the portal vein and the left hepatic vein aids in confirming the liver-up or liver-down signs. A coronal section with a high frequency transducer demonstrates the upturned thoracic left lobe of liver and it continuity with the intra-abdominal right lobe.
c. Mediastinal shift to the right side. The degree of mediastinal shift determines the extent of pulmonary hypoplasia and is assessed by the observed to expected lung head ratio (O/E LHR). The right lung is measured as the longest orthogonal diameters in the four-chamber view. These diameters, head circumference and the gestational age may be entered into the online calculator for computation of the O/E LHR.[4]
d. Paradoxical movement of the herniated content at the diaphragmatic level during fetal breathing is seen best in the coronal view.
e. In cases where there is no mediastinal shift and only intestinal herniation with intra-abdominal stomach, the diagnosis is solely on the nonhomogeneous nature of the 'left lung field' compared to the normal right lung. Presence of thoracic intestinal peristalsis is a confirmative finding and is typically seen in zoomed views.
f. Demonstration of cephalad direction of the superior mesenteric artery by color Doppler is helpful in these cases.
g. The residual left dome of diaphragm may be demonstrated in coronal views.
h. Scaphoid abdomen as recognized by a small abdominal circumference reflects the migration of abdominal contents into the thorax.
i. Polyhydramnios when present is possibly due pressure on esophagus or due to partial gastric outlet obstruction (as the stomach is flipped over, and there is gastroduodenal kinking).

Sonographic Features of Right CDH

The absence of intrathoracic stomach and the nearly same echopattern of liver and lung make the diagnosis challenging **(Figure 1B)**. Mediastinal shift to the left is the first clue. Presence of intrathoracic gallbladder or colon if recognized is a useful sign. Color Doppler landmarking of the right hepatic vein and the altered course of the portal vein clinch the diagnosis. Bilateral CDH are very rare and marked by an anterior or superior displacement of the cardia with the liver, stomach and intestines in both hemithoraces.

Prognostication

The extent of pulmonary hypoplasia is the most important factor determining the survival in isolated CDH. The O/E LHR is the most used

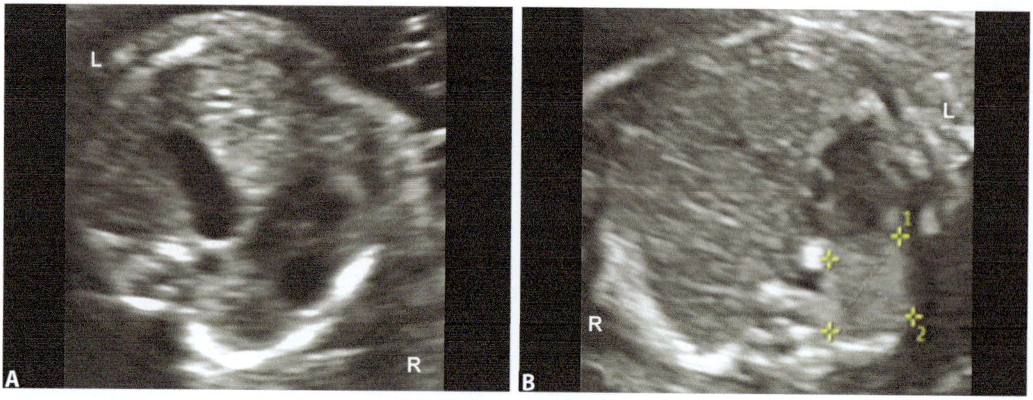

Figure 1: (A) Left congenital diaphragmatic hernia with mediastinal shift to the right. Liver is seen between the stomach and cardia; (B) Right congenital diaphragmatic hernia with liver in the right hemithorax and mediastinal shift to left

parameter to assess the extent of pulmonary hypoplasia. Prenatal prediction of survival is guided by the following classes as defined by the value of O/E LHR: Extreme—15% or lesser; Severe—15-25%; Moderate—26-35%; Mild—36% and above. In all categories the survival rates were poorer when liver was up.[5] In cases with liver-up position the ECMO rates double.[6] The outcome for the chromosomal and syndromal groups is uniformly poor. Trisomy 21 and 18 are the main associations. Syndromes that have CDH in their spectrum include Fryns, Beckwith-Wiedemann, Denys-Drach, Simpson-Golabi-Behmel and Pallister Killian. Fetal karyotyping and array CGH should be included in the workup of CDH. If all efforts draw blank isolated congenital diaphragmatic hernia is diagnosed.

Obstetric Management

Maturity of the fetus is important. Aim is to deliver as close to term as possible. There is no advantage in delivery by cesarean section.[7]

Fetal Therapy

Endotracheal balloon occlusion (fetendo) done fetoscopically is considered in cases with low O/E lung head ratios (<25% and with liver up position). The dilated balloon is left in situ for several weeks during which the elevated endotracheobronchial luminal pressure stimulates alveolar growth in the compressed lungs. The balloon is removed before delivery.

Postnatal Management

In utero transfer is recommended. Postnatal resuscitation and stabilization is crucial. This would entail monitoring blood gases, intubation with gentle ventilation or even extracorporeal membraneous oxygenation (ECMO). Pulmonary hypertension should be recognized or ruled out as this influences the time of surgery. After the neonate is stabilized surgery is planned. If the defect is small, direct closure is the method of choice. For larger defects, closure is by prosthetic patch. This may need revision as the child grows.

CONGENITAL PULMONARY AIRWAY MALFORMATION

Congenital pulmonary airway malformation (CPAM) is a lung mass with unorganized proliferation of terminal bronchi with deficient normal alveolar structures and typically involves one lung lobe. The ipsilateral uninvolved lobe/s are generally not seen as the lesion is expansive and occupies the hemithorax flattening and displacing it/them. CPAM is unilateral in 97% of cases. These lesions are generally sporadic and have no syndromal, genetic or chromosomal association. Histologically, three types have been described by Stocker.[8] Type I, with large cysts (2–10 cm); type II, with small cysts (0.5–2 cm); and type III, solid or microcystic (<0.5 cm). In varying proportion of cases, histopathology reveals presence of regions of pulmonary sequestration of segmentary bronchial atresia. These lesions are termed, hybrid.

Sonographic Features

The solid microcystic type is characterized by a hyperechoic lung with or without mediastinal shift. Well-defined macrocysts with posterior enhancement are seen in the other types **(Figure 2)**. A macrocyst is said to be dominant if it occupies more than one third the volume of the affected lung. Hydrops is more likely to occur if a dominant cyst is present.[9] The expansive nature of the lesion is reflected by mediastinal shift and inversion of the diaphragm. Direct arterial supply from the descending aorta is not demonstrated by color Doppler (optimize for low velocity flow detection). The volume of the lesion is assessed by computing the CPAM volume ratio (L × W × H × 0.52 of lesion in cm/head circumference in cm).[9] Hydrops was seen in 75% of cases in whom the CPAM volume ratio was 1.6 or more. Most lesions grow between 20 and 26 weeks and thereafter plateau. Serial scans at two to three weekly intervals is advised to follow the size of the lesion by the CPAM volume ratio and to look for hydrops. Since most lesions stabilize by 26 weeks the serial surveillance may be slackened later. A significant proportion of these lesions actually regress (10–20%) and even disappear in the third trimester. Disappearance of the lesion means that the lesion is isoechoic with the surrounding lung. In a proportion of these cases, MRI is able to still demonstrate the lesion.[9] Differential diagnosis would include left congenital diaphragmatic hernia if there is a macrocyst in the left lung lesion mimicking the stomach. Correct diagnosis is by the demonstration of the intra-abdominal stomach. A right congenital diaphragmatic hernia is differentiated from a right CPAM microcystic variety by the fact that the liver is less echogenic compared to the lung lesion. Color Doppler helps by recognizing the abnormal liver vascular landmarks. Color Doppler also helps by sorting out the differential diagnosis with pulmonary sequestration.

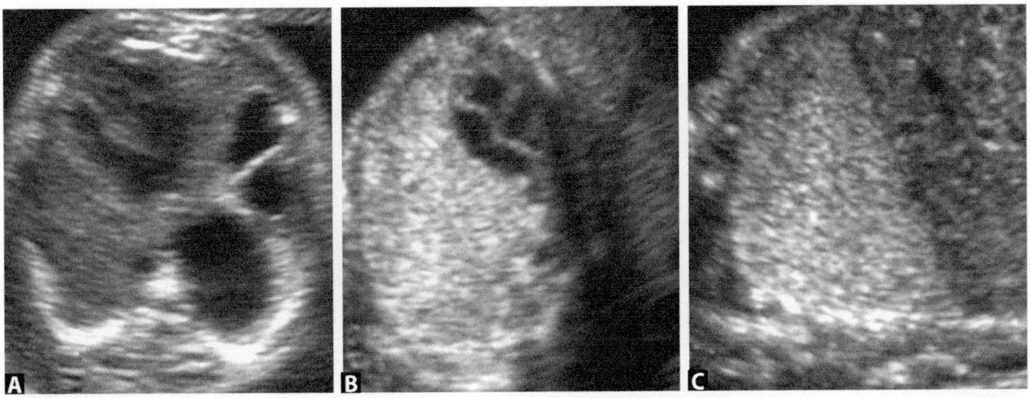

Figure 2: (A) Right congenital pulmonary airway malformation type I with subtle mediastinal shift to the left; (B) Right congenital pulmonary airway malformation type III with gross mediastinal shift to the left; (C) Parasagittal section showing right diaphragmatic flattening

Fetal Therapy

Single dominant macrocyst when associated with hydrops may benefit from needle aspiration or thoracoamniotic shunt. Two intramuscular injections of 12 mg betamethasone 24 hours apart has been tried in microcystic lesions with and without hydrops. Regression of the lesion (CPAM volume ratio) and hydrops has been demonstrated.[10] In select centers large, non-regressing lesions with hydrops presenting in the 26–32 weeks gestational age have been subjected to fetal surgery with good outcomes.

Obstetric Management

If there is no hydrops and lesion size is stable or regressing early delivery is not justified. Cesarean section does not influence the outcomes.

Postnatal management includes assessment with MRI and if the lesion is seen thoracotomy and lobectomy is done. This is to subvert recurrent infections and malignant transformation. If there is no hydrops and the lesion is not too huge the outcomes are excellent.

PULMONARY SEQUESTRATION

Pulmonary sequestration (PS) is a region of lung parenchyma that does not communicate with the bronchial system and is supplied from the systemic circulation (not pulmonary circulation). Most often the feeding artery arises from the descending thoracic or abdominal aorta. Venous drainage is into the azygos, hemiazygos veins or the cava in the extralobar type (75%) and into the pulmonary veins in the intralobar type (25%).[11] The former has its own pleural covering. It is the extralobar type that can be prenatally diagnosed. The lesion is unilateral and is seen in the lower lobe of the left lung in 90% of cases. 90% of lesions are supradiaphragmatic and the remaining are subdiaphragmatic. The cause is unknown. PS may be associated with CPAM and these are termed hybrid lesions (can be diagnosed only by histopathology).

Sonographic Features

The lesion is seen as a triangular or wedge-shaped hyperechoic region in the left lung lower lobe on the four-chamber view. Cystic components are not generally seen in PS. The arterial supply from the descending thoracic aorta may be demonstrated by power or color Doppler imaging **(Figure 3)**. Sagittal or parasagittal views enable recognition of subdiaphragmatic lesions as well as tracing the arterial supply from the abdominal aorta. Large lesions may be associated with pleural effusion and hydrops. Presence of pleural effusion literally rules

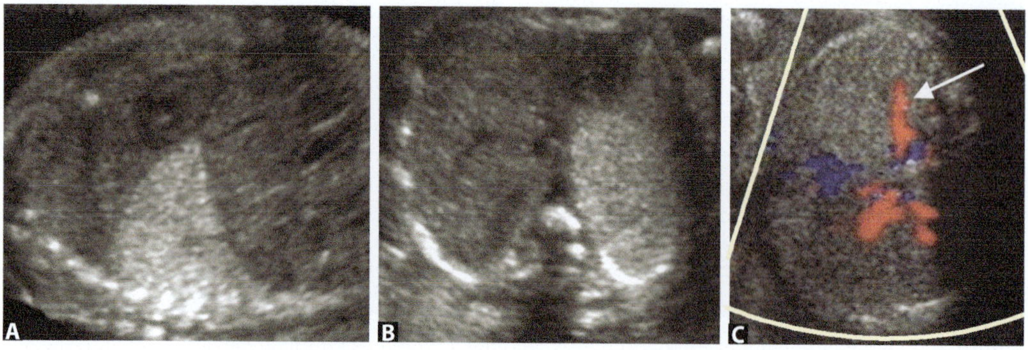

Figure 3: (A) Left lung lower lobe pulmonary sequestration—typical wedge-shaped hyperechoic lesion; (B) Axial section of the lesion; (C) Direct arterial supply from the descending thoracic aorta (arrow)

out CPAM. In 30% of cases, the lesion may regress with advancing gestational age.[12] Differential diagnosis includes microcystic type of CPAM. The triangular shape and the presence of the feeding artery from the descending aorta confirm PS. Hence it is important to examine any hyperechoic lung lesion with color Doppler for identification of any possible systemic arterial feeder. PS may be associated with other lesions like congenital diaphragmatic hernia or tracheoesophageal fistula or duplication cysts. Its association with CPAM has already been mentioned. Subdiaphragmatic lesions have to differentiated from adrenal or upper pole renal masses. This could be challenging.

Obstetric Management

Association with chromosomal anomalies is low, and hence, fetal karyotyping is not indicated in isolated lesions. Serial monitoring at three to four week intervals is recommended for follow up of lesional size and to identify hydrops. Hydrops is more common in those cases with a hypertensive hydrothorax. Pleuroamniotic shunt may mitigate the hydrops in such cases.

Postnatally surgical excision of the mass is the definitive treatment. Embolization of the feeder artery has been tried. Outcomes are excellent in nonhydropic cases.

CONGENITAL HIGH AIRWAY OBSTRUCTION SEQUENCE

Laryngeal (supraglottic, glottis or infraglottic) atresia (stenosis or web) or tracheal atresia are the causes of the typical phenotype of congenital high airway obstruction sequence (CHAOS).[13] There is increased intraluminal pressure due to entrapment of fluid in the tracheobronchial tree. This stimulates lung growth and the resultant hyperplastic lungs compress the cardia and esophagus resulting in ascites and polyhydramnios respectively. The condition is sporadic and is not associated with chromosomal abnormality. It may occur as a part of Fraser syndrome (autosomal recessive).

Sonographic Features

Bilateral hyperechoic and swollen lungs are a hallmark of CHAOS. The tumescent lungs cause the cardia to be compressed between them. Consequently the cardia appears small and centrally placed in the thorax. These findings are seen in the four chamber view. The diaphragmatic domes are flattened or inverted **(Figure 4)**. The fluid filled trachea and bronchi are dilated. These findings are best demonstrated in a coronal view. The abdomen is invariably dilated with ascites. There is really no differential diagnosis. The rare bilateral CPAM may be distinguished

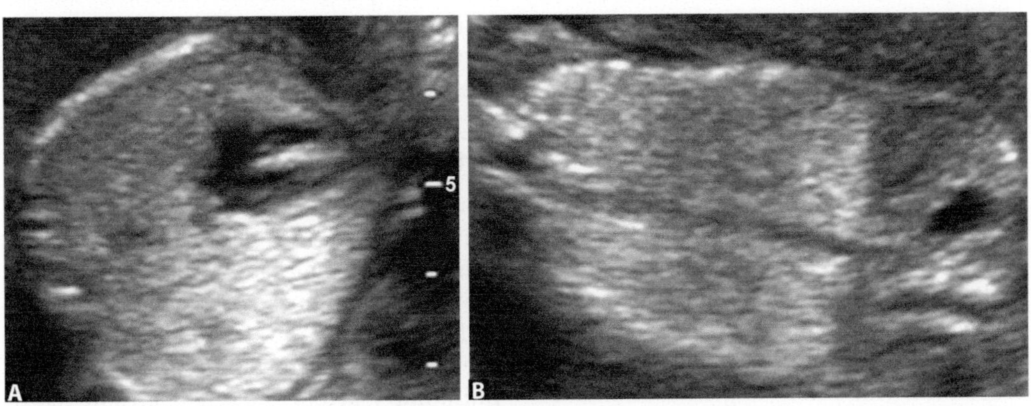

Figure 4: (A) Bilateral lung tumescence and hyperechogenicity with cardiac compression–CHAOS; (B) Coronal section showing flattening of diaphragmatic domes

from CHAOS by the absence of tumescent lungs and fluid-filled dilated trachea and bronchi. Associated bilateral renal agenesis, facial cleft, micro-ophthalmia or congenital heart disease could clinch the diagnosis of Fraser syndrome.

Obstetric Management

The outcome of CHAOS is uniformly dismal and termination of pregnancy is generally opted for.

PLEURAL EFFUSION/HYDROTHORAX

Pleural effusion (unilateral or bilateral) can occur in a plethora of conditions. It is termed secondary if the presence of pleural effusion is a part of general hydrops fetalis (immune or nonimmune). It is termed primary when seen as an isolated finding not associated with chromosomal or nonchromosomal abnormality. In this case, the effusion is due to atresia of the thoracic duct and is termed chylothorax.

Sonographic Features

Unilateral or bilateral presence of clear fluid in the pleural space surrounding the lung except at the hilum. If bilateral and when imaged from the posterior aspect the lungs typically show the bat's wing appearance. Unilateral pleural effusion under tension causes a mediastinal shift to the opposite side **(Figure 5)**. Such hypertensive effusions are generally chylothoraces.[14] If general hydrops is present thoracic subcutaneous edema may be seen.

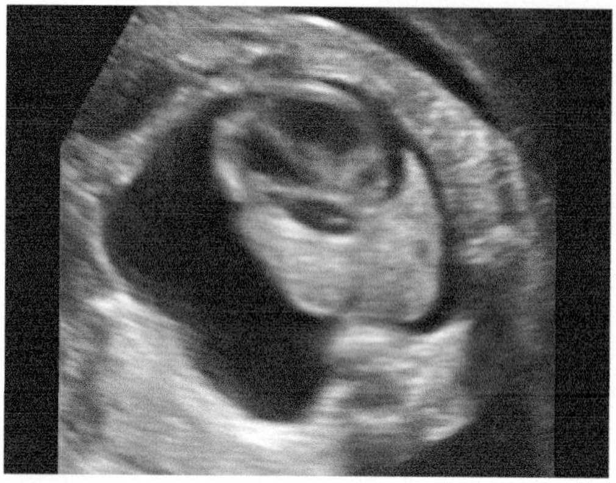

Figure 5: Left hypertensive pleural effusion with mediastinal shift to the right. Also present is mild right pleural effusion

Management

Pleural effusions associated with non immune hydrops or with chromosomal abnormality have a poor outcome. Fetal karyotyping is indicated. Outcome is also poor when associated with other congenital anomalies, e.g. congenital heart disease. Primary hypertensive pleural effusion may cause fetal hydrops. The hydropic changes regress when the effusion is decompressed. Decompression can be done by ultrasound-guided needle aspiration. If there is rapid reaccumulation, thoracoamniotic shunt may be planned.

PULMONARY AGENESIS

Pulmonary agenesis is absence of one or both lungs. Bilateral pulmonary agenesis is rare, and is incompatible with life. Unilateral pulmonary agenesis is relatively more common and is compatible with life. Associated anomalies are anomalous pulmonary venous drainage, tracheoesophageal fistula, hemivertebrae and ipsilateral radial ray defect. Chromosomal abnormality is not associated with pulmonary agenesis.

Sonographic Features

Ipsilateral mediastinal shift and diaphragmatic elevation are the major findings. The contralateral lung is enlarged and crosses the midline **(Figure 6)**. Associated scoliosis with concavity to the affected may be present even without a hemivertebra. The ipsilateral pulmonary artery branch is absent (color Doppler imaging). Differential diagnosis

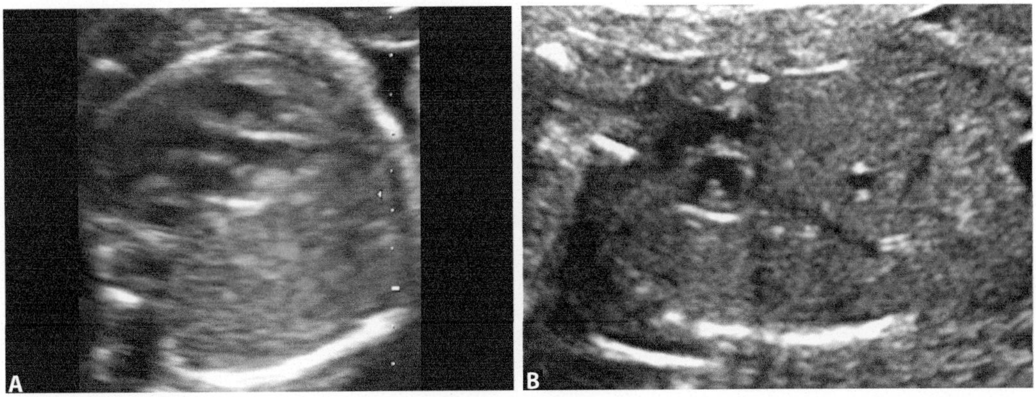

Figure 6: (A) Axial section showing mediastinal shift to right due to right pulmonary agenesis; (B) Coronal section showing an intact diaphragm

is mainly not to mistake a CDH or CPAM with contralateral mediastinal shift for the ipsilateral shift of unilateral pulmonary agenesis. Fetal MRI helps in confirming the diagnosis.

Obstetric Management

Delivery in a tertiary care center is recommended. Half of the children with pulmonary agenesis are either stillborn or die within a few months. The neonate is carefully examined for associated anomalies, including congenital heart disease. Long-term follow-up is necessary as these children have increased risk of infectious complications.

Thus, we see that prenatal ultrasound enables us to recognize thoracic lesions and follow them up. The fact that some lesions can actually regress with advancing gestational age should be borne in mind. Presence of hydrops with any of the described lesions worsens the prognosis. Some lesions like congenital diaphragmatic hernia and pleural effusion need fetal karyotyping. Select lesions may be treated in utero. Ultrasound findings help in counselling and planning obstetric management.

REFERENCES

1. Harrison MR, et al. Congenital diaphragmatic hernia: an unsolved problem. Semin Pediatr Surg. 1993;2:109-12.
2. Puri P, Gorman F. Lethal nonpulmonary anomalies associated with congenital diaphragmatic hernia: Implications for early intrauterine surgery. J Pediatr Surg. 1984; 19:29.
3. Manni M et al. Prenatal diagnosis of congenital diaphragmatic hernia: a retrospective analysis of 28 cases. Prenat Diagn. 1994;14:187.
4. Jani J, et al. Observed to expected lung area to head circumference in the prediction of survival in fetuses with isolated diaphragmatic hernni, Ultrasound Obstet Gynecol. 2007; 30:67-71
5. DePrest J, et al. Current consequences of prenatal diagnosis of congenital diaphragmatic hernia. J Pediatr Surg. 2006;41:423-30.
6. Geary M. Management of congenital diaphragmatic hernia diagnosed prenatally: an update. Prenat Diagn. 1998;18:1155-8.
7. Downward CD, Wilson JM. Current therapy of infants with congenital diaphragmatic hernia. Semin Neonatol. 2003;8:215-21.
8. Stocker JT, et al Congenital cystic adenomatoid malformation of the lung. Classification and morphologic spectrum. Hum Pathol. 1977;8: 155-71.
9. Crombleholme TM, et al. Cystic adenomatoid malformation volume ratio predicts outcome in prenatally diagnosed cystic adenomatoid malformation of the lung. J Pediatr Surg. 2002; 37:331-8.
10. Curran PF, Jelin EB, Rand L, et al. Prenatal steroids for microcystic congenital cystic adenomatoid malformations. J Pediatr Surg. 2010;45(1):145-50.

11. Johnson AM, et al. Congenital anomalies of fetal/neonatal chest. Semin Roentgenol. 2004;39:197.
12. Lopoo JB, et al. Fetal pulmonary sequestration: a favourable congenital lung lesion. Obstet Gynecol. 1999;94:567-71.
13. Lim FY, et al. Congenital high airway obstruction syndrome: Natural history and management. J Pediatr Sur. 2003;38:940.
14. Longaker MT, et al. Primary fetal hydrothorax: Natural history and management. Pediatr Surg. 1989;24:573-6.

7

CHAPTER

Fetal Cardiac Defects

BS Ramamurthy

INTRODUCTION

Congenital cardiac anomalies are one of the leading causes of neonatal morbidity and mortality. They are also one of the most commonly missed anomalies on antenatal scans.

The incidence of moderate to severe forms of CHD is about 6/1000 live births. If bicuspid aortic valves, small muscular ventricular septal defects (VSD) and other trivial defects are included the incidence is as great as 75/1000 live births.[1] The incidence of congenital cardiac anomalies is even greater prenatally considering pregnancy terminations and fetuses with severe cardiac malformations that may be still-born. This makes cardiac anomalies amongst the most common fetal defects.

Of these only 10 to 20% are found in high risk pregnancies with known risk factors for heart defects. The remaining 80 to 90% of cases are incidentally found in low risk pregnancies on routine antenatal screening. Hence it is important to thoroughly screen all pregnancies for cardiac anomalies in the basic antenatal ultrasound examination.

Multiple factors have been implicated in the pathogenesis of cardiac anomalies. They include chromosomal (trisomies 13, 18 and 21, Turner syndrome and 22q deletion), genetic (Holt Oram, Apert, Noonan and Ellis Van Creveld syndromes), teratogens (rubella, mumps, lithium, alcohol, phenytoin, and diabetes). Most cases have a multifactorial etiology. The recurrence of cardiac anomalies in future pregnancies increases if the cause is multifactorial. Recurrence rates quoted are 2–5% after one affected child, 5–10% after two affected children and 1–10% if one of the parents is affected.

There are two time-windows for the assessment of the fetal heart. The first is the early echocardiography done between 11 and 14 weeks. Increased NT, tricuspid regurgitation and ductus venosus late diastolic reversals are not only markers of aneuploidy but also of fetal cardiac defects. The other window is the mid-trimester anomaly scan period between 18 and 23 weeks. One can attempt to perform first trimester echocardiography only if one is well versed with mid-trimester echocardiography.

Image optimization is by using the highest transducer frequency possible, tissue harmonics, narrow imaging field, low persistence, high contrast, optimum zoom and a single focus. Color Doppler settings would include high velocity scale, high wall filter, just big enough color box and appropriate color gain and power settings.

The scheme adopted in this chapter is to highlight the *abnormality* that may be recognized by an examiner and how to proceed thereafter to arrive at a complete diagnosis. The following is the layout of this chapter:

A. Examine the heart as a whole organ: 1. Situs, 2. Size, 3. Axis, 4. Position.
B. Examine the heart as a set of chambers, vessels and their connections: 5. Four chamber view, 6. Left ventricular outflow tract and 7. Right ventricular outflow tract and 8. Three vessel trachea view.'

The heart should be first examined as a whole organ in terms of situs, size, axis, position and squeeze. One should then study the cardiac structure in terms of the chambers and vessels and their connections. Sequential segmental analysis is the term used to systematically examine the cardiac connections (venoatrial, atrioventricular and ventriculoarterial).

The sign of abnormality may be encountered at any of the following stages of examination:

SITUS ABNORMALITY

An abnormal situs is associated with a higher incidence of congenital heart defects. **Figure 1** describes the types of situs abnormalities and the association of congenital heart defects in each one of them.[2-4] Determination of situs is the first step in fetal echocardiography. An abnormal situs could be the first clue to a cardiac defect (which may range from a simple VSD to a complex cardiac defect) **(Figure 2)**. The upper abdominal transverse section is an integral view in assessment of situs and abnormalities thereof. Liver to right, stomach to the left, descending aorta to the left and inferior vena cava (IVC) to the right and anterior to the aorta is the normal spatial arrangement. Some of the abnormalities seen in this section are:

a. Mirror image arrangement seen in situs inversus totalis
b. Stomach to the right (heart and stomach on opposite sides), close to spine, midline large liver and absent spleen in heterotaxy.

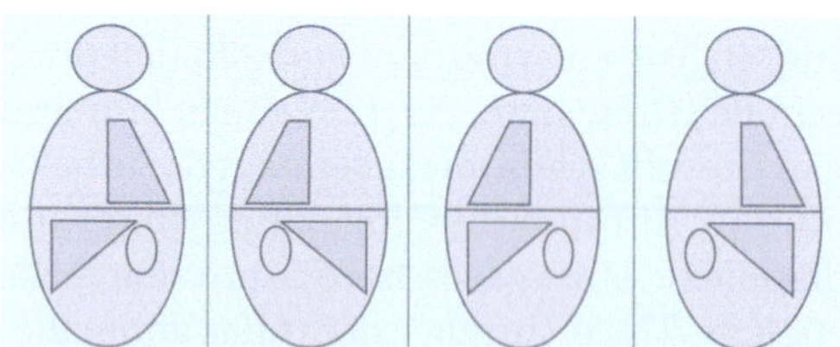

Situs solitus	Situs inversus totalis	Dextrocardia	Situs inversus with levocardia
0.6% live birth (1)	0.3 to 5% fetuses and newborns 2)	Very common (3, 4)	

Figure 1: Incidence of complex cardiac defects

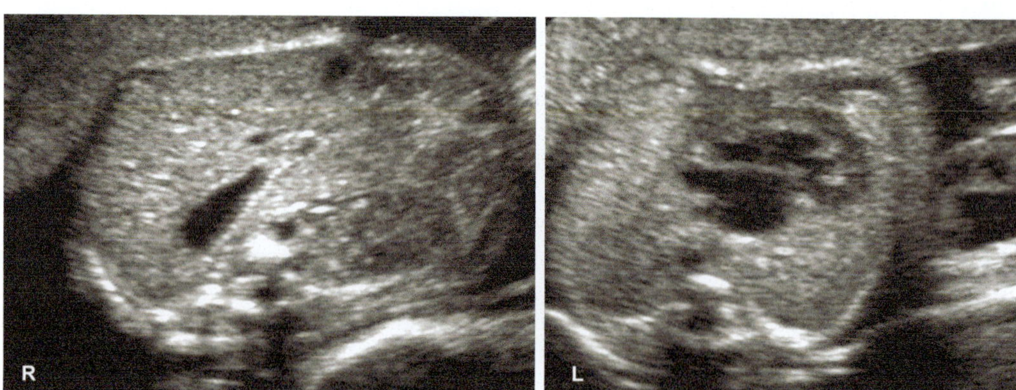

Figure 2: Situs inversus with levocardia (stomach to the right and apex of cardia to the left) note single inlet single ventricle (with malposed great arteries and pulmonary stenosis)

Occasionally the stomach is in the midline in heterotaxy.

c. Juxtaposed IVC (IVC anterior and on the same side of the aorta) is seen in right atrial isomerism.

d. Absent or interrupted IVC is seen in left atrial isomerism. This is accompanied by azygos prominence (see section on 'area behind the heart').

e. The absence of ductus venosus may be recognized in this upper abdominal plane. This is a rare anomaly. In subgroup I, the umbilical venous return bypasses the liver and directly drains into the IVC, iliac vein, renal vein, right atrium or the coronary sinus. There is cardiomegaly due to cardiac volume overload **(Figure 3)**. In subgroup II, the umbilical vein connects normally with

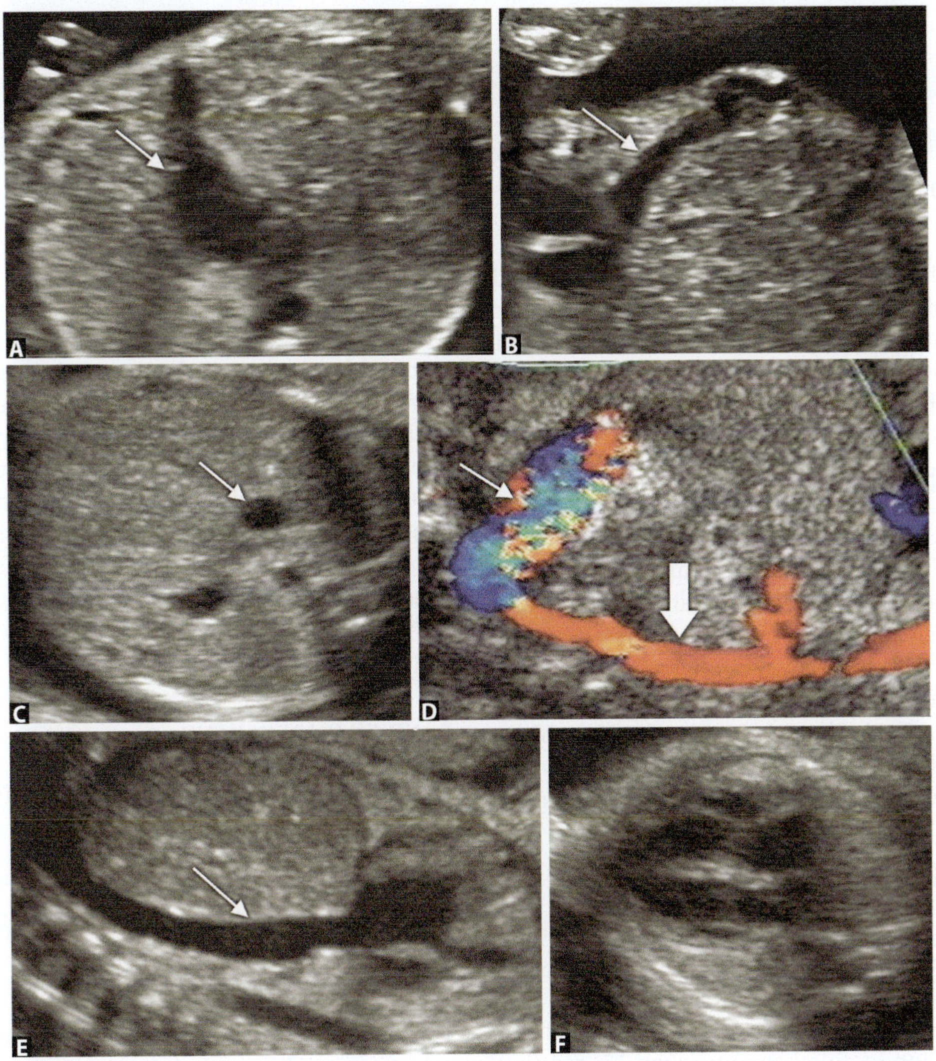

Figure 3: Absent ductus venosus with liver bypass; (A and B) Umbilical vein directly confluencing with the right atrium. Note the typical course of the umbilical vein anterior and superior to the liver; (C) DV not seen, IVC is dilated (arrow); (D) The umbilical vein (arrow) is draining into the right iliac vein consequently, IVC is dilated (solid arrow); (E) Dilated IVC in hammock view; (F) Cardiomegaly

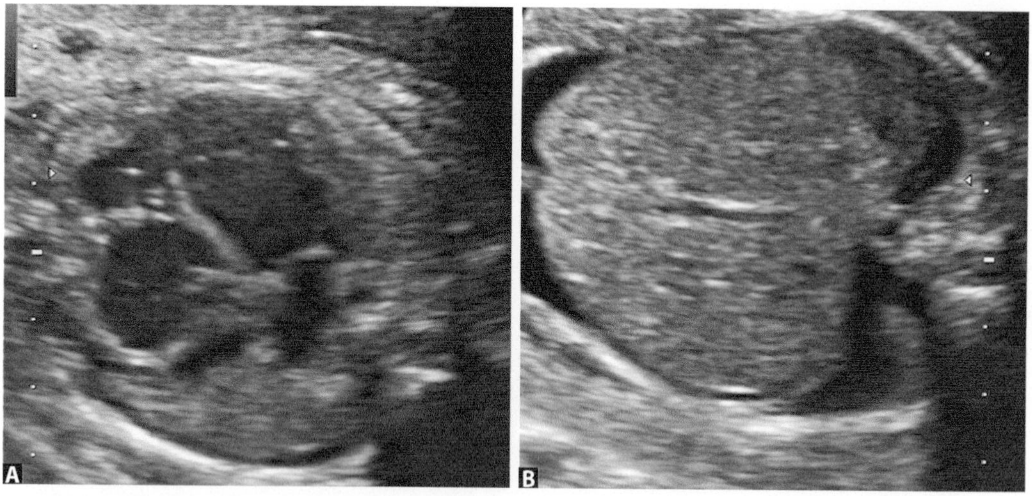

Figure 4: Obvious cardiomegaly in a case of dilated cardiomyopathy. The myocardial contractility was poor. Note the presence of early ascites and right pleural effusion indicating cardiac failure

the portal sinus but the ductus venosus is absent. Associated cardiac/extracardiac anomalies, syndromes (Noonan, VACTERL, Smith Lemli Opitz etc.) and aneuploidy should be looked for.

CARDIAC SIZE

Cardiac size is most often assessed subjectively. Objective assessment may be done by the cardiothoracic (CT) ratio. Area CT ratio and perimeter CT ratio of more than 35% and 50% respectively indicate cardiomegaly. Cardiomegaly could occur in valvular regurgitation (e.g. Ebstein anomaly), dilated cardiomyopathy, cardiac failure due to fetal acidemia, anemia or arrhythmia **(Figure 4)**.

CARDIAC AXIS

Left axis rotation is associated with outflow tract anomalies (tetralogy of Fallot), as also in Ebstein anomaly and coarctation of aorta **(Figure 5)**. In a series of 34 cases of left axis rotation (defined as more than 75° rotation) 61.7% association with cardiac anomalies was reported.[5]

CARDIAC POSITION

Any space occupying lesion or pathology in one hemithorax shifts the mediastinum (cardia) to the opposite side. Typical examples include congenital diaphragmatic hernia, congenital pulmonary airway malformation, pleural effusion and large bronchogenic cysts **(Figure 6A)**. Unilateral pulmonary aplasia or hypoplasia causes ipsilateral mediastinal shift **(Figure 6B)**. Cardiac shift to the right or left is referred to as dextroposition or levoposition respectively.

FOUR CHAMBER VIEW

a. Loss of atrioventricular valvular offset/absent crux.
b. Chamber disproportion.
c. Chamber attributes.
d. Area behind the heart.

Loss of AV Offset/Failure to Identify the Crux

The crux of the cardia is not seen in septum primum atrial septal defect (ASD), inlet ventricular septal defect (VSD), and complete atrioventricular septal defect (AVSD). There is

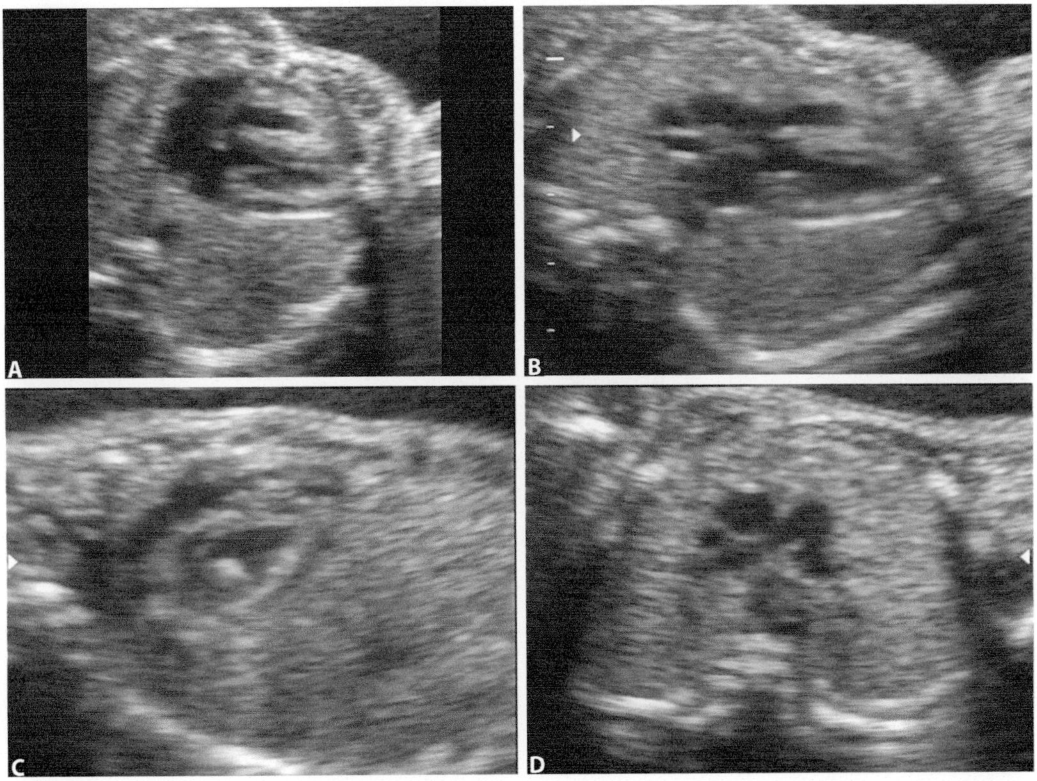

Figure 5: Left axis deviation (A), Malalignment ventricular septal defect and overriding aortic root (B), Narrow right Ventricular outflow tract (C) and narrow pulmonary artery, anterior placed aorta in three vessel view (D) in tetralogy of Fallot

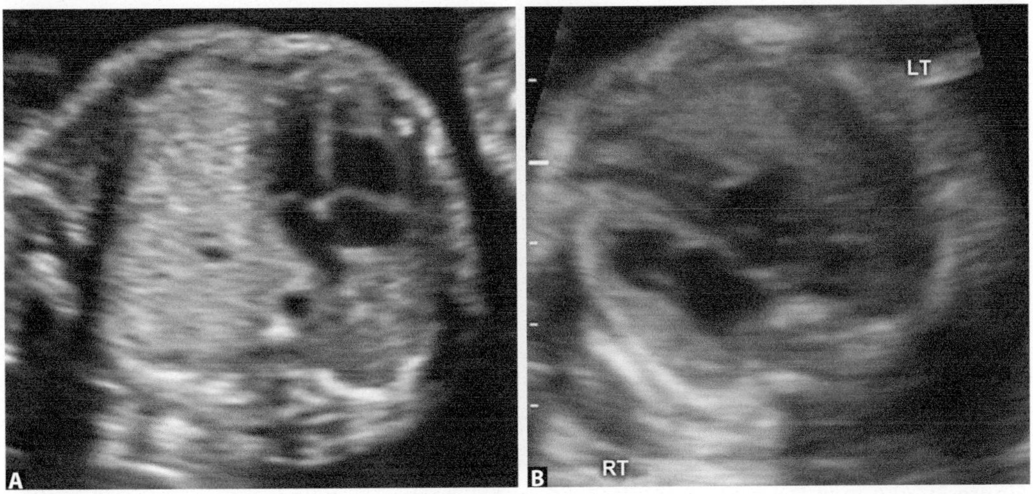

Figure 6: (A) Cardiac shift to the right due to left lung congenital pulmonary airway malformation, (B) Cardiac shift to the right due to right lung hypoplasia

loss of offset between the mitral and tricuspid valves (linear insertion) in all these instances. The crux is also not seen in single ventricle pathology and in cases of gross chamber disproportion.

Septum Primum ASD

There is a gap in the septum primum in the region of its attachment to the crux (**Figure 7**). In some instances, there may be a total absence of the septum primum. The mitral and tricuspid valve annuli are distinct. This lesion is also termed as partial (AVSD). A dilated coronary sinus due to persistent left superior vena cava is often misinterpreted as a septum primum ASD. Associated cardiac malformations include complete AVSD, single ventricle, anomalous pulmonary venous drainage, Ebstein anomaly, and pulmonary atresia with intact ventricular septum. Fetal karyotyping is indicated as septum primum ASD is a marker for Down syndrome.

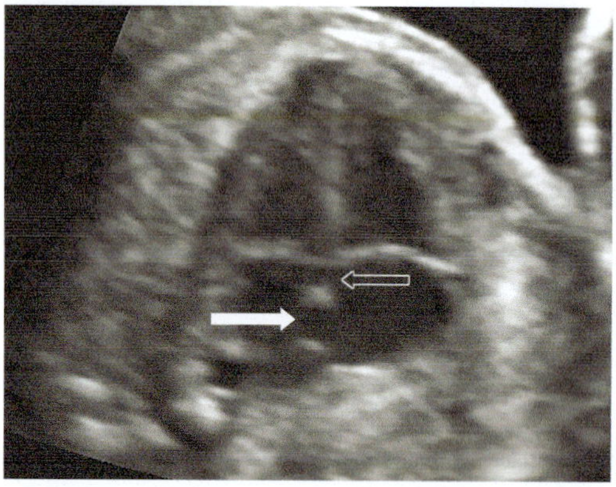

Figure 7: Gap in the septum primum (open arrow) in a fetus with septum primum ASD. Note the linear insertion of the mitral and tricuspid valve leaflets. The foramen ovale is marked by the solid arrow

Fossa ovalis ASDs though commonest cannot be reliably predicted prenatally. Sinus venosus ASD has not been diagnosed in utero.

Inlet VSD

Gap in the inlet ventricular septum at the crux seen in the four chamber view between the atrioventricular valves is diagnostic of a inlet VSD (**Figure 8**). These defects can sometimes be very subtle. Linear insertion of the atrioventricular valves may arouse suspicion of the lesion. The mitral and tricuspid valve annuli are distinct. This lesion is also classified as a partial AVSD. The ventricular

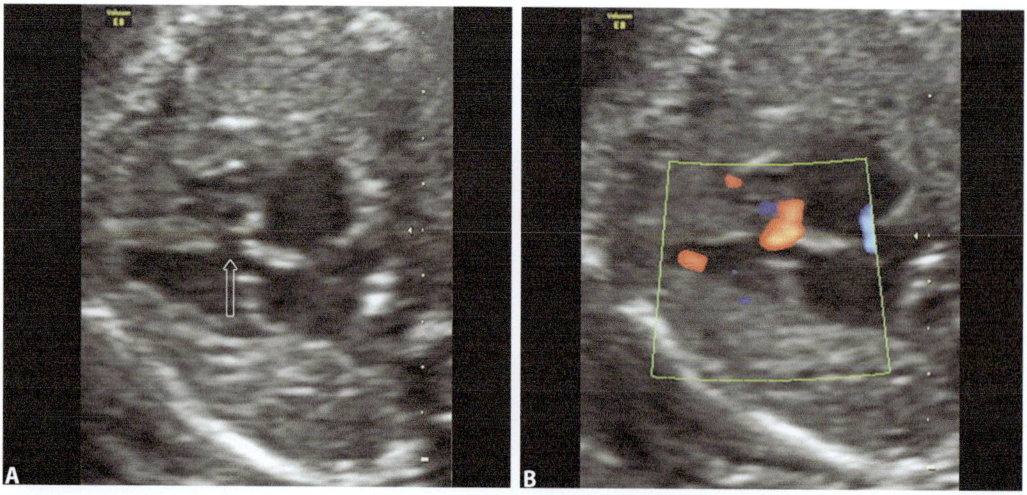

Figure 8: (A) Gap in the inlet ventricular septum (open arrow) in a fetus with inlet VSD. Since the defect is seen in the transverse four chamber view, the possibility of drop out artifact is ruled out; (B) Color Doppler flow across the defect

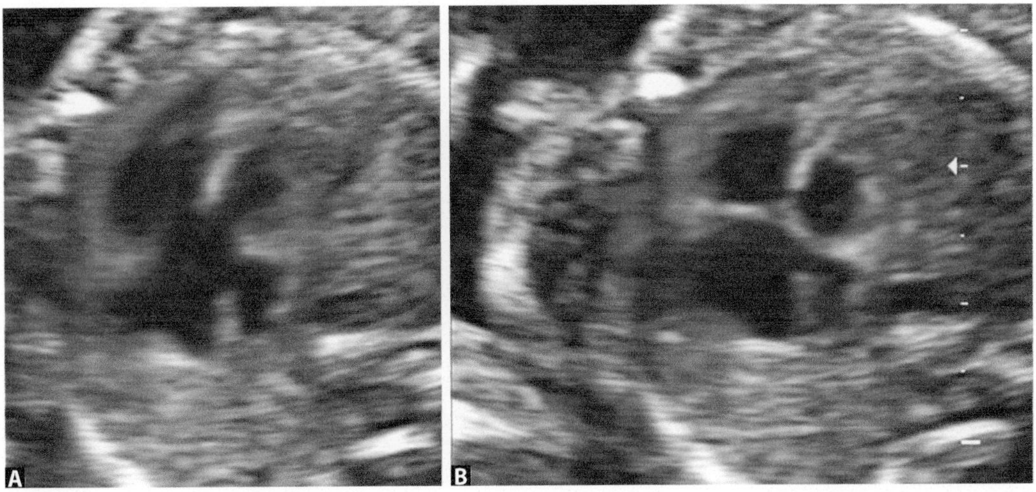

Figure 9: Complete balanced atrioventricular defect: (A) In diastole the single atrioventricular tract and absent crux are notable; (B) In systole the bar or boomerang linear form of the atrioventricular valve is well seen. The increased atrial length is evident

septal drop out artifact is a major pitfall. This may be resolved by a transverse or lateral four chamber view where the ventricular septum is seen to reach up to the crux in the case of drop out artifact. Over writing by color Doppler signals (bleeding artifact) may sometimes mimic the presence of a VSD. Proper equipment settings will correct the artifact. Inlet VSDs account for only a minority of all VSDs (5 to 8%).[6] Bidirectional flow in systole and diastole may be demonstrated by color Doppler in the lateral four chamber view. Fetal karyotyping is indicated mainly to rule out Down syndrome.

Atrioventricular Septal Defect (AVSD)

Septum primum ASD, inlet VSD and an abnormal common (single) atrioventricular annulus are the components of the complete form of AVSD. The single atrioventricular inflow may stream selectively into one of the ventricles resulting in ventricular disproportion resulting in unbalanced complete AVSD (cf balanced complete AVSD where the ventricles are equal in size). In systole there is loss of offset between the septal tricuspid leaflet and the anterior mitral leaflet. This results in a cycle bar or boomerang appearance of the valve leaflets. In diastole, there is a gap in the region of the crux due to absence of the septal structures **(Figure 9)**. The atrioventricular length (AVL) ratio is increased to more than 0.6 in 83% of cases.[7]

Subtle AVSDs may be missed on the lateral four chamber view but may be evident on apical four chamber view. Bradycardia should prompt the presence of an atrioventricular block and appropriate evaluation with M mode and spectral Doppler. AVSD may be recognized in the first trimester around 12 to 13 weeks. Association with a thick nuchal translucency may be extant. Single atrioventricular stream dividing over the crest of the ventricular septal defect can be demonstrated on color Doppler **(Figure 10A)**. Selective streaming into the dominant ventricle may be demonstrated in the unbalanced forms. Atrioventricular regurgitation if present may be demonstrated arising from the center of the atrioventricular valve **(Figure 10B)**. Differential diagnosis is single ventricle pathology.

Associated cardiac findings may include outflow abnormalities as double outlet right ventricle, conotruncal anomalies, right

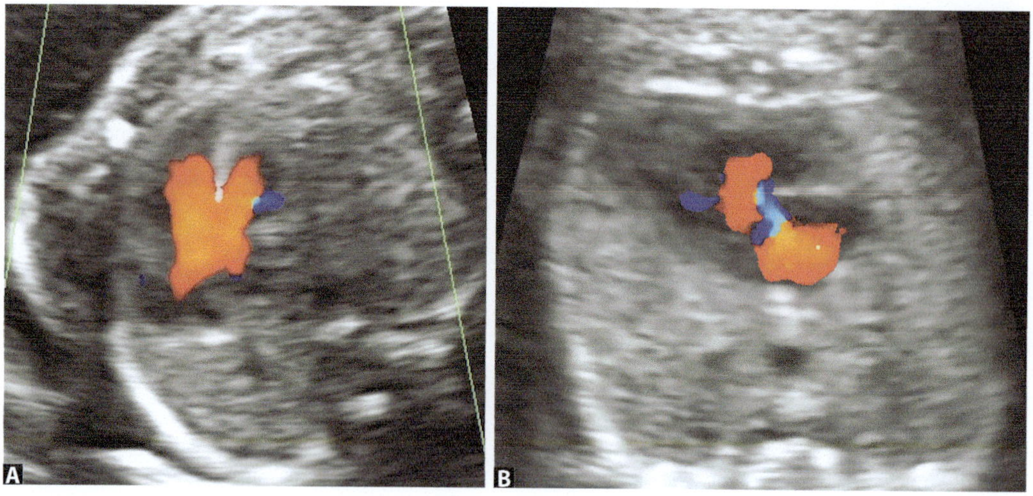

Figure 10: Complete balanced atrioventricular defect: (A) In diastole the single atrioventricular flow forking over the ventricular septal defect noted; (B) In systole the regurgitant stream is seen in blue with aliasing indicating high velocity

aortic arch, pulmonary and systemic vein anomalies. Unbalanced forms of AVSD may be associated with heterotaxy. Features which should suggest the presence of heterotaxy are situs abnormality (midline liver, asplenia), juxtaposed IVC, anomalous pulmonary venous connection and malposed great arteries.

Univentricular Atrioventricular Connection

Single functioning ventricle is the hallmark of this group of disorders. There could be two atria or one atrium connecting with the single ventricle through two or one patent atrioventricular valves resulting in either double inlet single ventricle or single inlet single ventricle **(Figures 11 and 12)**. Very rarely there could be two atria connecting with a single ventricle through a single atrioventricular valve. The single ventricle is commonly of left ventricular morphology (smooth interior) with a rudimentary right ventricle. Double inlet left ventricle (DILV) contributes to 80% of this group of disorders.[8] A small outlet right ventricle is seen supporting one of the great arteries. The outlet chamber communicates with the single ventricle through a bulboventricular foramen. The outlet chamber may not be seen in the typical 'four chamber view' but in a more cranial plane commonly to the left of the single ventricle. The great arteries are in D or L malposition. One or both great arteries may arise from the outlet chamber. Narrow caliber of one of the great arteries could be due to pulmonary stenosis or aortic coarctation. Heterotaxy should be ruled out. Chromosomal abnormality is unusual. Differential diagnosis for single ventricular pathology include pulmonary atresia with intact ventricular septum, hypoplastic left heart syndrome, unbalanced atrioventricular septal defect, tricuspid atresia with VSD and mitral atresia with VSD.

Chamber Disproportion

Chamber disproportion could be due to enlargement or reduction in size of a cardiac chamber. A fetal cardiac chamber fails to grow normally if the quantity of blood flowing through it is less or absent. This typically happens in valvular stenosis or atresia.

Valvular regurgitation on the other hand causes dilatation of the upstream chamber

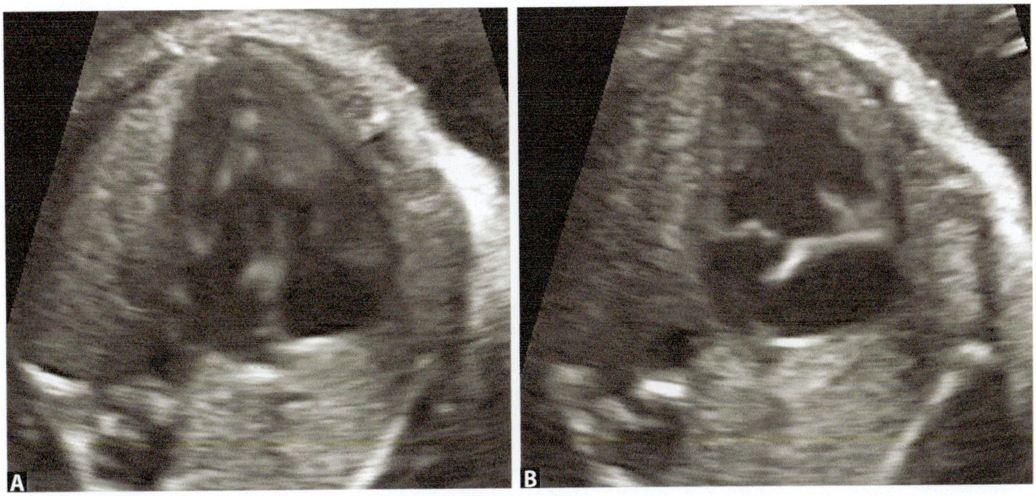

Figure 11: Double inlet single ventricle: (A) In diastole, the two atrioventricular valves are open; (B) In systole, the two atrioventricular valves are closed

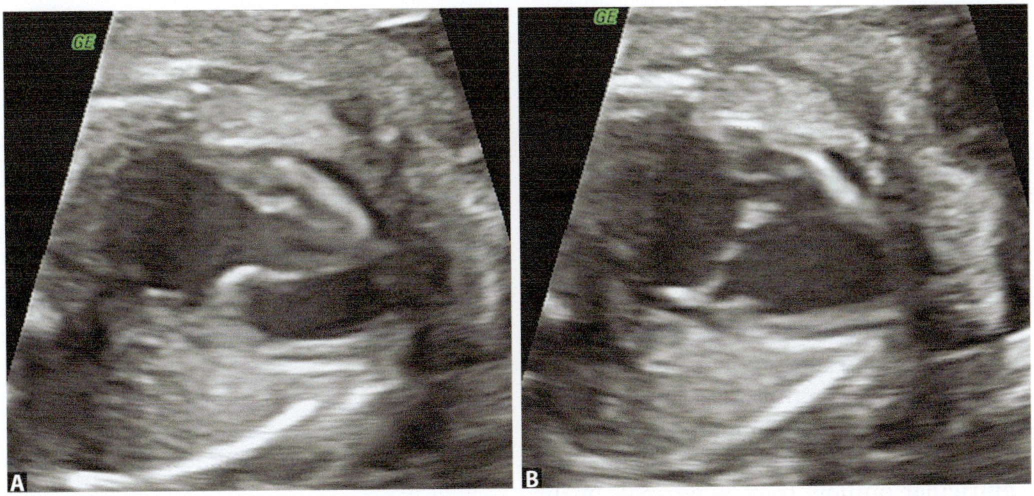

Figure 12: Single inlet single ventricle: (A) In diastole, the single atrio-ventricular valve is open; (B) In systole, the single atrioventricular valve is closed

primarily and the downstream chamber secondarily. The end result in valvular lesions is chamber disproportion. Atretic lesions of the mitral or aortic valves results in hypoplastic left heart syndrome.

Critical aortic stenosis also presents as reduced left sided chamber size. The only non-valvular lesion to cause diminution of the left sided chambers is coarctation of aorta.

Tricuspid atresia with VSD, pulmonary atresia with intact ventricular septum and critical pulmonary stenosis result in reduced right sided chamber size. Ebstein anomaly and tricuspid dysplasia result in tricuspid regurgitation and enlargement of the right sided chambers.

Hypoplastic Left Heart Syndrome

In the classical form there is atresia of the mitral and aortic valves with a very small or nearly absent left ventricle. In the other less common form the aortic valve is atretic but

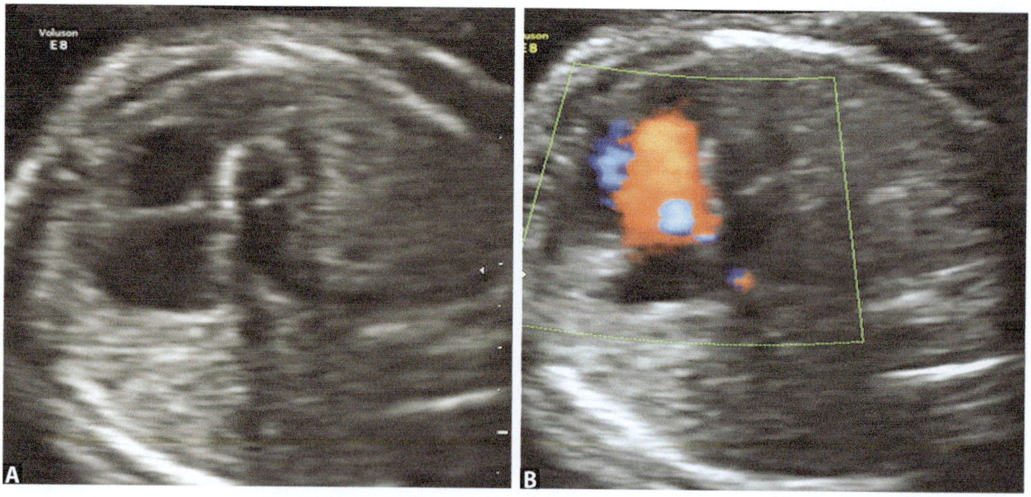

Figure 13: Four chamber view: (A) Smaller left atrium and left ventricle, hyperechoic interventricular septum and apex of the cardia by the right ventricle; (B) Absent transmitral and normal transtricuspid flow on color Doppler in diastole

the mitral valve is patent and dysplastic often with mitral regurgitation. The left ventricle is akinetic and globular with hyperechoic (endomyocardial fibroelastosis) walls. In the four chamber view, the apex is taken over by the right ventricle **(Figure 13)**. The foraminal flap bulges into the right atrium. The left atrium is generally smaller compared to the right atrium. In the presence of mitral regurgitation the left atrium is dilated. In the five chamber and left ventricular outflow tract views the aorta is either not identified or is very small in caliber (compared to the main pulmonary artery)**(Figure 14)**. The right ventricular outflow tract is normal. In the three vessel and three vessel trachea views the aorta is either not visualized or small in caliber **(Figure 15A)**. Color Doppler findings include absent transmitral flow, left to right transforaminal flow, and ductus dependent reversed fill of the aortic arch in the three vessel trachea view **(Figure 15B)**. Color Doppler may be the only way to identify the presence of aorta in the three vessel trachea view. In the forms were the mitral valve is dysplastic mitral regurgitation may be documented by color Doppler. Due to the presence of dramatic findings on the four chamber view hypoplastic left heart syndrome can be diagnosed in the first trimester (11 to 14 weeks) ultrasonography. Chromosomal abnormality should be ruled out. Associated conditions include Trisomy 13 or 18, Turner syndrome, Noonan syndrome or Holt Oram syndrome.

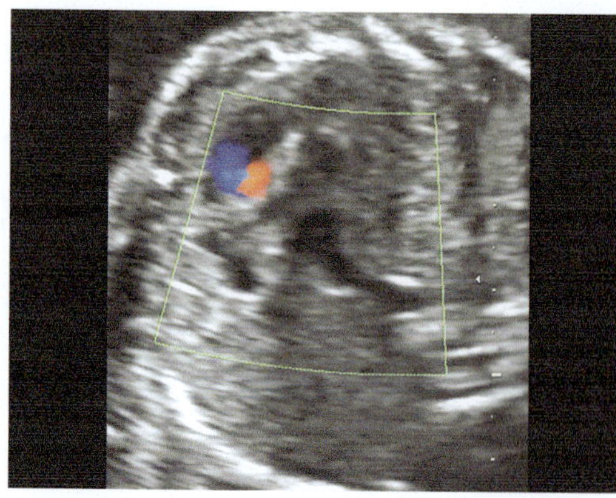

Figure 14: Left ventricular outflow tract – Narrow aorta with no forward flow on color Doppler

Critical Aortic Stenosis

Aortic stenosis in the fetus is usually valvular. The milder form does not produce any changes on the four chamber view and may be diagnosed by the presence of thickened aortic

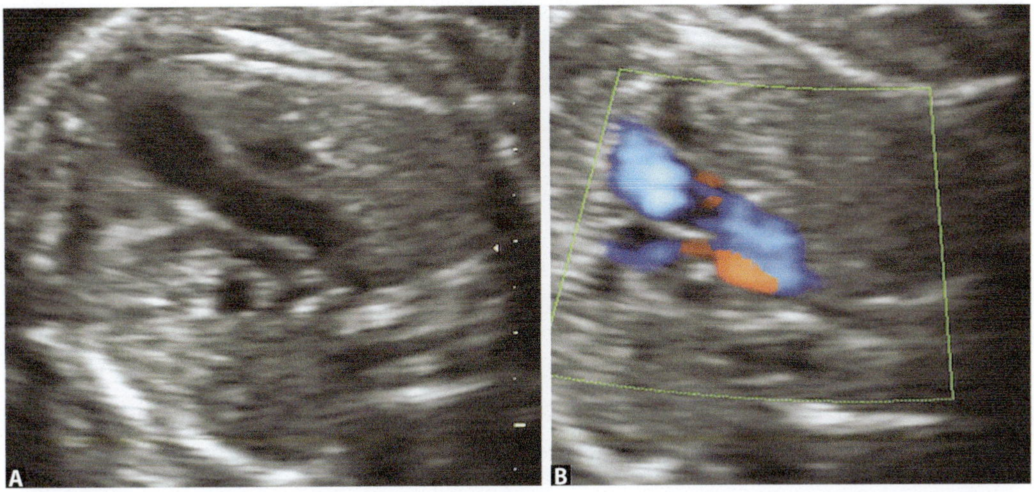

Figure 15: Three vessel trachea view: (A) Narrow aorta compared to the pulmonary artery, (B) Ductus dependant reverse fill of the aorta in red compared to forward flow in the pulmonary artery

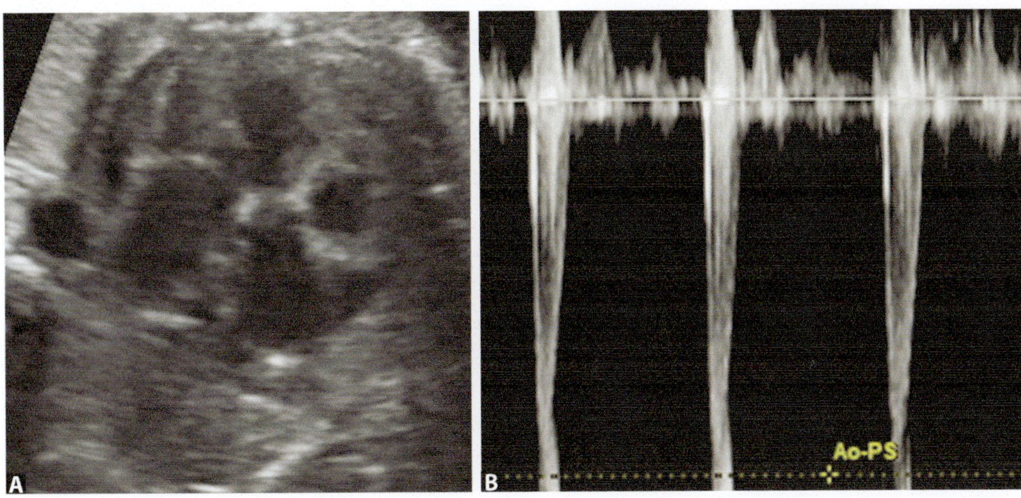

Figure 16: Severe aortic stenosis: (A) Left ventricular outflow tract showing thick aortic valve cusps, narrow aortic annulus and post stenotic dilatation; (B) Peak aortic systolic velocity of 194 cm/sec

valve cusps, poststenotic dilatation and systolic jetting (peak systolic velocity of 200 cm/sec or more)**(Figure 16)**. Critical form of aortic stenosis results in dilated left ventricle with reduced contractility and endomyocardial fibroelastosis. Forward transmitral flow is preserved. Presence of mitral regurgitation results in a dilated left atrium. In severe aortic stenosis the aortic velocities may be attenuated due to left ventricular failure.[9] Left to right foraminal flow and reverse flow through the ductus especially in diastole may be demonstrated on color Doppler. Follow up scans may demonstrate evolution into a full blown hypoplastic left heart syndrome.

Coarctation of Aorta

Implies discrete narrowing of the aortic isthmus (segment distal to the origin of the left subclavian artery and proximal to the

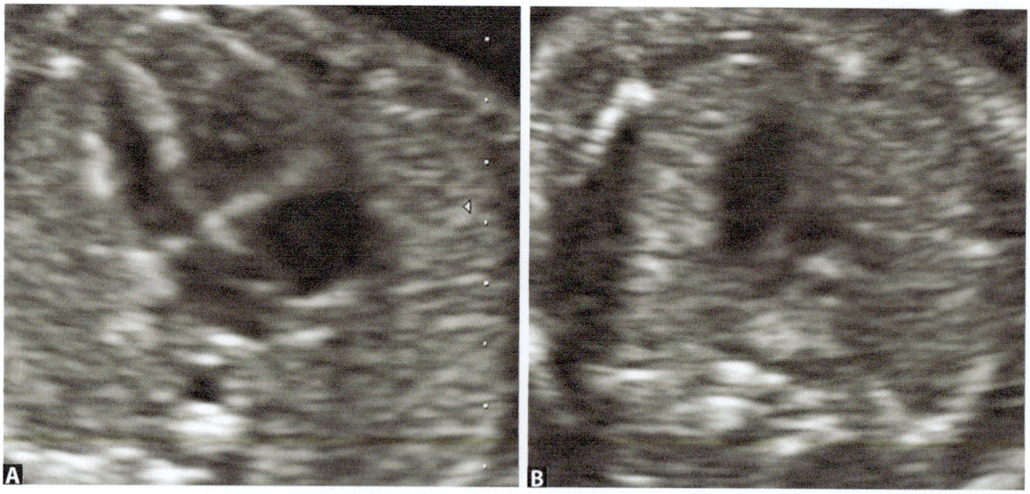

Figure 17: Coarctation of aorta: (A) Four chamber view with diminutive left sided chambers, (B) Three vessel trachea view with a narrow aortic arch compared to the ductus arch

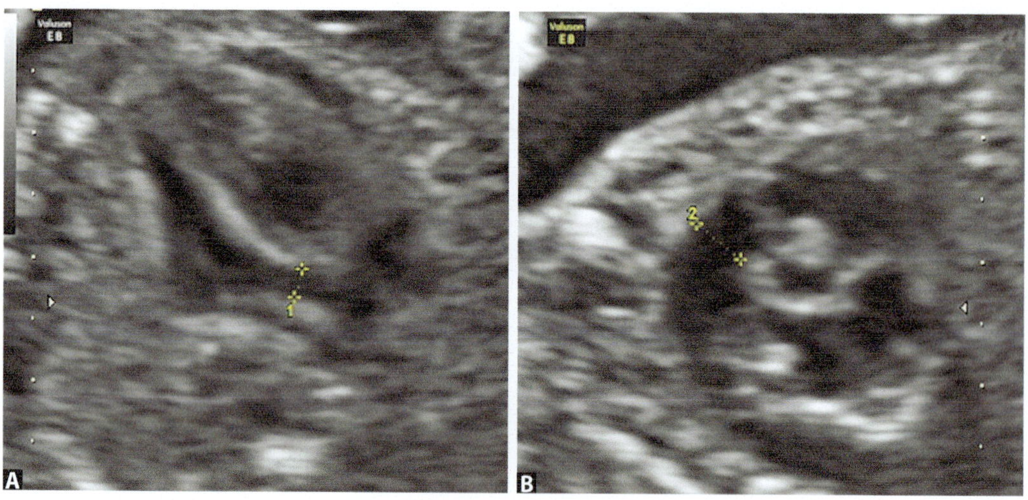

Figure 18: Coarctation of aorta; (A) Left ventricular outflow tract with narrow aorta; (B) Right ventricular outflow tract with normal pulmonary artery

ductus arteriosus. The severest form is tubular hypoplasia of the aortic arch. Presentation may be neonatal especially after the closure of the ductus. In a proportion of cases the presentation may be later in childhood or in adolescence. Chamber disproportion with predominance of the right sided chambers or rather the diminution of the left sided chambers is the first clue **(Figure 17)**. The aortic caliber is smaller compared to the main pulmonary artery **(Figure 18)**. The PA/Ao ratio has been described to be of value.[10] The aortic arch is small in caliber especially towards the isthmus in the three vessel trachea view. Color Doppler demonstrates forward flow across the mitral and aortic valves. In severe coarctation there could be a diastolic ductus dependent reverse fill. Direct evidence of coarctation is by the demonstration of the contraductal shelf in the isthmus region in

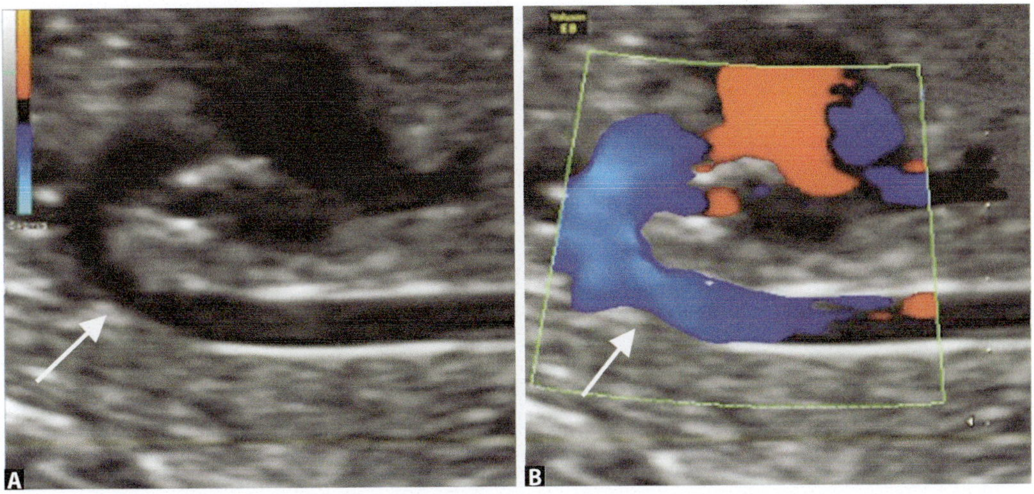

Figure 19: Coarctation of aorta: (A) Aortic arch with isthmial narrowing (arrow); (B) Color Doppler may overwrite the isthmus narrowing

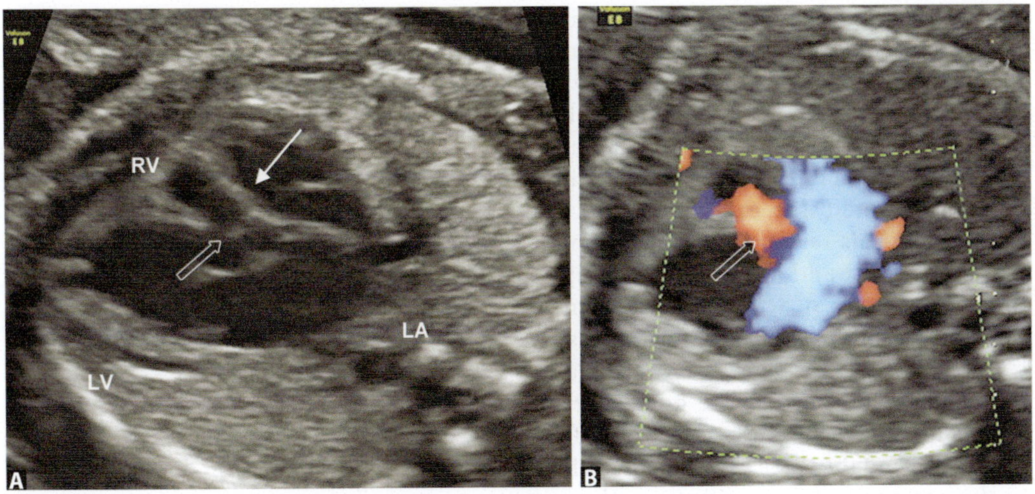

Figure 20: Tricuspid atresia with VSD: (A) Atretric tricuspid valve (solid arrow) small right ventricle and VSD (open arrow); (B) Color Doppler left to right flow through the VSD (open arrow) and exaggerated right to left flow across the foramen ovale in blue

the aortic arch view **(Figure 19)**. Left superior vena cava is associated with coarctation of aorta. Diagnosis is beset by high rates of false negatives and false positives. Differential diagnosis would include hypoplastic left heart syndrome, interrupted aortic arch and total anomalous pulmonary venous drainage (will be considered in the section of the area behind the heart). Chromosomal abnormality should be ruled out. Associated anomalies are common and should be looked for.

Tricupid Atresia with VSD

Understandably, the right ventricle is small. The tricuspid valve is atretic and thick membrane like with no leaflet excursions. The small right ventricle fills through an inlet VSD **(Figure 20A)**. The bigger the VSD larger

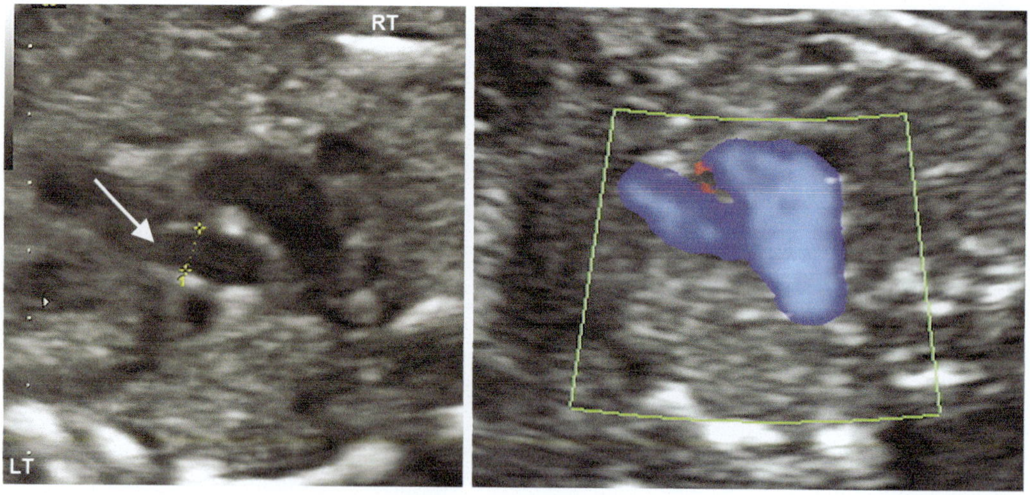

Figure 21: Three vessel view in tricuspid atresia with VSD showing smaller pulmonary artery (arrow) compared to aorta in gray scale and in color. Forward flow in pulmonary artery seen

is the size of the diminutive right ventricle. Right ventricular myocardial contractility is normal. The entire right atrial volume now has to egress out through the foramen ovale into the left atrium. Consequently, the foramen is wide, the septum bulges into the left atrium with exaggerated flap excursions into the left atrium. This results in a malalignment of the interatrial and interventricular septa. In type I the great arterial orientation is normal (common). D-transposition and L-transposition are seen in types II and III respectively (rare).[11] The great arterial arrangement may be assessed by the outflow tract views and the three vessel trachea view. In the commonest type with normal great arterial orientation the pulmonary artery arises from the right ventricle and its size depends on the size of the VSD and the right ventricle. The great arterial size discrepancy may be well demonstrated in the three vessel trachea view. Color Doppler shows absent transtricuspid flow with the right ventricle filling through the VSD **(Figure 20B)**. The VSD therefore shows a left to right flow direction. Since the transforaminal flow and hence the transmitral flow is increased there is aliasing seen across the mitral valve. Normal forward ductus flow is noted **(Figure 21)**. Severe pulmonary stenosis or atresia would cause a ductus dependent pulmonary circulation with reverse filling of the pulmonary artery.

Karyotyping and FISH for 22q11 del may be offered.

Pulmonary Atresia with Intact Interventricular Septum

Majority of these cases present as a small right ventricle or even thick walled right ventricle with no lumen **(Figure 22A)**. The tricuspid valve is without function. Less common is the form which presents as tricuspid regurgitation where the right ventricle is intact and dilated but hypokinetic. The narrow pulmonary artery is seen in the right ventricular outflow tract and the three vessel trachea views. On occasion it may not be possible to visualize the pulmonary artery on gray scale. It presence may only be confirmed by color Doppler which demonstrates the narrow caliber and also a ductus dependant reverse filling in the three vessel trachea view. Occasionally, the smaller pulmonary artery may demonstrate ductus dependant to and fro fill **(Figures 23 and 24)**. Absent filling of the right ventricle may be seen in the four chamber view

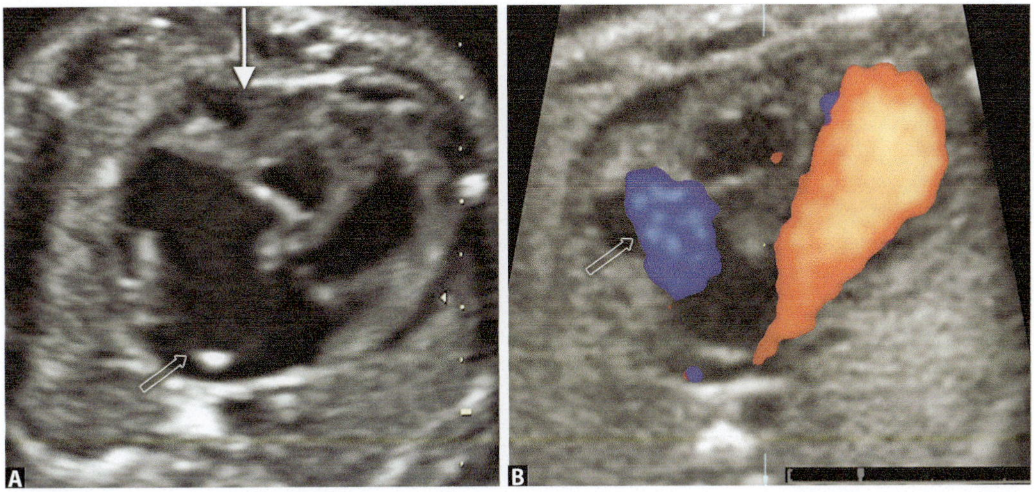

Figure 22: Four chamber view in pulmonary atresia with intact ventricular septum: (A) Small thick walled right ventricle (solid arrow) with a foraminal flap reaching far into the left atrium (open arrow); (B) Absent transtricuspid flow with exaggerated transforaminal right to left flow (open arrow)

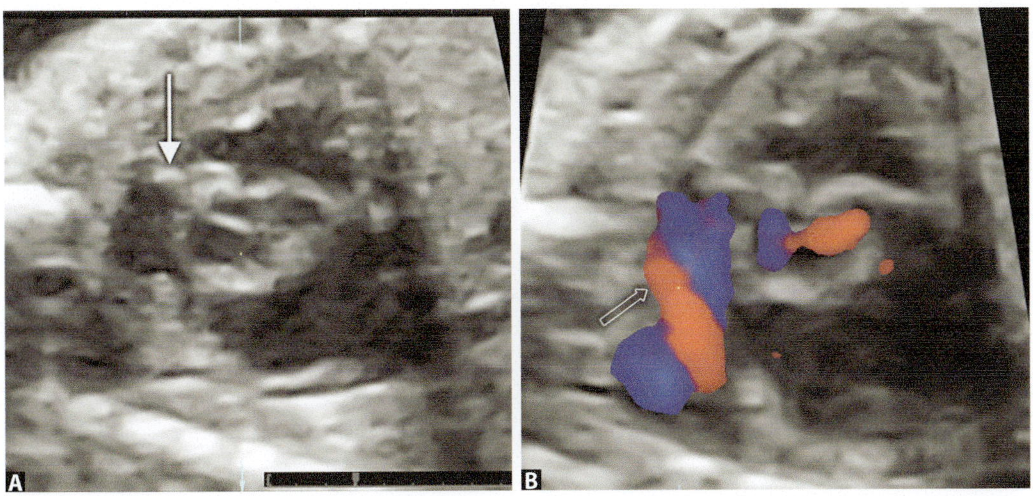

Figure 23: Right ventricular outflow tract in pulmonary atresia with intact ventricular septum: (A) Thick atretic pulmonary valve (solid arrow); (B) Ductus dependant to and fro flow in the main pulmonary artery (open arrow)

(Figure 22B). In the forms where there is a dilated right ventricle forward transtriscuspid flow and holosystolic regurgitation are present. In those instances with a reasonably sized right ventricle and transtricuspid forward diastolic flow without tricuspid regurgitation the presence of ventriculocoronary shunt/s should be sought for color Doppler. Major aortopulmonary collaterals are not a feature of pulmonary atresia with intact ventricular septum. Chromosomal abnormalities and associated anomalies are rare.

Pulmonary Stenosis

Pulmonary stenosis in the fetus is valvular. In the four chamber view, the only finding may be one of right ventricular myocardial thickening with ventricular septal bulging into the left

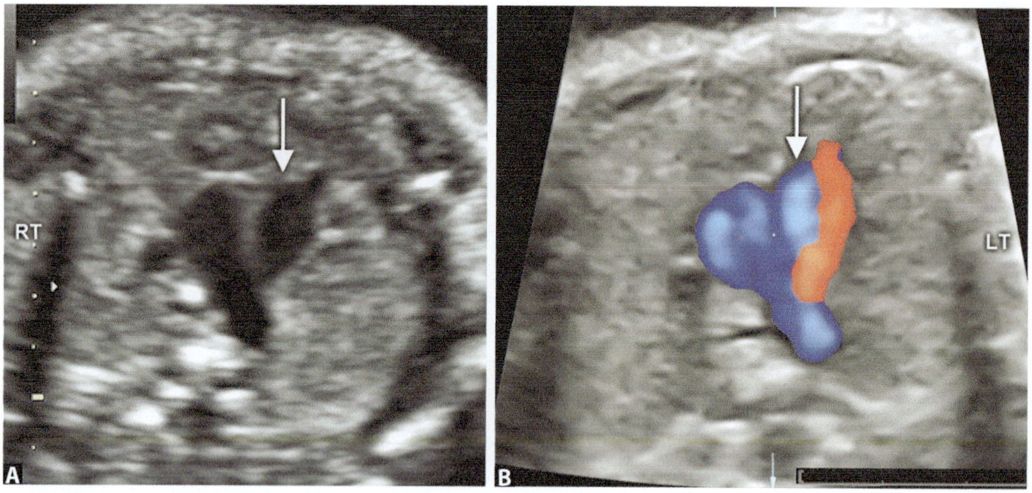

Figure 24: Three vessel view in pulmonary atresia with intact ventricular septum: (A) Smaller pulmonary artery (arrow) compared to aorta; (B) Ductus dependent to and fro flow in pulmonary artery (arrow)

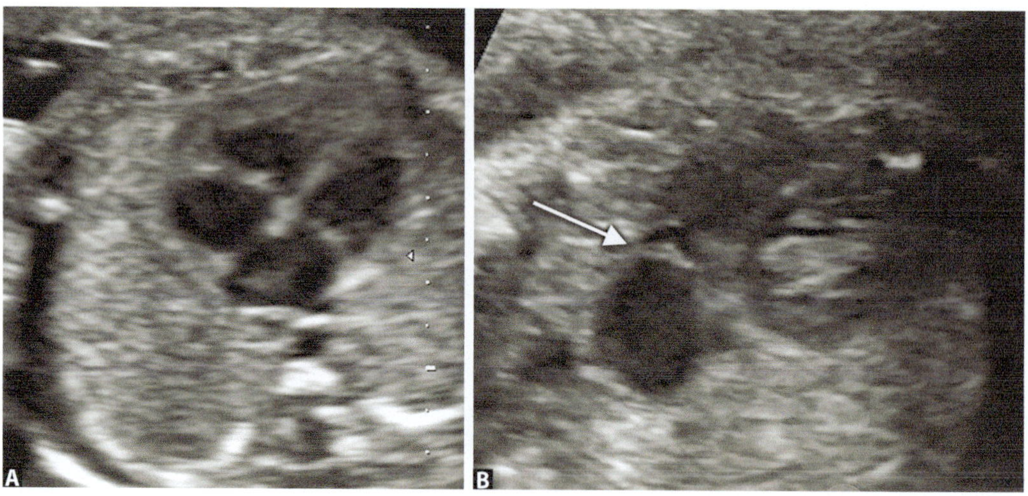

Figure 25: Subcritical pulmonary stenosis: (A) Four chamber view is unremarkable; (B) Right ventricular outflow tract with narrownannulus and thick pulmonary valve leaflets (arrow) and post valvular dilatation

ventricle (third trimester). Right ventricular contractility and tricuspid excursions are normal. Direct visualization of the pulmonary valve in the right ventricular outflow view reveals thickening and doming of the cusps during systole **(Figure 25)**. Normally the valve cusps are seen only in diastole and not in systole. Post stenotic dilatation and turbulent high velocity flow across the pulmonary valve are noted in the right ventricular outflow tract as well as in the three vessel trachea view **(Figure 26)**. Peak systolic velocity exceeds 200 cm/sec. Forward ductus flow noted. Evolution to pulmonary atresia is indicated by reversed ductus flow and the appearance of tricuspid regurgitation.[12] Pulmonary regurgitation due to valve dysplasia may be seen and Noonan syndrome should be suspected in these cases.

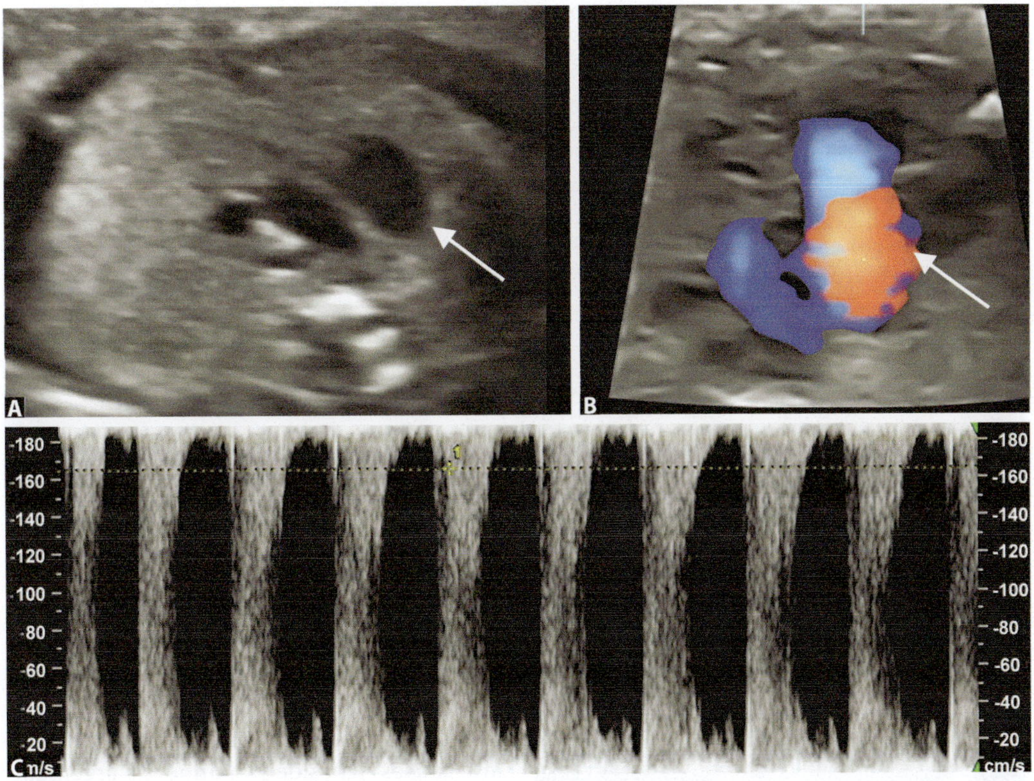

Figure 26: Subcritical pulmonary stenosis: (A) Three vessel view shows pulmonary artery dilatation (arrow); (B) Aliasing in the pulmonary artery (arrow); (C) Pulmonary artery peak systolic velocity of close to 200 cm/sec with turbulence

Ebstein Anomaly

Abnormal apical attachment of the septal and posterior tricuspid leaflets results atrialization of a part of the right ventricle **(Figure 27A)**. This may vary from a subtle to severe displacement. Cardiomegaly is mainly due to the right atrial dilatation especially in the third trimester.[13] This could be subtle in the second trimester. Pulmonary hypoplasia may occur due to the cardiomegaly. The apically displaced attachment of the tricuspid valve leaflets may be demonstrated in the four chamber view. This helps in differentiating from tricuspid dysplasia. Right atrial dilatation may result in an atrial septal defect. The pulmonary artery is small compared to aorta and is most often due to functional atresia. The holosystolic tricuspid regurgitation (200 cm/sec) may be demonstrated even before atrial dilatation is manifest **(Figure 27B)**. Forward flow through a narrow pulmonary artery or ductus dependant reversed fill may be demonstrated **(Figure 28)**. The latter represents functional atresia of the pulmonary valve.

Tricuspid Valve Dysplasia

Thickened but normally inserted tricuspid valve leaflets constitute this anomaly. Typically the thickened tricuspid leaflets do not close properly in systole. The right atrium is enlarged in the four chamber view due to tricuspid regurgitation which can be demonstrated on color Doppler study **(Figure 29)**. The pulmonary artery is narrow with forward flow or ductus dependant reverse flow indicating functional atresia.

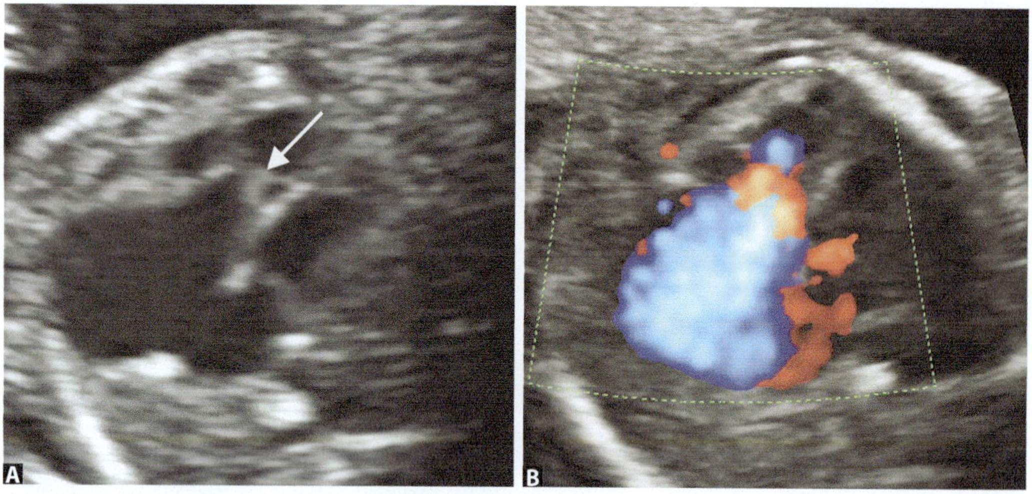

Figure 27: Ebstein anomaly: (A) Right atrial dilatation with apical insertion of the septal leaflet of triscuspid valve (arrow); (B) Tricuspid regurgitation

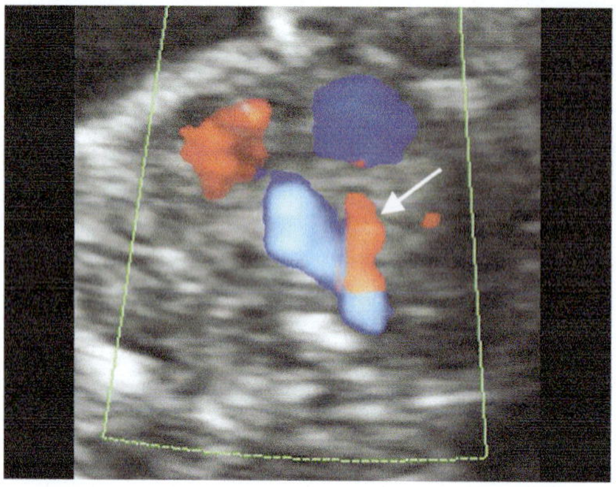

Figure 28: Ebstein anomaly—Three vessel view with ductus dependent reverse pulmonary artery fill indicating functional atresia. Also note the narrower pulmonary caliber compared to the aorta

Chromosomal abnormality and associated congenital anomalies are unlikely.

Chamber disproportion could also be seen due to non-valvular causes. In total anomalous pulmonary venous drainage, the pulmonary venous return is channelized into the right atrium and hence there is a right sided chamber dominance. This condition will be considered in the section dealing with the area behind the heart. Increased venous return to the heart (increased preload) as in chorioangioma, vein of Galen aneurysm, fetal tumor or fetal anemia result in right sided chamber enlargement. Raised fetoplacental resistance and premature constriction of the ductus result in increased afterload which also causes right sided chamber enlargement.

Chamber Attributes

The presence of atrioventricular discordance may be detected in the four chamber view as the moderator band and the normal apically inserted tricuspid septal leaflet are now seen in the left sided ventricle. This happens in the congenitally corrected transposition of the great arteries and will be dealt later.

Area Behind the Heart

The area behind the heart refers to the region between the posterior wall of the left atrium and the spine. The descending aorta is the only structure seen in this region. The left atrium almost touches the descending aorta. The fluid filled esophagus may be transiently seen between the left atrium and the descending aorta. The vertical vein in total anomalous pulmonary venous drainage and the enlarged azygous vein in IVC interruption

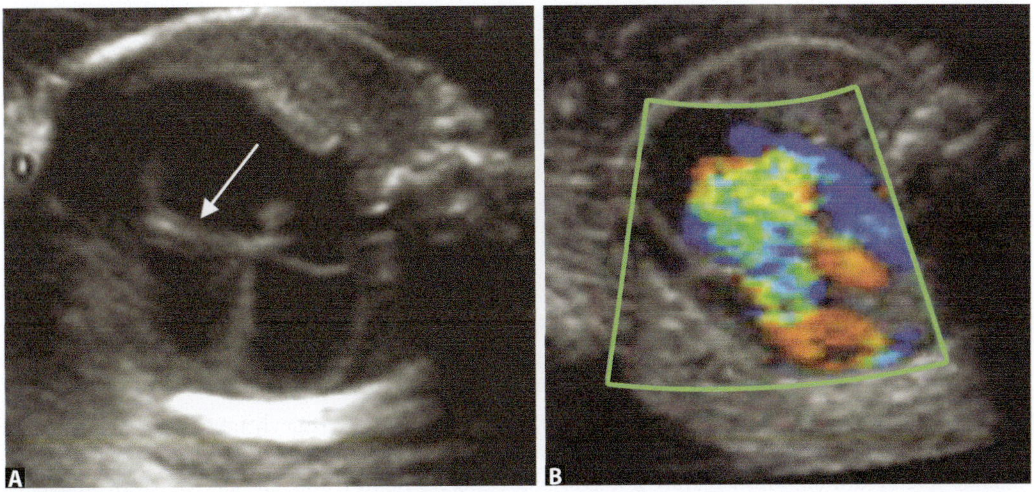

Figure 29: Tricuspid dysplasia: (A) Four chamber view with right atrial enlargement and thickened but normally attached tricuspid valve leaflet; (B) Tricuspid regurgitation

are the two pathological situations related to the cardia that may be potentially recognized in the area behind the heart. The presence of any of these vessels is termed the 'Double vessel sign.'[14] The azygos vein is the right and subtly posterior to the descending aorta. The vertical vein in TAPVD is seen anterior to the descending aorta. The presence of right sided aortic arch in levocardia or left sided aortic arch in dextrocardia may be easily suspected by noting the position of the descending aorta in relation to the spine. Non-cardiac lesions like an esophageal duplication cyst or a neurenteric cyst may be occasionally be seen.

Total Anomalous Pulmonary Venous Drainage

All four pulmonary veins drain directly or indirectly into the right atrium. The area behind the heart does not show the normal pulmonary venous connection with the left atrium **(Figure 30A)**. The left atrial posterior wall is rounded in contour. The distance between the descending aorta and the left atrium (post LA space) is increased **(Figure 30A)**.[15] The four pulmonary veins converge to form a vertical vein in the area behind the heart **(Figure 30B)**. In the supracardiac type of TAPVD this vertical vein courses superiorly to drain into the left innominate vein. In the three vessel trachea view, the vertical vein is seen as the fourth vessel to the left of the pulmonary artery **(Figure 30C)**. The superior vena cava is larger in caliber. Color Doppler cardiofugal direction of flow will help in differentiating from left superior vena cava which has cardiopetal flow. In the infracardiac type, the vertical vein courses inferiorly along the esophagus, through the diaphragm, to drain into the portal venous system. Obstruction to the vertical vein is common in the infracardiac type. The Doppler waveforms from the vertical vein is abnormal and lacks the normal pulsatility. The pulmonary veins drain into the coronary sinus in the cardiac type resulting in a dilated coronary sinus. Dilated coronary sinus in the absence of a persistent left superior vena cava should raise the suspicion for cardiac type of TAPVC. The pulmonary veins may directly connect with the posterior wall of the right atrium. Right sided chamber dominance is noted as the pulmonary venous return is directly or indirectly into the right atrium. TAPVC is commonly seen in cases of right atrial isomerism.

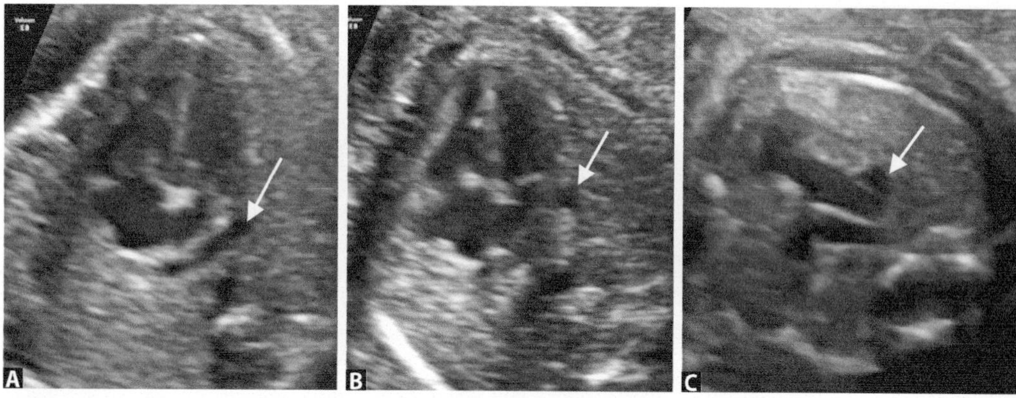

Figure 30: Supracardiac total anomalous pulmonary venous drainage: (A) Four chamber view with increased post LA space and pulmonary veins not confluencing with left atrium (arrow); (B) Vertical vein axial section at four chamber level (arrow); (C) Vertical vein at the level of three vessel view (arrow). The superior vena cava is prominent

WHEN ONE ROTATES THE TRANSDUCER FROM THE FOUR CHAMBER VIEW TO OBTAIN THE LEFT VENTRICULAR TRACT ONE OF THE FOLLOWING MAY BE ENCOUNTERED

a. Aorta overriding a malalignment VSD.
b. Parallel great arteries.

Overriding Aorta

A malalignment ventricular septal defect is diagnosed when there is an aortoseptal discontinuity with the aortic root overriding the septal defect. The aorta now receives output from both ventricles. This is a finding and not the final diagnosis. The status of the pulmonary artery yields the final diagnosis. The pulmonary artery could be i. narrow, or ii. atretic, or iii. the branch arteries are dilated or iv. it (pulmonary artery) arises from a common trunk.

i. The pulmonary artery is narrow—*Tetralogy of Fallot*: Four chamber view is basically normal. There could however be a left axis rotation **(Figure 31A)**. However in the five chamber or left ventricular outflow tract view the malalignment VSD and aortic root overriding the VSD are visualized **(Figure 31B)**. The long axis of the ascending aorta is collinear with the interventricular septum. In the right ventricular outflow tract view and in the three vessel view the pulmonary artery is narrow in caliber (compared to the aorta) **(Figure 32A)**. This difference in caliber increases with advancing gestational age. Demonstration of the pulmonary artery bifurcation is necessary for prognostication. In addition to the great arterial size discrepancy the anteriorly placed aorta is seen in the three vessel view. The three vessel trachea view should also be used to rule out or confirm a right aortic arch. Aortic commitance to both ventricles can be demonstrated by color Doppler in the apical five chamber view **(Figure 31C)**. Forward flow through the narrow pulmonary artery must be demonstrated to rule out pulmonary atresia **(Figure 32B)**. Reversed ductus dependant filling of the pulmonary artery could also occur in severe pulmonary stenosis. Invasive testing for chromosomal abnormalities and FISH for 22q11 deletion should be done. Thymic hypoplasia may be quantified by the thymic thoracic ratio.[16] Associated extracardiac congenital

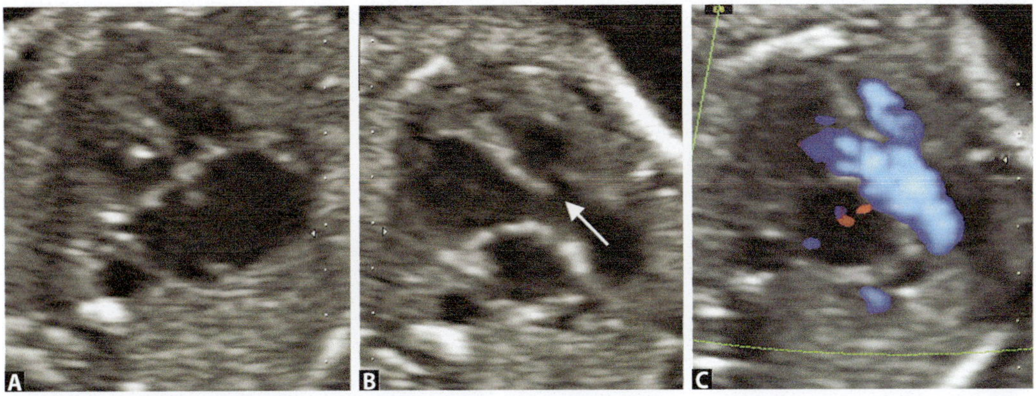

Figure 31: Tetralogy of Fallot: (A) Four chamber view with left axis rotation; (B) Left ventricular tract view with malalignment VSD and overriding aortic root (arrow); (C) Color Doppler of left ventricular outflow tract—aorta committed to both ventricles

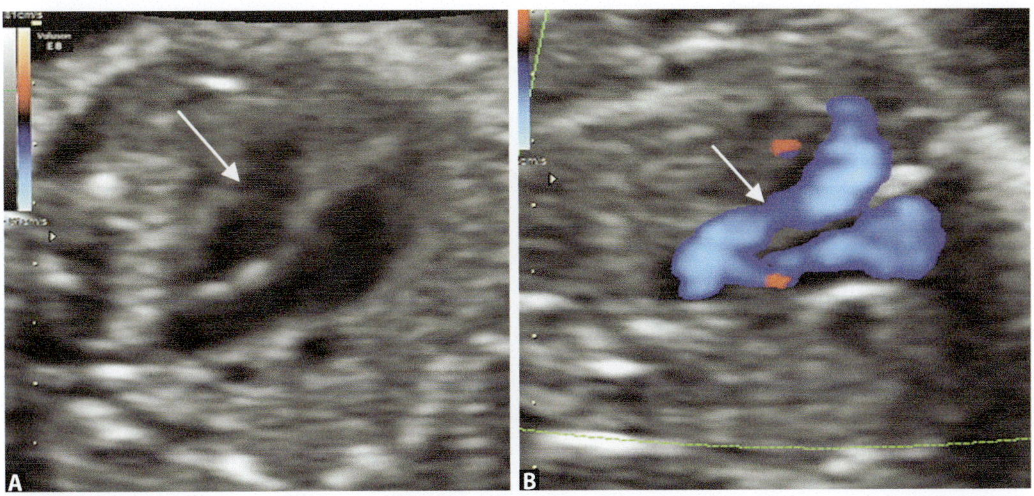

Figure 32: Tetralogy of Fallot—Three vessel trachea view: (A) Gray scale—Pulmonary artery (arrow) is narrower than aorta; (B) Color Doppler—Forward flow in pulmonary artery (arrow)

anomalies must be looked for. Follow up scans every four weeks is necessary to monitor the pulmonary caliber and flow direction. Increasing aortopulmonary discrepancy is of poor prognosis.

ii. The pulmonary artery is not seen—*Pulmonary atresia with VSD*: The pulmonary artery is not visualized. Blood supply to the lungs is through the ductus or directly from the descending aorta (major aortopulmonary collaterals—MAPCA's). The four chamber view is unremarkable **(Figure 33A)**. The five chamber and the left ventricular outflow tract view show a large artery (aorta) overriding a malalignment VSD **(Figure 33B)**. The aorta is larger than in tetralogy of Fallot as the entire output of both ventricles pass through it given that the pulmonary artery is atretic. The only vessels to be seen in the three vessel view are the aorta and SVC **(Figure 34A)**. Right aortic arch and thymic

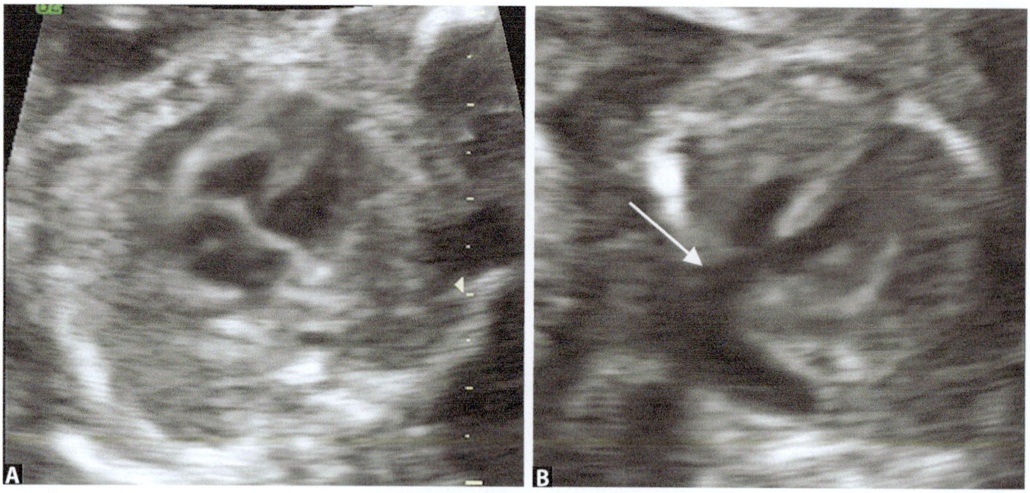

Figure 33: Pulmonary atresia with VSD: (A) Normal four chamber view; (B) Overriding large aorta on a malalignment VSD (arrow)

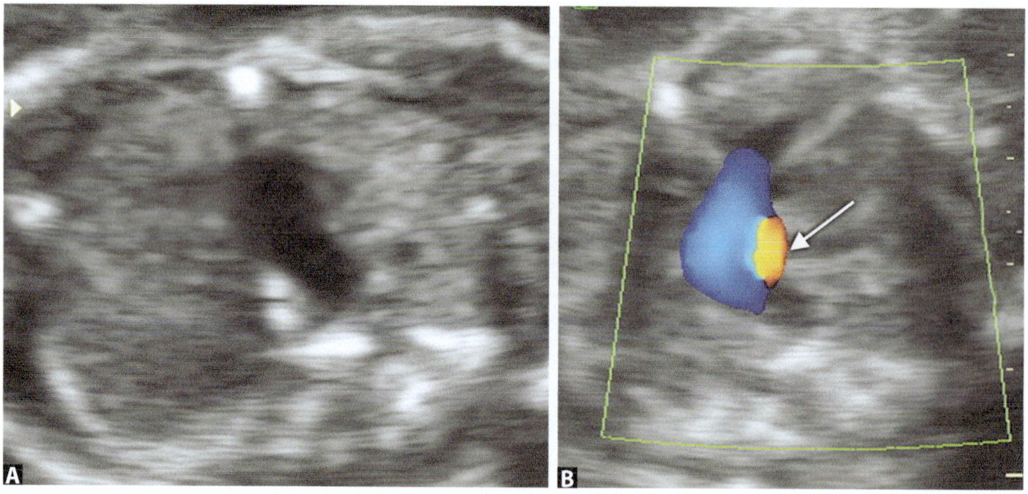

Figure 34: Pulmonary atresia with VSD: (A) Only aorta and SVC are seen in the three vessel view; (B) Small pulmonary artery with reverse ductus dependant fill in red (arrow) on color Doppler

hypoplasia should be looked for. On color Doppler the aorta is committed to both ventricles. The right ventricular tract is not demonstrable. A thin pulmonary artery with retrograde fill from the ductus may be identified in the three vessel view **(Figure 34B)**. Occasionally, the pulmonary valve is atretic but distal to the valve the pulmonary artery is well seen and is of reasonable caliber. In these cases, there is a to and fro movement of blood in the main pulmonary artery (ductus dependant). The descending aorta should be carefully studied with color Doppler in the transverse and coronal planes to look for major aortopulmonary collaterals especially in those cases where there is no ductus dependant pulmonary artery fill. Karyotyping and FISH for 22q11 deletion may be planned.

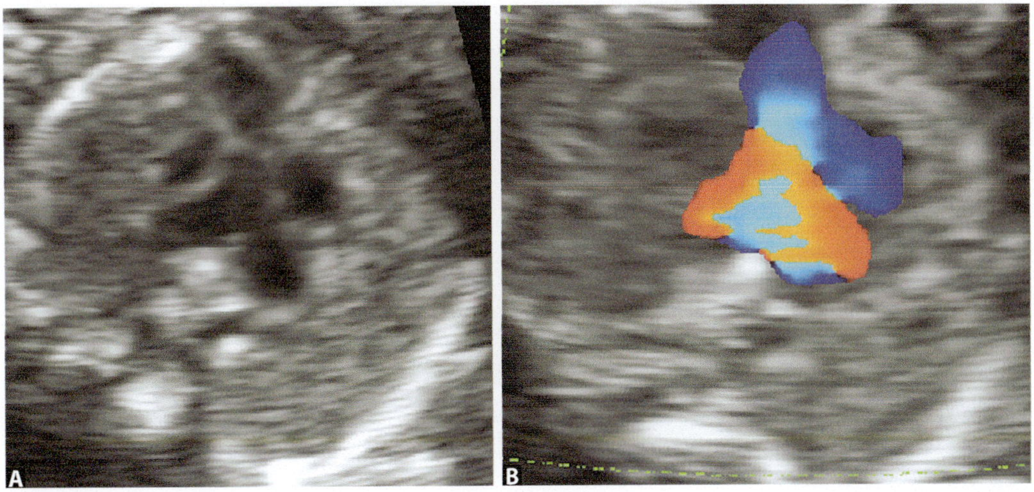

Figure 35: Absent pulmonary valve syndrome: (A) Short axis right ventricular outflow tract with relatively narrow pulmonary annulus and dilated branch pulmonary arteries; (B) Color Doppler fill of the dilated branch pulmonary arteries. The ductus arteriosus is absent

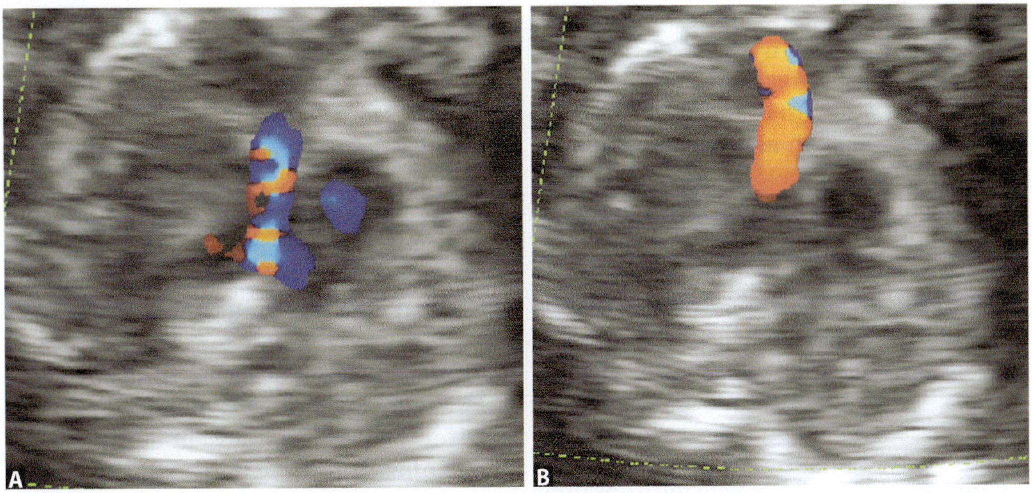

Figure 36: Absent pulmonary valve syndrome: (A) Forward flow in pulmonary artery in systole with Doppler aliasing indicating stenosis at the valve; (B) Reverse flow in diastole indicating pulmonary regurgitation. The ductus arteriosus is absent

iii. The branch pulmonary arteries are markedly dilated—*Absent pulmonary valve syndrome*: The pulmonary valve cusps are rudimentary or absent. Consequently, there is a free unhindered to and fro movement of blood across the pulmonary annulus **(Figure 36)**. The main, right and left pulmonary arteries are severely dilated **(Figure 35)**. The ductus arteriosus may be absent **(Figure 35)**. The pulmonary annulus itself may be narrow **(Figure 35)**. The aorta root is over-riding a malalignment VSD. The dilated pulmonary arteries may cause airway compression. This condition is a subtype of Tetralogy of Fallot. The four chamber view shows a right ventricular dominance due to the

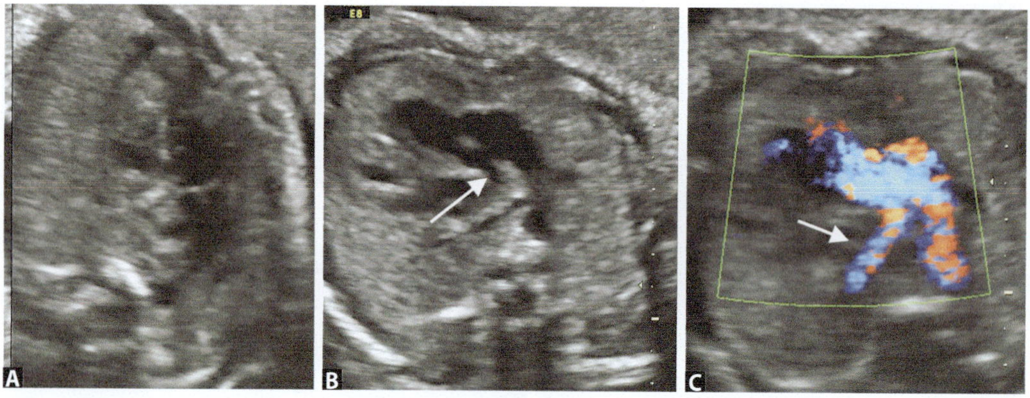

Figure 37: Common arterial trunk: (A) Large single outflow tract overriding the malalignment VSD, truncal valve closed; (B) pulmonary artery arising from trunk just distal to the truncal valve closed (arrow); (C) Pulmonary artery arising from the trunk (arrow) on Color Doppler

pulmonary regurgitation. The three vessel and short axis view shows dramatically dilated (three to four fold) aneurysmal branch pulmonary arteries. Right aortic arch and thymic hypoplasia should be sought for. Spectral Doppler peak systolic velocity across the pulmonary annulus could be as high as 200 to 250 cm/sec. Karyotyping and FISH for 22q11 deletion must be offered.

iv. The pulmonary artery and the aorta arise from a common trunk—*Common arterial trunk*: The common arterial trunk overrides a malalignment VSD and hence the trunk is committed to both ventricles. Occasionally, the common trunk arises solely from the right ventricle. Depending on the anatomic origin of the pulmonary artery/ies from the trunk three types are described. Type I is when there is a pulmonary trunk arising from the common arterial trunk. The pulmonary trunk bifurcates into the right and left pulmonary arteries. In types II and III, the right and left pulmonary arteries arise independently from the common trunk either close to each other (type II) or at a distance from each other (type III). The previously categorized type IV (pulmonary artery arising from the isthmial segment of the common truncal arch) is now considered as pulmonary atresia with VSD. The four chamber view appears normal. On moving to the five chamber and left ventricular outflow tract views the malalignment VSD and an overriding large artery are detected **(Figure 37A)**. Demonstration of the pulmonary artery/ies arising from the large outflow tract just beyond the annulus confirms it to be the common arterial trunk (rules out pulmonary atresia with VSD)**(Figure 37B)**. The truncal valves are often thickened and may be tricuspid or tetracuspid.[17] Only two vessels are seen in the three vessel view. Right aortic arch and thymic hypoplasia should be sought for. The ductus is absent in most cases. Color Doppler confirms the common trunk committed to both ventricles and may help in tracing the pulmonary arteries **(Figure 37C)**.

Truncal regurgitation if present may be detected. Non-specific extracardiac anomalies should be ruled out and a karyotype and FISH for 22q11 del must be planned.

Parallel Great Arteries

The great arteries run parallel to each other. This can happen in two groups of

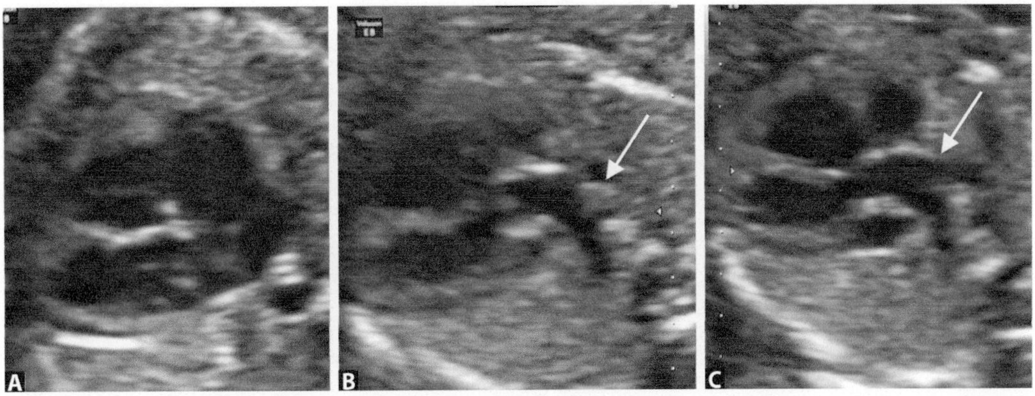

Figure 38: Complete transposition of great arteries: (A) Normal four chamber view; (B) Left ventricular outflow tract showing the artery to abruptly turn and point to the spine (arrow); (C) Left ventricular outflow tract is bifurcating in the axial plane (arrow) indicating that it is the pulmonary artery

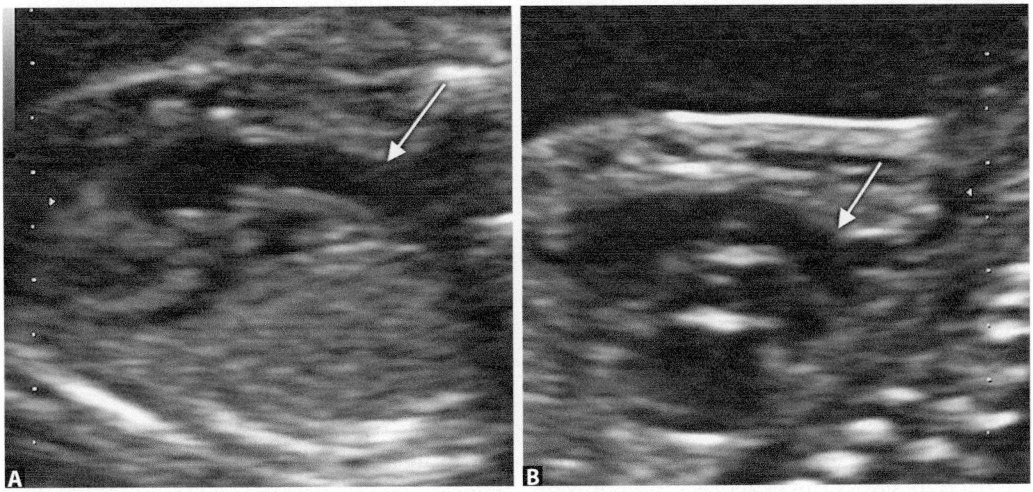

Figure 39: Complete transposition of great arteries: (A) The arching outflow tract (aorta) arising from the substernal right ventricle (arrow); (B) Parallel course of the great arteries on the oblique view

conditions i. Ventriculoarterial discordance—Transposition of great arteries (complete or congenitally corrected) and ii. Both arteries majorly arise from the right ventricle—Double outlet right ventricle.

Complete Transposition of Great Arteries

Venoatrial and atrioventricular connections are normal. The ventriculoarterial connections are discordant, i.e. the aorta and pulmonary artery arise from the right and left ventricles respectively. The great arteries course parallel to each other the aorta being anterior and to the right of the pulmonary artery. VSD and pulmonary stenosis are the associated cardiac anomalies. The four chamber view is typically normal **(Figure 38A)**. The pulmonary artery is seen to arise from the left ventricle in the five chamber and left ventricular outflow tract views. It bifurcates shortly after its origin **(Figures 38B and C)**. The aorta arises from the right ventricle and courses anterior and parallel to the pulmonary artery (seen in an oblique plane)**(Figure 39)**. The three vessel

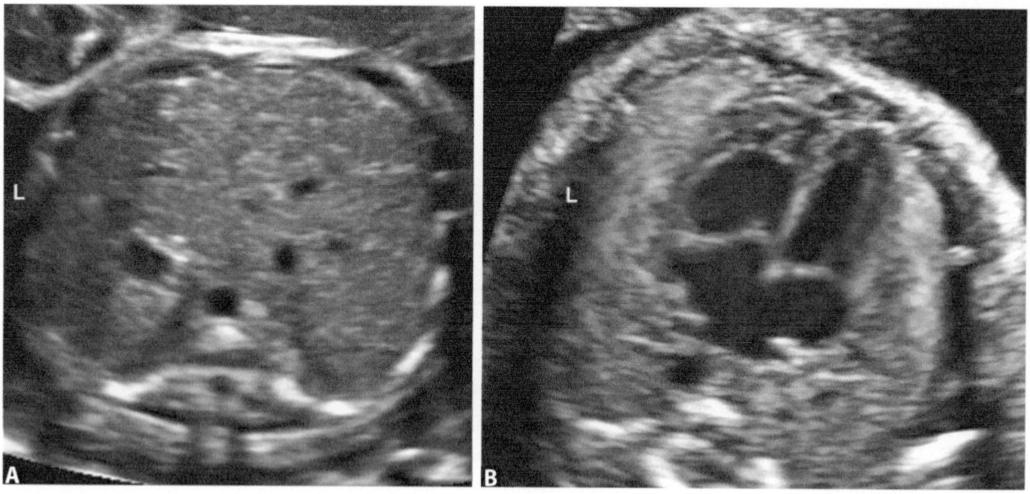

Figure 40: Congenitally corrected transposition of great arteries: (A) Upper abdominal plane with stomach to the left side; (B) Mesocardia with apex substernal, the left sided atrium is the left atrium marked by the pulmonary venous connection, the left sided ventricle is the morphological right ventricle marked by the apical insertion of the tricuspid valve and the moderator band, this clearly demonstrates atrioventricular discordance

trachea view shows a single large artery i.e. the aorta with the superior vena cava. The pulmonary artery is not seen in this plane as it is inferior to the aorta. The aortic arch is broad and its origin is anteriorly placed. Color Doppler displays the parallel relation of the great arteries. It also helps to assess ventricular defect[18] and pulmonary stenosis. The 4D (STIC) coronal view of the atrioventricular and semilunar orifices may be used to assess the exact relation between the origins of the great arteries. A side-to-side relation has a high association with coronary artery abnormalities. Associated extracardiac anomalies are rare. Karyotyping is not indicated. FISH for 22q11 del may be offered.

Congenitally Corrected Transposition of Great Arteries

Venoatrial connections are normal. The atrioventricular and ventriculoarterial connections are discordant. This results in the systemic venous blood reaching the pulmonary circulation and the pulmonary venous blood reaching the systemic circulation. Dextrocardia or mesocardia are a common association **(Figure 40B)**.[19] The morphologic left atrium (pulmonary venous drainage) connects with the morphologic right ventricle (moderator band, apically attached atrioventricular valve, and septal chorda tendinae). The morphologic right atrium (systemic venous drainage) connects with the morphologic left ventricle (apex forming, absent moderator band and absent septal chorda tendinae)**(Figure 40B)**. The morphological left ventricle supports an axially branching pulmonary artery **(Figure 41A)**. The arching aorta arises from the morphological right ventricle **(Figure 41B)**. The great arteries are parallel to each other with the aorta anterior and to the left of the pulmonary artery **(Figure 42)**. On the five chamber view the first outflow tract to be seen is from the morphological left ventricle (right sided) pointing to the left of the spine. This artery branches and is hence the pulmonary artery. The aorta arises from the morphological right ventricle (left sided) and courses parallel and to the left of the pulmonary artery.

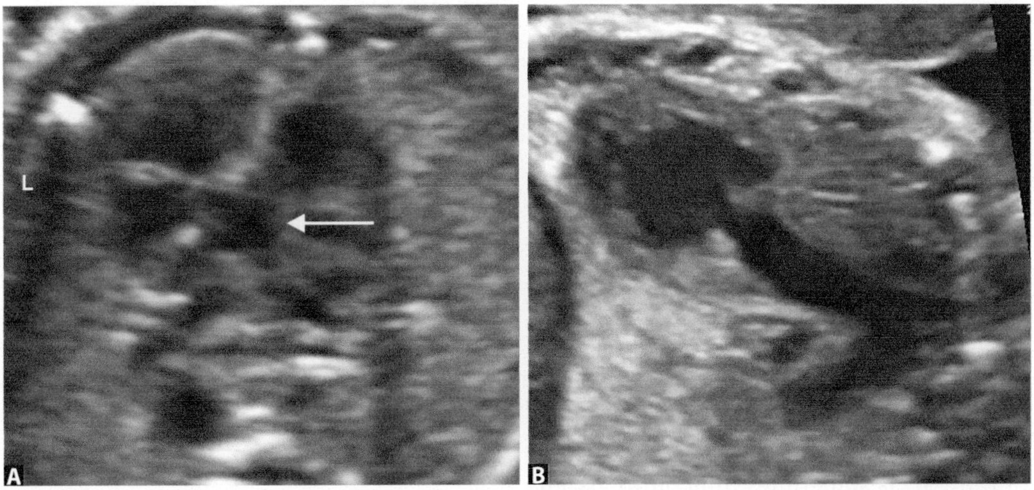

Figure 41: Congenitally corrected transposition of great arteries: (A) Cephalad angulation from four chamber view shows the dividing pulmonary artery (arrow) to arise from the right sided morphological left ventricle; (B) The morphological right ventricle is seen to support the aorta, indicating ventriculoarterial discordance

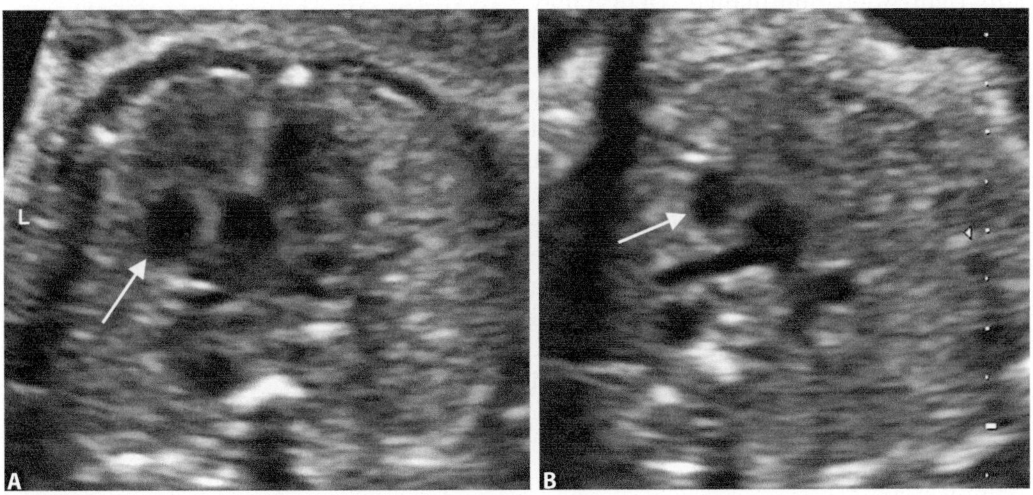

Figure 42: Congenitally corrected transposition of great arteries: (A) The short axis of both great arteries seen side to side with the aorta (arrow) being to the left of the pulmonary artery; (B) The aorta (arrow) seen to the left of the pulmonary artery (dividing) in the three vessel view

Sequential segmental approach thus helps in reaching the correct diagnosis. Color Doppler aids in the diagnosis of ventricular septal defect, tricuspid regurgitation and pulmonary stenosis which may coexist. It is also useful in demonstrating the parallel course of the great arteries. Extracardiac abnormalities are rare. Karyotype is normal as a rule. FISH for 22q11 del is recommended particularly if there are associated anomalies.

Double Outlet Right Ventricle (DORV)

This term encompasses a group of anomalies where both the aorta and the pulmonary artery arise wholly or predominantly from the morphological right ventricle. A ventricular septal defect is almost always present. There may be associated aortic or pulmonary stenosis. The great arterial origins may bear any of the following relationships:

a. Aortic valve to the right of the pulmonary valve (side-to-side type)
b. Aortic valve is anterior and to the right of the pulmonary valve (D-transposition type)
c. Aortic valve is posterior and to the right of the pulmonary valve (Tetralogy of Fallot type), and
d. Aortic valve is anterior and to the left of the pulmonary valve (L-transposition type).[20]

The VSD may be subaortic, subpulmonary, remote or doubly committed. Exact position of the VSD is sometimes difficult to assign. The four chamber view of the heart may be unremarkable. There may be ventricular disproportion due to left-sided smallness and right-sided dominance. DORV may be associated with atrioventricular septal defect, mitral atresia or double inlet ventricle. In these instances, the four chamber view will obviously be abnormal. Aorto-septal discontinuity is seen on the five chamber view/left ventricular outflow view. Both the great arteries arising from the right ventricle (substernal chamber) is also seen in the same views. Parallelism of the great arteries can be demonstrated by angling the probe cephalad towards the three vessel view **(Figure 43)**. The arterial calibers should be recorded to detect stenosis. A right sided aortic arch which may be associated with DORV can be picked up on the three vessel trachea view. Due to the malposition of the arteries, only one artery (commonly the aortic arch) may be seen on the three vessel trachea view (with the pulmonary artery coursing at an inferior plane). Color Doppler helps in demonstrating:

i. Left to right flow across the VSD
ii. Blood flow into both great arteries from the right ventricle
iii. Presence of great arterial stenosis (turbulence).
iv. Reversed flow in either great artery in the case of atresia.

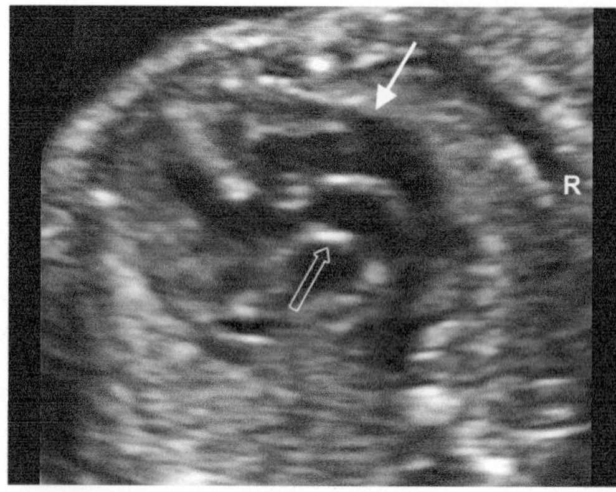

Figure 43: Double outlet right ventricle—Both great arteries are arising from the right ventricle and are parallel to each other (malposed) the aortic origin (arrow) being to the right and anterior to the pulmonary artery origin (open arrow) (D TGA type), the VSD is subpulmonic

IN THE PLANE OF THE THREE VESSEL VIEW OR THREE VESSEL TRACHEA VIEW ONE MAY ENCOUNTER ANY ONE OF THE FOLLOWING FINDINGS:

a. Size abnormality of any of the vessels
b. Abnormal flow direction in any of the vessels
c. Abnormal spatial arrangement of the vessels
d. Abnormality in the number of the vessels
e. Miscellaneous abnormalities.

Size Abnormality of Any of the Vessels

Normally the aorta is slightly smaller in caliber compared to the pulmonary artery. The aorta is significantly small in caliber in aortic coarctation **(Figure 44)** and hypoplastic left heart syndrome. The pulmonary artery is small in caliber in tricuspid atresia, pulmonary atresia with intact ventricular septum, tetralogy of Fallot and pulmonary atresia with ventricular septal defect. These entities have already been dealt with.

Abnormal Flow Direction in Any of the Vessels

The aorta and the pulmonary artery display the same flow direction on color Doppler

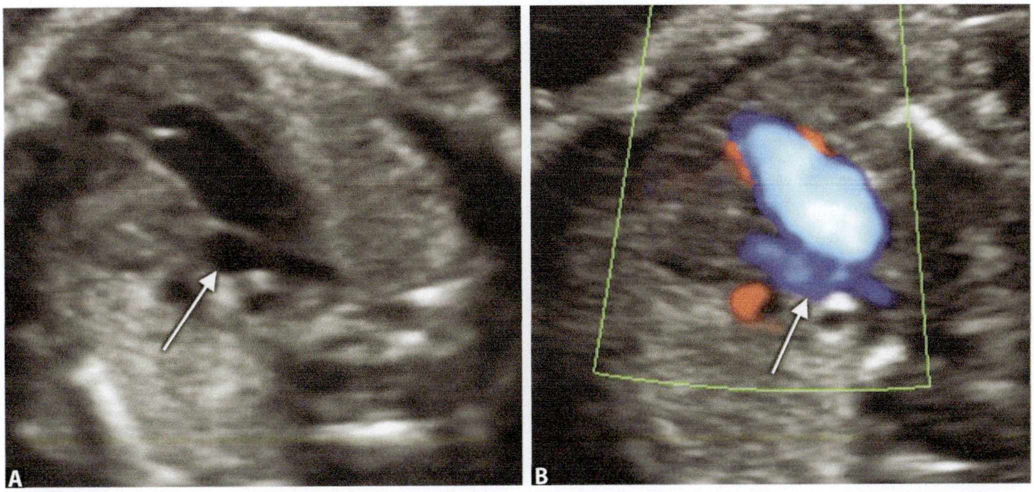

Figure 44: Coarctation of aorta: (A) The aorta (arrow) is much smaller compared to the pulmonary artery; (B) Forward flow noted in the aorta in the three vessel trachea view

examination in the three vessel trachea view (normal). In hypoplastic left heart syndrome the aorta is small in caliber and displays retrograde (ductus dependent) flow direction **(see Figure 15)**. In pulmonary atresia, the pulmonary artery is small in caliber and displays retrograde (ductus dependent) flow direction **(see Figure 34B)**. In absent pulmonary valve syndrome there is to and fro movement of blood in systole and diastole respectively indicating free pulmonary regurgitation.

Abnormal Spatial Arrangement of the Vessels

Spatial Arrangement Abnormality Amongst the Vessels

Typically seen in tetralogy of Fallot or in double outlet right ventricle (tetralogy of Fallot type) where the aorta is anteriorly placed in relation to the superior vena cava and pulmonary artery **(Figure 45)**.

Spatial Arrangement Abnormality in Relation to the Trachea

The 'V' configuration of the great arteries in the three vessel trachea view has its apex to the left of the trachea and points to the left of the spine indicating a normal left sided aortic and ductus arch. In right aortic arch with right ductus arch the apex of the 'V' is to the right of the trachea and points to right of the spine **(Figure 46A)**. In right aortic arch with left ductus arch the great arteries are in a 'U' configuration forming a loose sling around the trachea and the esophagus **(Figure 46B)**. In double aortic arch, a tight vascular ring is formed around the trachea and oesophagus with the left aortic arch passing anteriorly and right aortic arch passing posteriorly to converge posterior to trachea and esophagus. Situs abnormalities (including heterotaxy) and 22q11 del are associated with aortic arch anomalies. Left aortic arch with aberrant right subclavian artery (ARSA) is a common variant where the right subclavian artery is the last artery to arise from the aortic arch (normally the right subclavian artery is a branch of the brachiocephalic trunk which is the first branch of the aortic arch). It then courses posterior to the trachea and esophagus from the apex of the 'V' in the three vessel trachea towards the right shoulder **(Figure 47)**. ARSA is best sought for in the three vessel trachea view with a lower PRF and higher gain setting. Presence of ARSA with other markers of

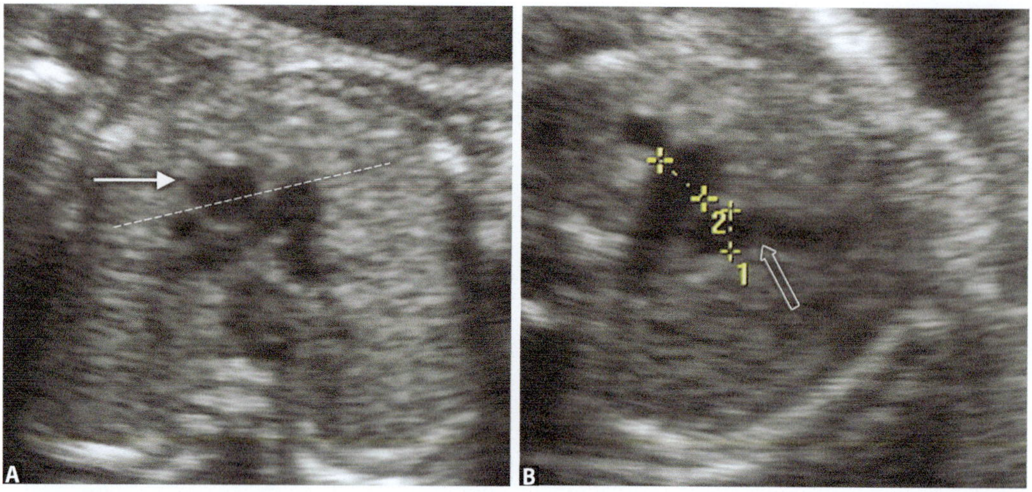

Figure 45: Tetralogy of Fallot: (A) The aorta (solid arrow) is anteriorly placed in relation to the pulmonary and superior vena cava in the three vessel view; (B) The pulmonary artery (open arrow) is smaller in caliber

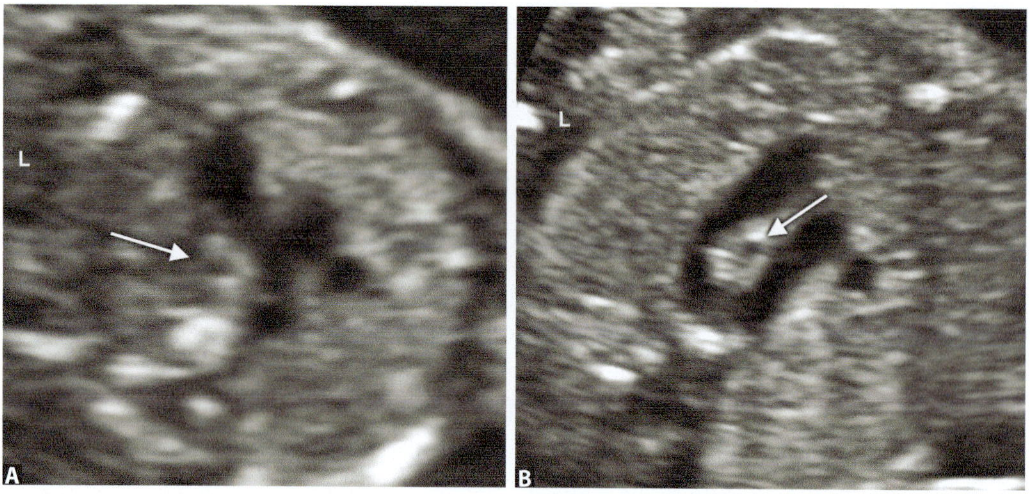

Figure 46: (A) Right aortic arch with right ductus arch—V to the right sign (arrow indicates the trachea) (B) Right aortic arch with left ductus arch—U sign forming a sling around the trachea (arrow) and esophagus

aneuploidy necessitates fetal karyotyping. ARSA with a conotruncal anomaly increases the risk for 22q11 del.

Spatial Arrangement Abnormality in Relation to the Sternum

When the thymus is hypoplastic or absent the vessels in the three vessel trachea view are too close to the sternum **(Figure 48)**. This should prompt the presence of possible 22q11 del.

Abnormality in the Number of Vessels

There may be only two vessels seen in the three vessel trachea view. This happens in common arterial trunk where there is only one great arterial trunk arising from the ventricles **(Figure 49A)**. In complete transposition of great arteries, the pulmonary artery and the ductus arch are inferior to the aortic arch and hence in the three vessel trachea view only the aorta is seen. The aorta and pulmonary

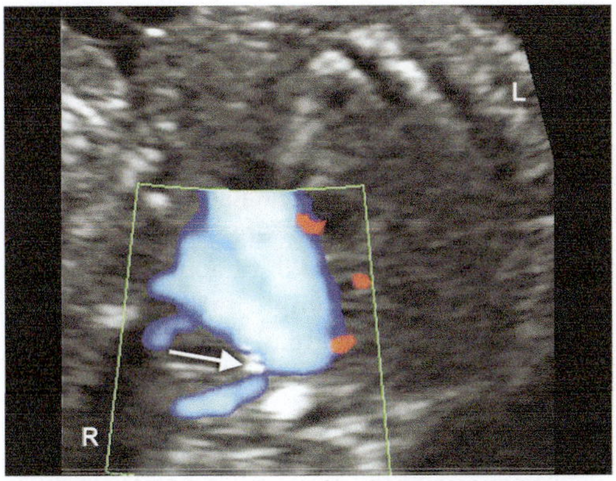

Figure 47: Left aortic arch with aberrant right subclavian artery. Three vessel trachea view with ARSA seen arising from the apex of the 'V' and coursing to the right side. The trachea is marked by arrow

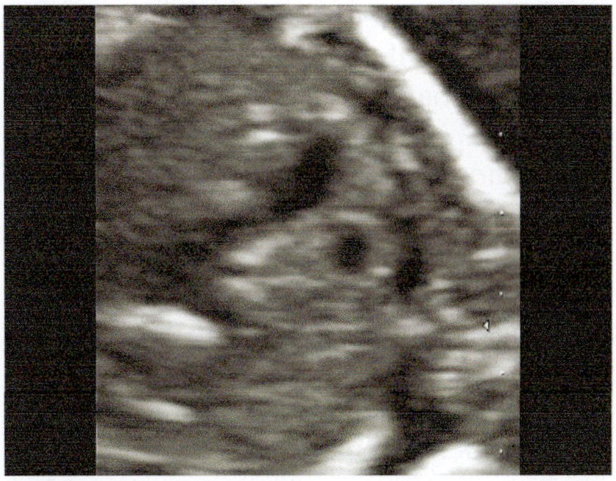

Figure 48: The great vessels in the three vessel view are placed too close to the anterior chest wall in this case of double outlet right ventricle. The thymus is either absent or grossly hypoplastic

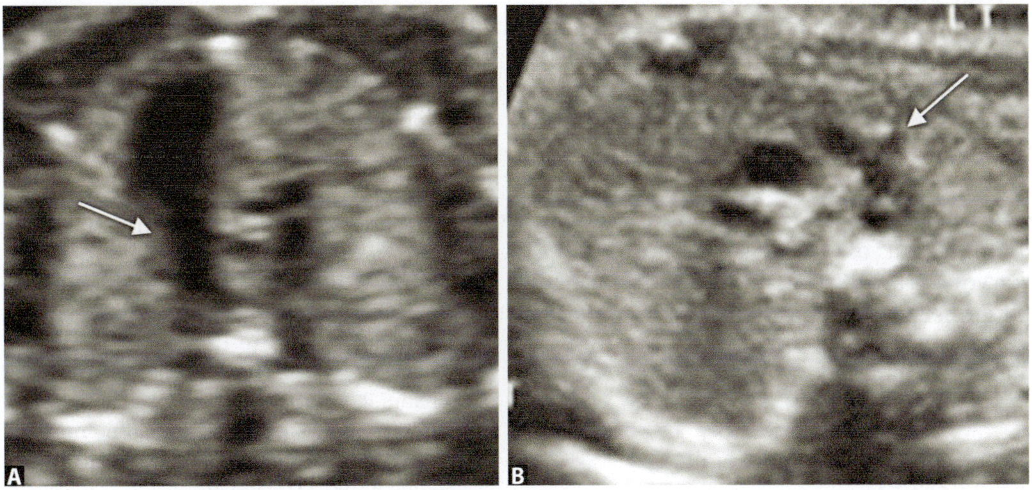

Figure 49: (A) Single artery (aorta–arrow) seen in the three vessel view in a case of common arterial trunk; (B) Persistent left superior vena cava (arrow) in the three vessel view is the fourth vessel

artery in hypoplastic left heart syndrome and pulmonary atresia with intact ventricular septum respectively may be so small in caliber that they may not be identified by gray scale ultrasound thus causing only two vessels to be seen in the three vessel trachea view. Color Doppler helps in identifying the vessel.

There may be four vessels seen in the three vessel trachea view. This happens in persistent left superior vena cava (SVC).

Persistent Left SVC

This is the most common venous variant in the thorax. Coexisting cardiac malformation (heterotaxy, conotruncal abnormalities and left ventricular outflow tract obstruction) is seen in about 5% of cases. The right superior vena cava may or may not be present. The left superior vena cava is identified as an extra vessel to the left of the pulmonary artery in the three vessel view **(Figure 49B)**. It may also be identified in the left atrioventricular groove in the four chamber view. The coronary sinus (into which it drains) is prominent (3 to 7 mm)[21] and can be recognized when the probe is angled caudally from the four chamber view. Differential diagnosis is the vertical vein in supracardiac total anomalous venous drainage. Color Doppler will demonstrate caudocranial flow direction in a vertical vein (in contrast to craniocaudal flow direction in the left superior vena cava).

Miscellaneous Abnormalities

Tracheal dilatation may be recognized in the three vessel view in congenital high airway obstruction sequence (CHAOS). An esophageal duplication cyst or a neurenteric cyst may be picked up in the three vessel view.

Thus we see that a systematic examination using the standard planes of section is necessary for the recognition of findings. Integrating these findings together yields the final diagnosis. Complementation by recognition of extracardiac anomalies, karyotype and FISH results in a total fetal diagnosis. The pediatric cardiologist is thus equipped with the whole information which is vital for counseling and for further management.

REFERENCES

1. Hoffman J, Kaplan S. The incidence of congenital heart disease. J Am Coll Cardiol. 2002;39(12):1890-900.
2. De Vore GR, et al. Prenatal diagnosis of cardiovascular malformations in the fetus with situs inversus viscerum during the second trimester of pregnancy. J Clin Ultrasound. 1986;14:454-7.
3. Vijaykumar V, Brandt T. Prolonged survival with isolated levocardia and situs inversus. Cleve clin J Med. 1991;58(3):243-7.
4. Gindes L et al. Isolated levocardia - Prenatal diagnosis, clinical importance, and literature review. J Ultrasound Med. 2007;26:361-5.
5. Smith RS et al. Ultrasonographic left cardiac axis deviation - a marker of fetal anomalies. Obstet Gynecol. 1995;85(2):187-91.
6. Lincoln C, Jamieson S, Shinebourne E, et al. Transatrial repair of ventricular septal defects with reference to their anatomic classification. J Thoracic Cardiovasc Surg. 1977;74:183-90.
7. Machlitt A, Heling KS, Chaoui R. Increased atrioventricular length ratio in fetal four chamber view:a new marker for atrioventricular septal defect. Ultrasound Obstet Gynecol. 2004;24(6):618-22.
8. Van Praagh R, Van Praagh S, Vlad P, et al. Diagnosis of the anatomic types of single or common ventricle. Am J Cardiol. 1965;15:345-66.
9. Hornberger LS, Sanders SP, Rein AJ, et al, Left heart obstructive lesions and left ventricular growth in the mid trimester fetus. A Longitudinal study. Circulation 1995;92(6):1533-8.
10. Wong SF, Ward C, Lee-Tannock A, Le S, Chan FY. Pulmonary artery/aorta ratio in simple screening for fetal outflow tract abnormalities during the second trimester. Ultrasound Obstet Gynecol. 2007;30: 275-80.
11. Tandon R, Edwards JE. Tricuspid atresia: a re-evaluation and classification. J Thorac Cardiavasc Surg. 1974;67:530-42.
12. Todros T, Paladini D, Chiappa E, et al. Pulmonary stenosis and atresia with intact ventricular septum during prenatal life. Ultrasound Obstet Gynecol. 2003;21(3):228-33.
13. Chaoui R, Bollmann R, Goldner B, et al. Fetal cardiomegaly - echocardiographic findings and outcome in 19 cases. Ultrasound Obstet Gynecol. 2003;21(1):81-93.
14. Berg C, Georgiadis M, Geipel A, Gembruch U. The area behind the heart in the four-chamber view and the quest for congenital heart defects. Ultrasound Obstet Gynecol. 2007; 30:721-7.
15. Kawazu Y, Inamura N, Shiono N, Kanagawa N, Narita J, Hamamichi Y, et al. 'Post-LA space index' as a potential novel marker for the prenatal diagnosis of isolated total anomalous pulmonary venous connection. Ultrasound Obstet Gynecol. 2014;44:682-7.
16. Chaoui R, Heling KS, Sarut Lopez A, Thiel G, Karl K. The thymic-thoracic ratio in fetal heart defects: a simple way to identify fetuses at high risk for microdeletion 22q11. Ultrasound Obstet Gynecol. 2011;37:397-403.

17. Fuglestad S, Puga G, Danielson G. Surgical pathology of the truncal valve: A study of twelve cases. Am J Cardiovasc Pathol. 1988;2:39-47.
18. Kirklin JW, Barratt-Boyes BG. Complete transposition of great arteries. In: Kirklin JW, Barrat-Boyes BG (Eds). Cardiac surgery. New York: Churchill Livingstone. 1993:2; 1383-467.
19. Losekoot TG, Becker AE. Discordant atrioventricular connection and congenitally corrected transposition. In: Anderson RH, Macartney FJ, Shinebourne EA, et al. (Eds.). Pediatric Cardiology. Edinburgh: Churchill Livingstone. 1987:94;867-88.
20. Sridaromont S, Feldt RH, Ritter DG, et al. Double-outlet right ventricle: Hemodynamic and anatomic correlations. Am J Cardiol. 1976:38; 85.
21. Chaoui R, Heling KS, Kalache KD. Caliber of the coronary sinus in fetuses with cardiac defects with and without left persistent superior vena cava and in growth restricted fetuses with heart sparing effect. Prenat Diagn. 2003;23: 552-7.

8
CHAPTER
Gastrointestinal Tract Abnormalities and Anterior Abdominal Wall Defects

Sonal Panchal, Chaitanya Nagori

INTRODUCTION

Gastrointestinal tract assessment during the intrauterine life may be considered to be difficult and challenging as compared to most other systems of the fetal body. This is because of the ongoing development causing changes in the appearances as the gestation advances and also because of the fetal swallowing of amniotic fluid, bowel peristalsis and evacuation of the fluid through the anus. It is therefore essential that in the fetuses at high risk of gastrointestinal tract abnormalities, or having any other associated abnormalities, repeated scans till third trimester must be pursued. More over it is also essential to be aware of the changing appearances due to physiological changes.

THE NORMAL APPEARANCES

The gastrointestinal tract abnormalities when mentioned, it includes the assessment of the entire tract starting from the lips, palate and tongue to the anus and hepatobiliary tract. Though abnormalities of lips, palate and tongue are discussed with the facial abnormalities and we shall not discuss in this chapter. Taking a swift look at the normal appearances of all other structures and the variations in their appearances in normal physiological states, is therefore required before the discussion on abnormalities and their ultrasound diagnosis.

Hypopharynx

It is seen as a round, hypo to anechoic area posterior to the palate and the tongue on axial section. It shows opening and closing with the fetal swallowing starting from about 16–18 weeks onwards, till term. On sagittal section it is seen as an anechoic area, usually trianglish in shape posterior to the base of the tongue **(Figure 1)**.

Esophagus is best evaluated on the midsagittal section of the neck and the thorax as a pair of parallel hyperechoic lines running from the hypopharynx to the stomach. It may show peristalsis with fetal swallowing. It is at this time that it may show a transient fluid passage in between two lines **(Figure 2)**.

Diaphragm

It is seen as anechoic curved line with convexity cranially separating a slightly hyperechoic lung from the liver in parasagittal sections of the trunk **(Figure 3)**.

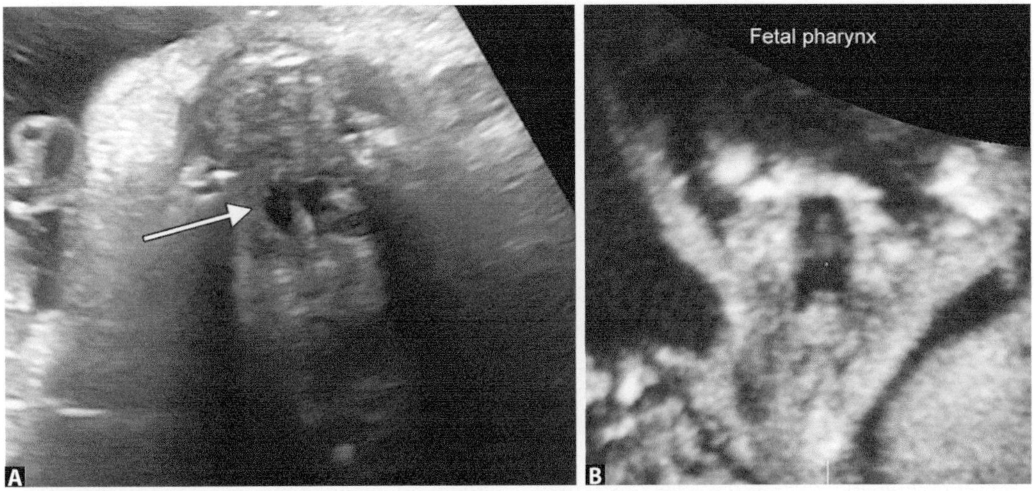

Figure 1: B-mode ultrasound image of hypopharynx on axial section and coronal section respectively

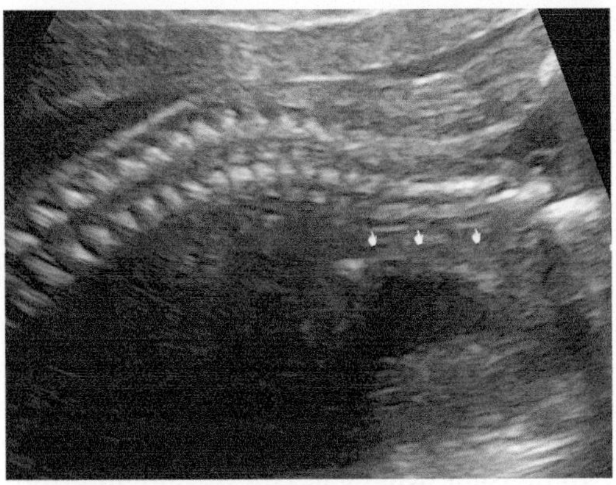

Figure 2: B-mode ultrasound image of esophagus on midsagittal section of the fetus

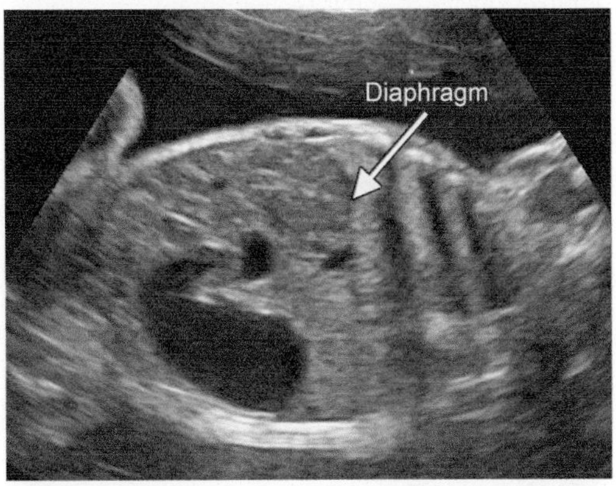

Figure 3: Diaphragm seen on parasagittal section of fetus on B-mode ultrasound image

Stomach

It can be seen as anechoic round or oval structure at all ages of gestation after 12 weeks of pregnancy on left parasagittal section of the trunk. Stomach can also be seen on the axial section of the upper abdomen, in the left hemi-abdomen posteriorly. Stomach does fill up when fetus swallows the amniotic fluid and empties at a periodic cycle of 30–90 minutes **(Figure 4)**. Therefore when not seen on one examination, a repeat scan after 30–45 minutes must be done.

Liver

It is seen as a triangular hypoechoic structure on the right parasagittal section of the trunk, just under the diaphragm. On the axial section, same as that for the stomach, the entire right side of this section is filled with liver appearing as a hypoechoic structure **(Figure 4)**.

Gallbladder

On the axial section of the upper abdomen, same as the level of stomach, a pear-shaped anechoic structure is seen anteriorly and on

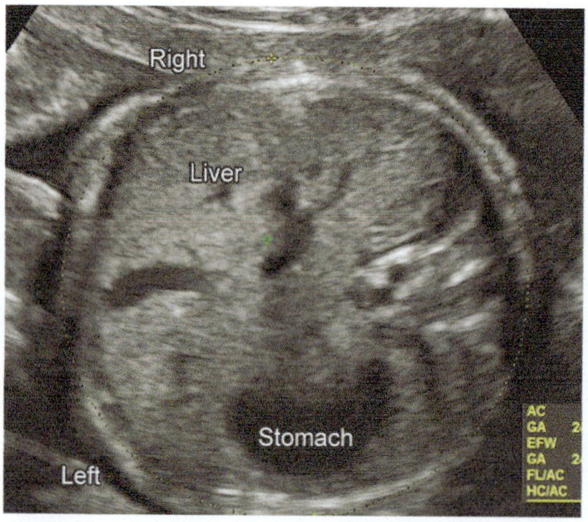

Figure 4: B-mode ultrasound image of transverse section of fetal abdomen at the level of stomach showing stomach on left side and liver filling up approximately half of this section area

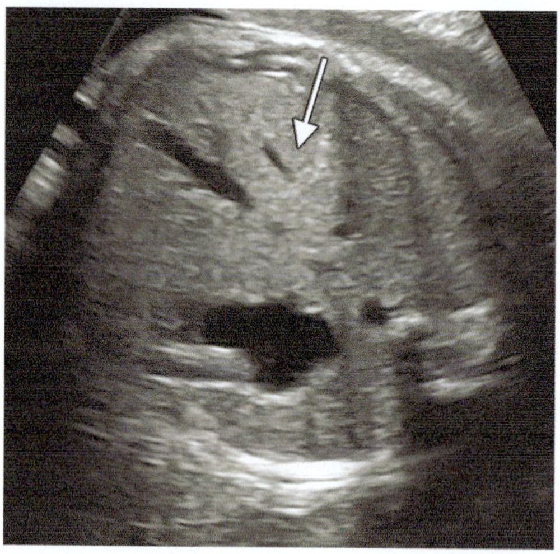

Figure 5: Gallbladder is seen on the right side anteriorly, on B-mode ultrasound image of the transverse section of abdomen

the right side of the abdomen, at about 7–7.15 o'clock position, if spine is considered at 12 o'clock **(Figure 5)**.

Small Bowel

On sagittal or parasagittal sections of the abdomen, hyperehoic area is seen inferior to the liver. On zoomed images this hyperechoic

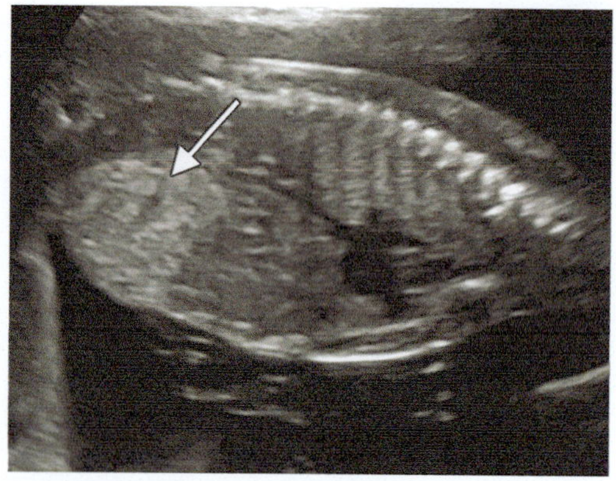

Figure 6: Sagittal section of the fetus trunk on B-mode ultrasound image shows mildly hyperechoic small bowel

area is formed of multiple small bowel loops, each of which appears as a hyperechoic double line formed by bowel walls and central anechoic line which represents the lumen **(Figure 6)**.

Colon

It is usually seen as an irregular tubular structure with thin echogenic walls, the lumen of which is filled with hypoechoic content. It can be seen usually in late second and third trimester and can be traced along its normal anatomical position as ascending, transverse and descending colon. Though it is true that it is usually not seen entirely on all scans. Its maximum diameter is 10 mm in the third trimester **(Figure 7)**.

Rectum

On the midsagittal section of the lower abdomen as well as on the transverse section of the lower abdomen, rectum is seen behind the bladder respectively as anechoic oval/tubular and a rounded structure **(Figure 8A)** Anal sphincter is seen as a target sign on the perineum **(Figure 8B)**.

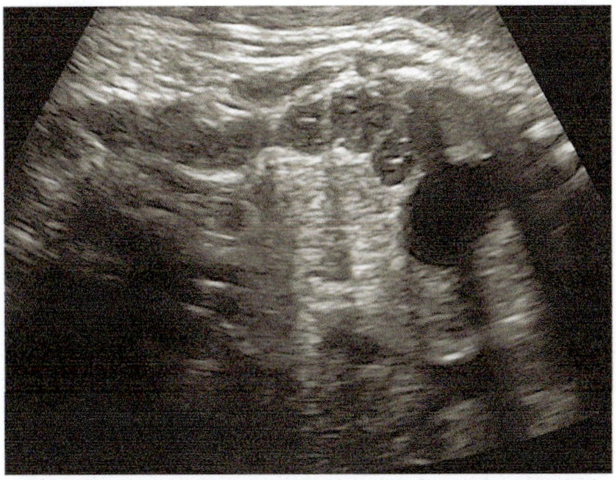

Figure 7: Coronal section of fetal abdomen showing tubular large bowel on B-mode ultrasound image

Abdominal Wall and Insertion of Umbilical Cord

The assessment of the anterior abdominal wall is done by a sweep of the probe from upper to lower abdomen with the abdomen seen on image in a transverse section and another sweep from one to another side of the fetus with fetus seen in sagittal plane **(Figure 9)**.

Gastrointestinal tract anomalies can be divided into four groups:

1. Bowel abnormalities
2. Non-bowel anomalies.
3. Anterior abdominal wall defects
4. Diaphragmatic defects

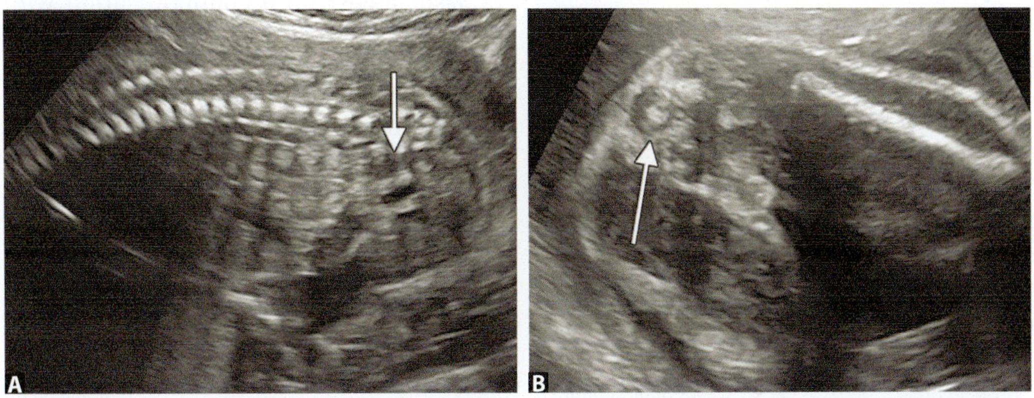

Figure 8: (A) Rectum is seen as hypoechoic to anechoic tubular area in front of the sacrum on sagittal section image of B-mode ultrasound; (B) Anal sphincter demonstrated on the B-mode image of the perineum

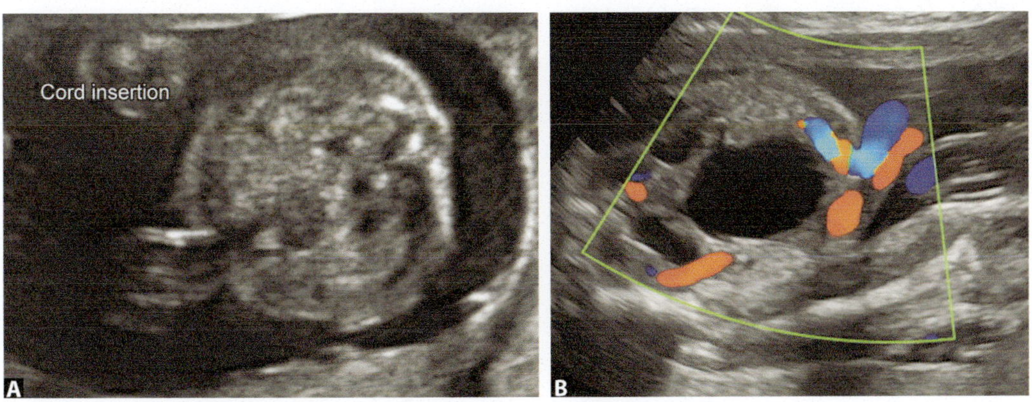

Figure 9: B-mode ultrasound images of cord insertion in fetal abdomen

BOWEL ABNORMALITIES

Esophageal Atresia

Interruption of blood supply to the esophagus during its development leads to non-communication between the proximal and distal part of the esophagus. Its incidence is highly variable in different studies and has been described to be between 1 in 2,500–4,000 live births.

It develops as early as 8 weeks of gestation. It is at this stage of embryonic development that the primitive foregut may not divide into ventral tracheobronchial part and dorsal digestive part and this may lead to tracheo-esophageal fistula. Tracheoesophageal fistula is associated in 86–90% of cases of esophageal atresia.

Esophageal atresias have been divided into five types, and this is known as Gross classification **(Figure 10)**.[1]

- Type A: No fistula (8%)
- Type B: Fistula with the proximal stump (1%, and these are most commonly associated with Down's syndrome)
- Type C: Fistula with the distal stump (88%)
- Type D: Double fistula with both stumps (1%)
- Type E: Fistula without concomitant esophageal atresia (1%).

Diagnosis

Though a persistently absent stomach bubble is considered to be the surest sign for the diagnosis of esophageal atresia, it is not found in about 90% of cases.[2] This is so because, in about 90% of the cases, esophageal atresia is associated with a communication with the trachea (tracheoesophageal fistula). In cases of tracheoesophageal fistula, the communication of the trachea is with the distal stump of the esophagus. This allows some amniotic fluid to flow from the trachea

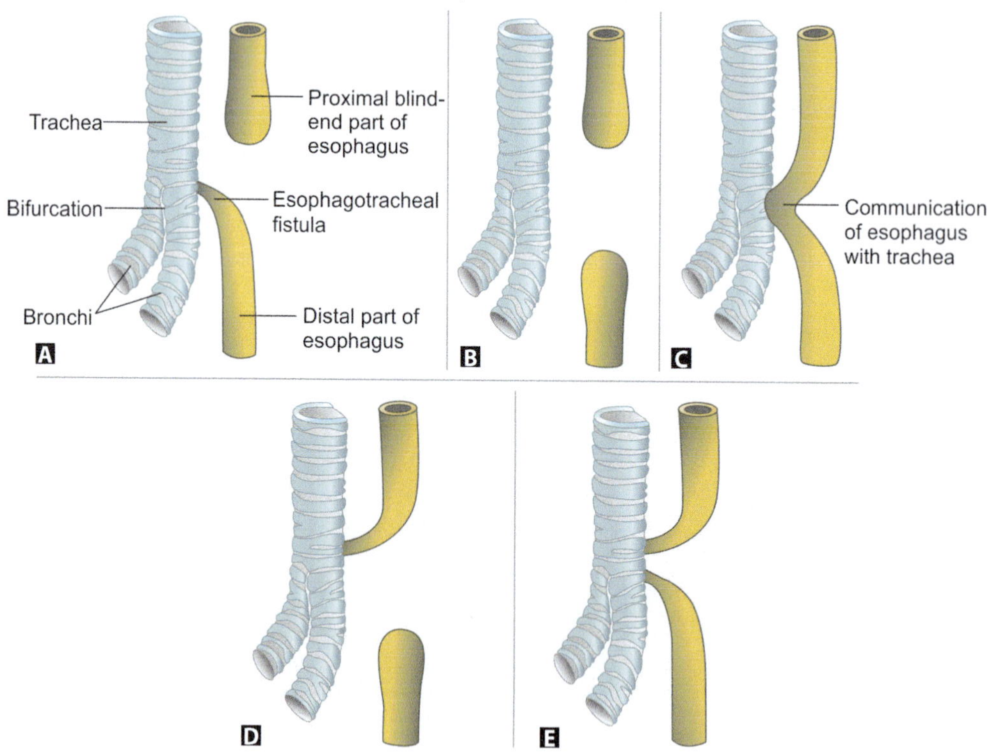

Figure 10: Diagrammatic representation of different types of tracheoesophageal fistulae

through the fistula to the stomach. This leads to filling and visualization of the stomach bubble and makes the diagnosis of tracheo-esophageal fistula extremely difficult in most cases. Though persistently small stomach, **(Figure 11)** polyhydramnios and esophageal pouch **(Figure 12)** if seen, may be the most reliable sign trio for the diagnosis of tracheo-esophageal fistula.[3] The esophageal pouch is a fluid filled proximal blind stump of the esophagus, between the trachea and the spine.

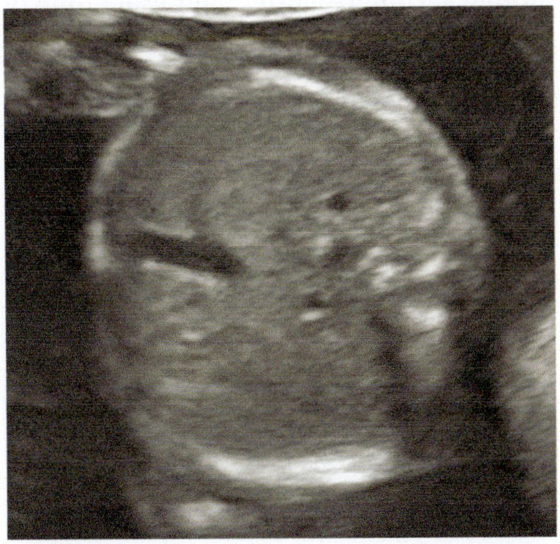

Figure 11: Absent or small stomach bubble on B-mode ultrasound image of transverse section of abdomen suggestive of tracheoesophageal fistula

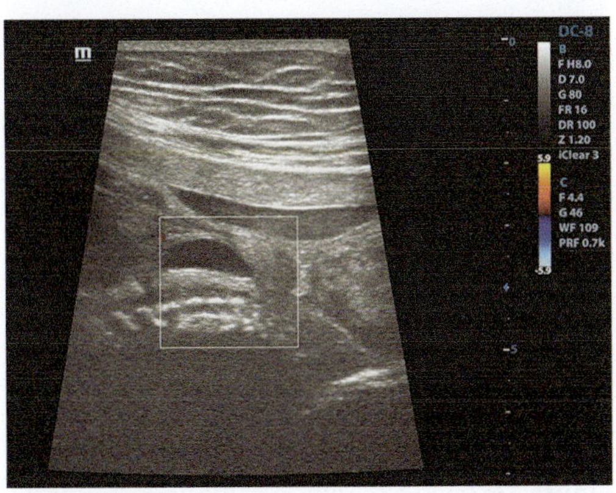

Figure 12: Blind esophageal pouch seen on sagittal section ultrasound image suggestive of tracheoesophageal fistula

Though at times this may be seen transiently when the fetus swallows amniotic fluid, but if it remains persistent it is a sign of blind esophageal pouch. Putting all these signs together, still the overall detection rate of esophageal atresia is only 24–42%.[4]

Differential Diagnosis

The most indicative sign of esophageal atresia is absent stomach, but is not a specific sign for the same. Absent stomach bubble is also seen in any condition that leads to severe oligohydramnios or anhydramnios. The causes of which may be premature rupture of membranes, severe pregnancy-induced hypertension and fetal growth retardation and bilateral renal agenesis. But if the amniotic fluid is normal in quantity and still the stomach bubble is not seen, a more detailed assessment of the fetus is required to rule out other abnormalities like congenital diaphragmatic hernia, displacing the stomach in the thorax or cleft lip and palate where swallowing may be a problem, congenital high airway obstruction (CHAOS) and fetal akinesia sequence. If everything else is normal of course, the possibility may not be structural, it may be impaired deglutition.

When fetal growth retardation is found, it is usually associated with oligohydramnios, but in esophageal atresia it is usually polyhydramnios. So a combination of polyhydramnios with fetal growth retardation is strongly indicative of esophageal atresia. In the fetuses with esophageal atresia, fetal growth retardation is due to reduced intestinal absorption of amniotic fluid proteins from the stomach and bowel which should be about 2 g per day at term.[5,6]

However, the prognosis is related to the associated abnormalities.

Associated Abnormalities

In 40–70% of cases, esophageal atresia is associated with other major abnormalities. It may be associated with other gastrointestinal abnormalities in abut 28% of cases, with cardiovascular defects in 24% of cases, with genitourinary abnormalities in 13% and musculoskeletal abnormalities in 11% of cases. VACTERL as it is known is the commonest association with multi-organ involvement which includes vertebral anomalies (scoliosis and hemivertebrae), anorectal atresia, cardiac defects (ventricular septal defect), tracheoesophageal fistula, renal anomalies (dysplasia, ectopia, etc) and limb abnormalities (radial aplasia). It may also be a part of CHARGE syndrome (coloboma of the eye, heart anomaly, choanal atresia, mental retardation, microphallus and ear abnormalities).

The risk of chromosomal abnormalities is 20–44%, with highest prevalence of trisomy 21 and trisomy 18 and it is the commonest with type A esophageal atresia.

Obstetric Management

Detailed scan to rule out other abnormalities and karyotyping to rule out chromosomal abnormalities is required.

Delivery in NICU set up, especially for the high risk of fetal growth retardation, prematurity, associated abnormalities and specialized feeding needs of the newborn.

Surgical correction is the final answer, but it depends on the presence or absence of fistula and the length of the blind gap as to what surgical procedure/procedures may be required. Though even after best surgical corrections, severe gastroesophageal reflux is a common complication. Prognosis of any corrective procedures is also dependent on associated abnormalities.

Duodenal Atresia or Stenosis

It is a non-canalized part of the bowel between proximal and distal part of duodenum. In about 80% of cases it is complete atresia, distal to the ampulla of Vater. But in 20% of cases presenting as duodenal atresia, it is a diaphragm or a membrane in the lumen of the duodenum, leading to complete or partial stenosis. Another possible etiology is focal ischemia with consequent segmental infarction. Its incidence is 1 in 2,500 to 1 in 10,000.

Ultrasound Diagnosis

Classical diagnosis of duodenal atresia is a double bubble sign, **(Figure 13)** wherein instead of a single stomach bubble, two anechoic shadows are seen on the axial section of the abdomen for abdominal circumference. This becomes evident around second trimester[7] and exact time of appearance depends on the severity of lesion. Initially there is only dilatation of the stomach, before the actual double-bubble sign appears **(Figure 13)**. It is important to confirm the continuation between the two bubbles to confirm the second bubble is duodenal bubble. It is only by this that the duodenal atresia can be differentiated from the other rare abnormalities like enteric duplication cyst or other cystic lesions of abdomen. The development of the polyhydramnios also has a progressive development. It is for this reason that duodenal atresia may be often missed on early anomaly scan.

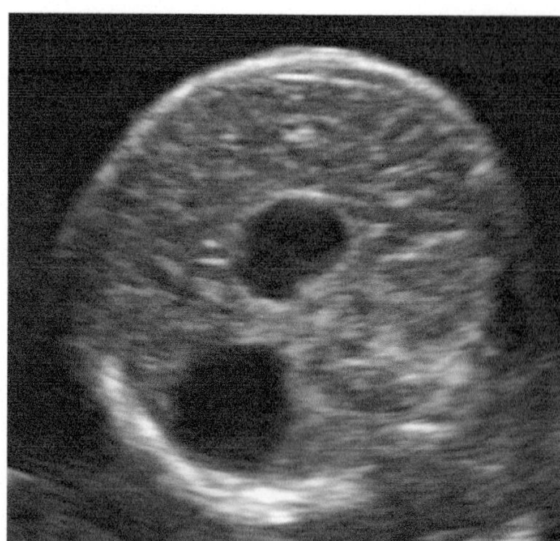

Figure 13: Transverse section of the abdomen at the level of the stomach shows two anechoic bubbles—double-bubble sign of duodenal atresia

Though rarely but when duodenal atresia is associated with esophageal atresia the two bubbles are massive in size. Prognosis of duodenal atresia is generally good in absence of associated abnormalities.

Differential Diagnosis

The duodenal bubble especially needs to be differentiated from choledochal cysts, hepatic cysts and enteric duplication cyst and as mentioned earlier the diagnostic confirmation of duodenal atresia is only the communication between the two bubbles.

Associated Abnormalities

About 40–50% of cases of duodenal atresia are associated with other major fetal anomalies of gastrointestinal tract, vertebral anomalies (33%) and cardiac anomalies (30%). Among the gastrointestinal anomalies are malrotation of the intestines, biliary tract anomalies and annular pancreas. But all these three lesions are markedly difficult to diagnose on antenatal ultrasound. Duodenal atresia is seen in 5–15% of trisomy 21 neonates. Overall 40% of cases of duodenal atresia are associated with trisomy 21. Though unlike esophageal atresia, duodenal atresia is not commonly associated with non-chromosomal syndromes.

Obstetric Management

Due to its high association with trisomy 21, karyotyping is a must apart from a detailed ultrasound scan to rule out associated abnormalities. Watch on the amniotic fluid index is essential to predict the possibility of preterm labor. These neonates require surgical correction and often may be multiple surgeries. The surgical outcome is good (90%) generally except for the cases associated with biliary abnormality and this leads to 20–40% neonatal mortality.

But the actually surgical results are very good with mortality rates of only 3–6%.[8] Late consequences of the surgery may consist of mega-duodenum, duodenogastroesphageal reflux and peptic ulcers[8].

Small Bowel Atresia

Like duodenal atresia, even small bowel atresia may be because of atresia or a diaphragm or a membrane in the small bowel. The sites where atresia may occur in the small bowel are jejunum in 50%, ileus in 43% and both in 7%. Depending on the cause and patho-anatomy it can be divided into four types.

- Type I: Intraluminal diaphragm or membrane (20%)
- Type II: Fibrous string connecting the two blind-ending stumps (32%)
- Type III: Complete separation of two stumps without any fibrous connection (48%)
- Type IIIB: In which the bowel shows the so called apple peel aspect (11%).
- Type IV: Atresia at multiple sites (17%). It is difficult to identify the types on antenatal ultrasound scans. Its incidence is 1 in 2,500 to 1 in 5,000. The probable causative factors for atresia of the small bowel are also the same as for duodenal atresia, vascular insult at the time of organogenesis.

Ultrasound Diagnosis

It usually presents late in pregnancy, commonly after 25 weeks. In the early pregnancy there is a single small bowel loop dilatation commonly in the central abdomen on axial section of the abdomen. The normal maximum diameter of the small bowel in 2nd and 3rd trimester is 7 mm.[10] This dilated loop shows echogenic contents **(Figure 14)** and hyperperistalsis[11] may be only after about 25 weeks polyhydramnios develops.[12,13] It is nearly the same age of gestation that severe dilatation of intestinal loops may be seen. Ileal loops have a high tendency to rupture and jejunal loops lead to more severe dilatation of loops.

Differential Diagnosis

Small bowel atresia is very difficult to differentiate from large bowel abnormalities of the fetus like Hirschsprung's disease and volvulus. Volvulus may be differentiated from small bowel atresia only by observing

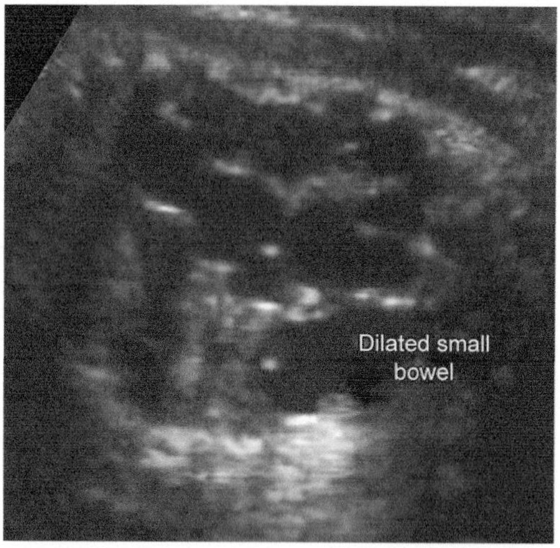

Figure 14: Dilated bowel loops with echogenic contents seen on B mode scan suggestive of bowel obstruction

the previous scan to assess the time taken for development of the lesion. It is a gradual development in small bowel atresia and in case of volvulus it is comparatively sudden (3–4 days). Meconium is another abnormality that needs to be differentiated from small bowel atresia, and this is done by echogenic bowel content and if at all perforation occurs there are diffuse calcifications in the abdomen (peritoneum).

Prognosis

Prognosis is bad in cases in perforation occurs and there is development of meconium peritonitis. Cystic fibrosis is one of the most adverse associations. The prognosis is also adversely affected in cases with polyhydramnios.

Associated Malformations

Small bowel atresia is not commonly associated with other malformations or chromosomal and non-chromosomal syndromes. More distal the obstruction is, better is the prognosis. Though associated gastrointestinal abnormalities like malrotation of the gut, esophageal atresia, microcolon and intestinal duplication may be of prognostic importance.

Obstetric Management

Due to polyhydramnios, there is a risk of premature delivery and amniodrainage may be done to deal with this complication. Polyhydramnios may also lead to abnormal fetal presentations and therefore the incidence of cesarean section is increased. In most cases surgery is to be done almost immediately after delivery so delivery is preferred in tertiary centers. The surgical outcome is generally good except in type IIIb and IV atresias and the major problem in these cases would be short bowel syndrome (malabsorption syndrome). Associated abnormalities like volvulus also affects the prognosis adversely.

Meconium Ileus

Mechanical obstruction of the ileus by inspissated thick meconium is named as meconium ileus. The meconium becomes thicker because of high protein content and also because of impaired bowel secretions. The commonest cause is cystic fibrosis (90%). Severe obstruction may lead to severe dilatation of the ileum and in turn may lead to perforation leading to meconium peritonitis.

Ultrasound Diagnosis

Bowel loops dilatation is seen with hyperechoic content and hyperechoic walls. Hyperechoic bowel may be the first sign[13] **(Figure 15)**. It usually becomes evident in late second trimester after 24–25 weeks. In some cases meconium fluid levels may be seen. Meconium peritonitis presents as diffuse intra-abdominal calcifications. The bowel distal to the bstruction is not seen. Magnetic resonance imaging (MRI) may be a useful additional investigation for confirmation of diagnosis.[14]

Differential Diagnosis

Hyperechoic bowel may also be seen in fetuses with trisomy 21 and fetal growth restriction with ileal ischemia.

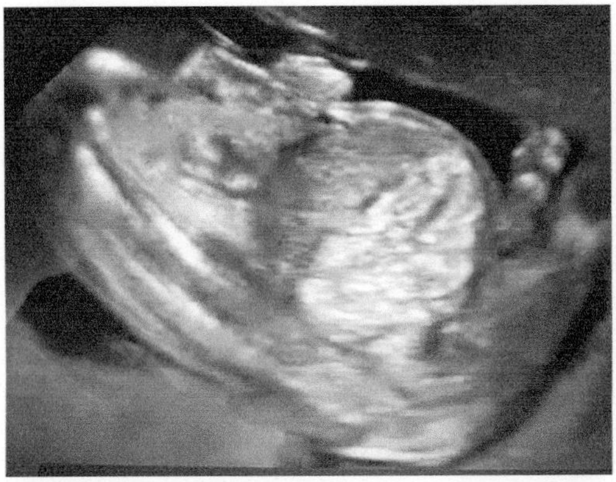

Figure 15: Hyperechoic bowel loops indicative of meconium ileus are seen on B-mode ultrasound image of abdomen

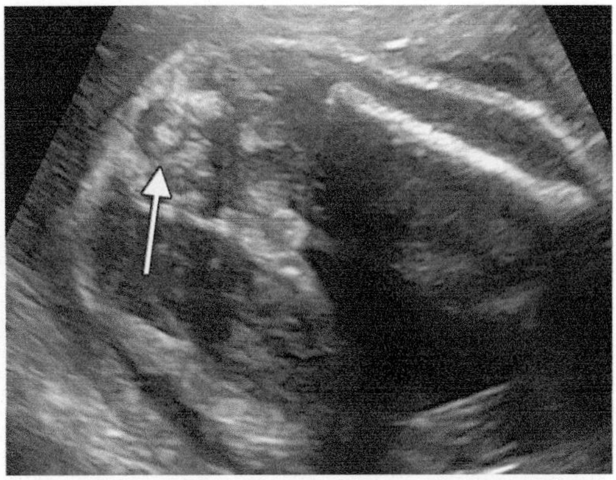

Figure 16: Normal anal sphincter on the B- mode image that is seen as a target sign on the perineum

Prognosis in these cases is usually bad, especially due to its association with cystic fibrosis.

Obstetric Management

Amniocentesis and deoxyribonucleic acid (DNA) testing for cystic fibrosis and karyotype for trisomy 21 are the two most essential investigations. Survival and quality of life depend directly on severity of cystic fibrosis.

Anorectal Anomalies

These may be divided into external malformations, internal malformations and mixed malformations.

a. *External malformations*: Imperforate anus with/without fistula. This occurs due to abnormalities of development and fusion of external perineal layers.
b. *Internal malformations*: Rectal atresia with or without fistula. It occurs due to developmental anomaly of primary partition of cloaca by urogenital septum.
c. *Mixed malformations*: Including all possible sites of ectopic anus.

Ultrasound Diagnosis

These anomalies are generally difficult to diagnose on antenatal ultrasound. Anus can be seen on the fetal perineum as a target sign. The anal sphincter appearing as a central hyperechoic area and the sphincter muscle as an anechoic rim **(Figure 16)**. Imperforate anus appears as an absence of this target sign that is replaced by a hyperechoic rim extending from anterior to posterior aspect of the perineum **(Figure 17A)**. Anorectal atresia may be possible to detect antenatally. The positive sign is rectal overdistention that may be evident only in the third trimester **(Figure 17B)**. The rectal diameter matches that of bladder or may be larger than the bladder and rectum may also appear bilobed in anorectal atresia. Sometimes this may be filled with hyperechoic meconium. When this is associated with rectovesical fistula it may be associated with oligohydramnios. These anomalies may share the ultrasound appearances of other distal bowel obstructions.

Associated Anomalies

About 70–90% of cases of anorectal atresias are associated with other anomalies, the commonest being urogenital malformations, because of their common embryological origin. But associations with other gastrointestinal tract, skeletal and central nervous system anomalies is also well documented. Anorectal anomalies are also present in fetuses with trisomy 18 and 21. Apart from

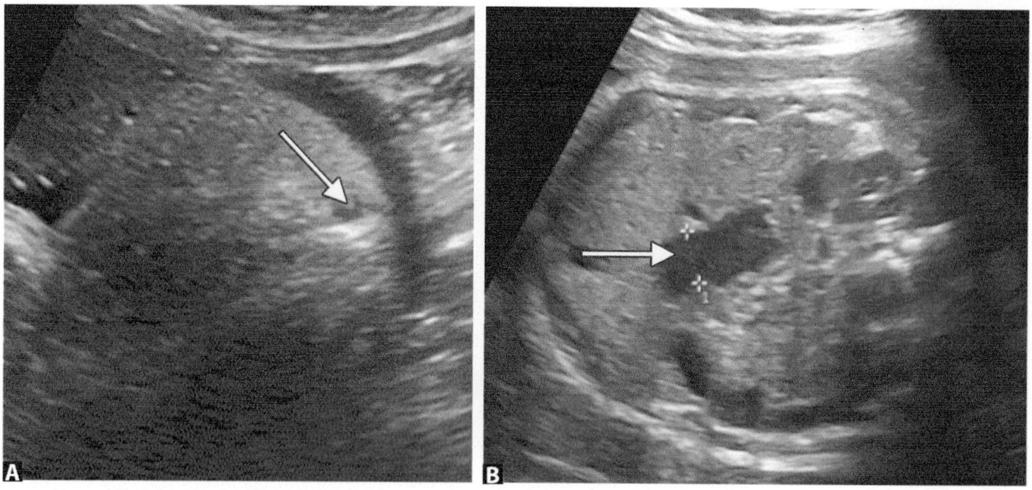

Figure 17: (A) Absent anal sphincter—imperforate anus seen as a linear shadow on the B mode image of the perineum; (B) B-mode ultrasound image of over-distended large bowel

this, anorectal anomalies are also a part of non-chromosomal syndromes like VACTERL syndrome, caudal regression syndrome and sirenomelia. VACTERL syndrome has already been described earlier. Apart from anorectal malformation, the anomalies seen in caudal regression syndrome are renal agenesis, sacral agenesis, lumbar vertebral anomalies, femoral hypoplasia and talipes equinovarus. Whereas anomalies seen in sirenomelia, along with anorectal malformations are fusion of lower limbs, renal agenesis, severe vertebral anomalies and genital anomalies.

Obstetric Management

If all associated anomalies are excluded, surgical option may be considered. Sagittal anorectal plasty is the surgical procedure required and has good results in experienced hands.

NON-BOWEL ABNORMALITIES

Choledochal Cyst

It is a rare congenital dilatation of common bile duct or intra-or extrahepatic portion of the biliary tree. The cystic lesions may be single or multiple.[15] It can be divided into four types:

1. Fusiform dilatation of common bile duct.
2. Diverticular dilatation of the common bile duct.
3. Intramural dilatation of the common bile duct.
4. Intrahepatic biliary dilatation.

Its incidence is about 1:2000 live births.

On ultrasound it is seen as a cystic lesion in the upper right abdomen with dilated proximal ducts **(Figure 18)**.[17]

It needs to be differentiated from duodenal atresia, hepatic cyst, dilated gallbladder, mesenteric cyst and ovarian cyst.

The cystic lesion in duodenal atresia is more close to the midline in the upper or mid abdomen, hepatic cyst is not related to the biliary tree, gallbladder is usually seen more anteriorly and usually at the level of the stomach, mesenteric cyst may change position and ovarian cyst usually lies lower in the pelvis.

The prognosis depends on the size of the cystic lesion and associated obstruction.

Mesenteric and Omental Cyst

These cystic lesions may be in the mesentery of large or small bowel or in the omentum. These are thin walled unilocular or multilocular cysts **(Figure 19)**. The differential diagnosis

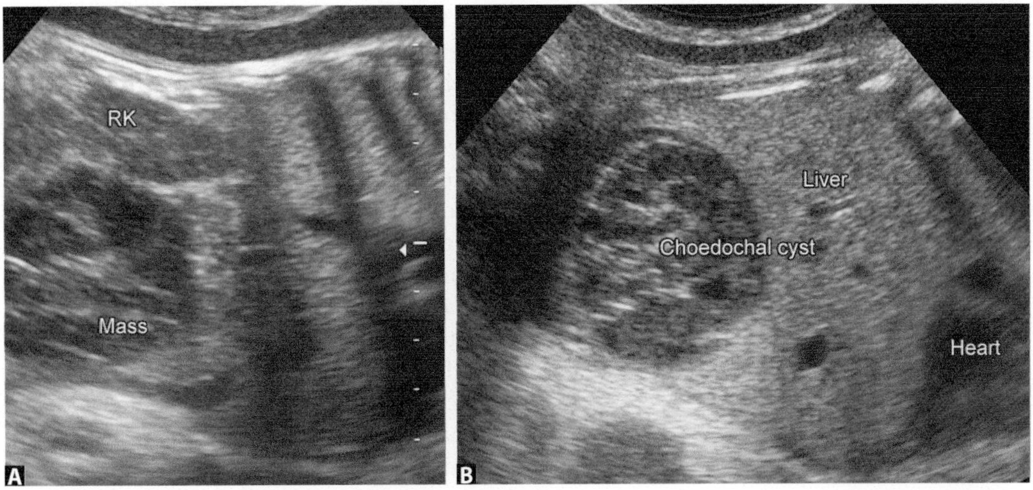

Figure 18: B-mode image showing a cystic area in right upper abdomen, that might be because of choledochal cyst

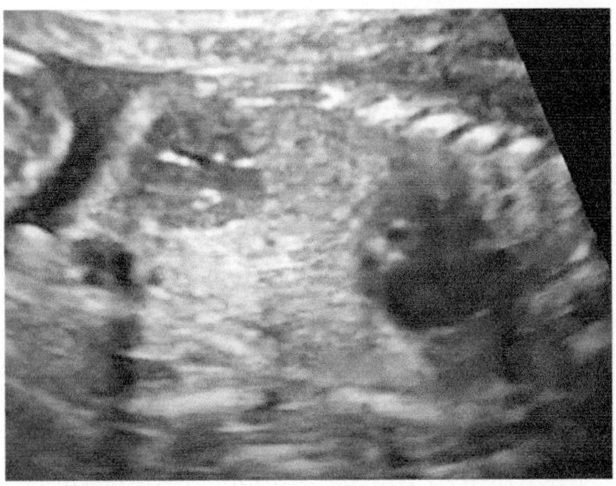

Figure 19: Mesenteric cyst seen on antenatal B mode ultrasound scan of fetus

is by exclusion of other cystic lesions of the abdomen. The prognosis for small lesions is very good and no surgical intervention is required.

Hepatosplenomegaly

Enlargement of liver and spleen are respectively named as hepatomegaly and splenomegaly. Commonest cause of hepato-splenomegaly is intrauterine fetal infections.

Etiopathology

Apart from the infections (of which cytomegalovirus is one of the commonest), hepatosplenomegaly is also seen in fetuses with Down's syndrome, because of the associated myoproliferative disease. Tumors like hemangiomas or hepatoblastoma may be the cause. In fact any condition that leads to overload on the heart and cardiac failure may cause venous congestion and therefore hepatomegaly. Hepatomegaly may also be seen with Beckwith-Weidemann syndrome (hepatosplenomegaly, omphalocele, body hemihypertrophy, macroglossia) and Zellweger syndrome (hepatosplenomegaly, polycystic kidney, agenesis of corpus callosum). Splenomegaly may be seen with storage diseases like Gaucher's and Neimann-Pick syndrome. Though these later two cause splenomegaly towards the end of the pregnancy, close to the full term.

Ultrasound Diagnosis

Ultrasound diagnosis is almost always subjective where liver and spleen, fills up the entire transverse section of the abdomen. In

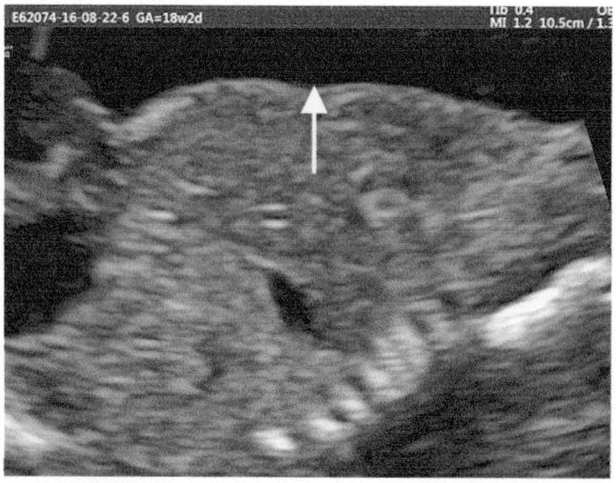

Figure 20: Sagittal section of fetal abdomen on B-mode ultrasound section shows a notch at the thoracoabdominal junction, indicating an over-distended abdomen

severe cases of hepatomegaly, the anterior abdominal wall may be pushed anteriorly and on sagittal section this shows as a dip at thoracoabdominal junction **(Figure 20)**.

The enlargement can be documented as largest maximum diameter by B-mode ultrasound or a largest volumes. Nomograms for either can be used for confirming the enlargement.[18]

Ascites may often be present and may enhance the contrast to better evaluate the size of both liver and spleen.

Differential Diagnosis

The appearance of thoracoabdominal dip matches that of thoracic hypoplasia, where because of small thorax, abdomen appears evidently large and therefore there is a thoraco-abdominal dip. There is a rare possibility that a normal left lobe of liver, which is markedly larger than in adulthood may be mistaken for an enlarged spleen.

Prognosis and Obstetric Management

It is very important to understand here that hepatosplenomegaly is only presentation of some underlying disease process and therefore the prognosis depends on the presence of other signs and symptoms present due to that underlying disease. Evidently in cases of infection, presence of ascites and cerebral calcifications are the two important factors that would lead to worse prognosis. Whenever; therefore, hepatosplenomegaly is documented, it is important to assess the other fetal systems carefully to exclude, infections (also by serological studies), trisomy 21, Beckwith-Weidemann syndrome and Zellweger syndrome.

Storage diseases are lethal in first few years of life and severe cytomegalovirus (CMV) infection leads to hearing loss, neurological damage and also at times early perinatal demise.

Hepatic Masses

The most common amongst the hepatic masses are hemangioma and hamartomas. Mesenchymal hamartomas appear like irregular hyperechoic masses in liver.[19] Hemangiomas are well defined, usually round hypoechoic, hyperechoic or mixed echogenic lesion depending on the degree of fibrosis and stage of involution.

Hepatoblastomas and adenomas have a solid looking appearance. Polyhydramnios is often associated with these tumors.

Hepatic calcifications may be seen in cases of intrauterine infections like cytomegalovirus, parovirus B19, herpes, rubella, toxoplasmosis, Varicella) or vascular accidents like thrombosis or ischemic disorders.

ANTERIOR ABDOMINAL WALL DEFECTS

- Omphalocele
- Gastroschisis
- Body-stalk abnormalities

Omphalocele

It is an anterior abdominal wall defect due to incomplete development of abdominal muscles, fascia and skin involving the cord insertion. It may be because of abnormality in the process of body infolding. Through this defect there is herniation of the abdominal organs and the herniated products are covered by peritoneum and amnion. It may contain liver or bowel and both have a different embryogenetic basis and also different prognosis. Documented incidence of omphalocele is 1 in 4,000 live births. Though it is mostly sporadic, a familial occurrence with sex-linked or autosomal pattern of inheritance has been reported.

Ultrasound Diagnosis

It appears as a bulge or out-pouching from the anterior abdominal wall that can be appreciated both on transverse section and sagittal section. The cord is always seen arising from the top of the bulge **(Figure 21)**. Presence of the umbilical vein in the omphalocele is an indirect sign representing that it is a primary closure defect of the abdominal wall. In small omphalocele the content may only be the omentum.

If the bowel is the content, the narrow neck of the herniation sac may lead to bowel obstruction and polyhydramnios. This may be seen in about 1/3rd of cases.

When the bowel is contained in the herniation sac, the sac contents are hyperechoic than the abdominal contents and when liver is contained in the herniation sac, the sac contents are hypoechoic to the abdominal contents.

Though omphalocele can be diagnosed in the end of the first trimester, it must be remembered that before 11 weeks, 4 days of gestation, it may be a normal finding. Therefore, ideally the diagnosis must be confirmed only around 13 weeks. But even before that if the neck of the omphalocele is larger than 7 mm or on the transverse section at the level of umbilicus of the fetus, the herniation sac appears larger than the transverse section of the abdomen, it is considered pathological.

Differential Diagnosis

Gastroschisis is the closest similar. The cord arising from the convexity of the herniated products and double layered covering the strong differentiating points. In gastroschisis the bowel loops are floating in amniotic fluid and the cord arises from the side of the herniation. The diagnosis is especially difficult when the covering membrane may occasionally disrupt.

Omphalocele if associated with ascites, it may give an appearance similar to that of gastroschisis because of floating bowel

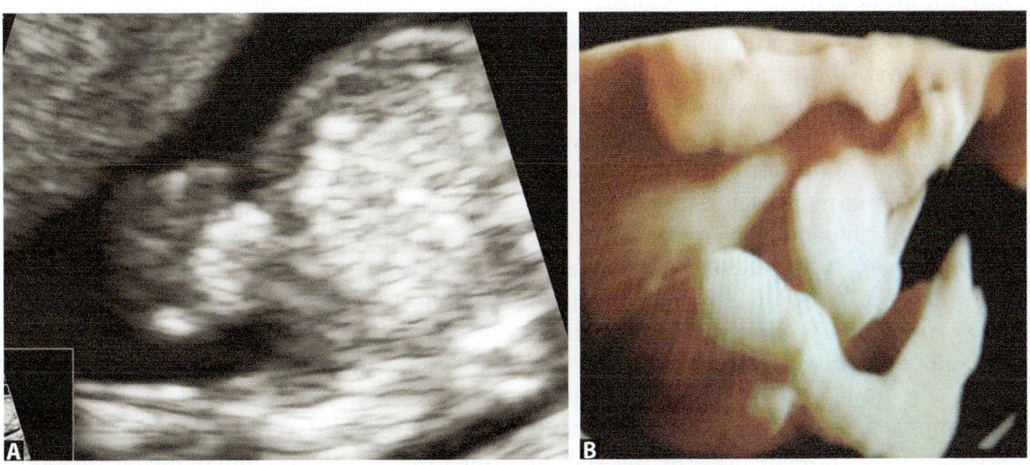

Figure 21: B-mode ultrasound image of the fetal abdomen showing the bulge out from the anterior abdominal surface with umbilical cord arising from its convexity suggesting omphalocele

loops in ascitic fluid. Presence of some intra-abdominal fluid as well as the membrane (double-layered) covering the local fluid collection in the herniation sac, confirms the diagnosis.

When it is a large omphalocele with major part of the liver herniating, it should be differentiated from limb-body-wall complex. Though in the later condition there is also associated scoliosis, limb and skull abnormalities. It is often because of amniotic band. It is important to differentiate omphalocele from cloacal extrophy. This median anterior abdominal wall defect extends caudally with bladder extrophy and also abnormalities of external genitalia. Confirming normal bladder in the abdominal cavity excludes this abnormality.

Bowel, containing omphaloceles are often associated with gastrointestinal, genitourinary and cardiac malformations. It is also considered a marker for trisomy 13, 18 commonly and less commonly triploidy, trisomy 21 and Turner's syndrome.

Omphalocele is a component of Beckwith-Weidemann syndrome (mentioned earlier) and pentalogy of Cantrell (omphalocele, diaphragmatic hernia, sternal fusion defects, ectopia cordis and cleft lip and palate).

Obstetric Management and Prognosis

In all cases of bowel-containing omphalocele chromosomal studies are a must. Detailed scan to exclude other abnormalities in the fetus is essential in all cases with omphalocele. Omphalocele is associated with other abnormalities in 50–70% of cases and with chromosomal disorders in about 30% of cases.[20,21] Amongst the associated malformations, cardiac are seen in up to 47%, genitourinary abnormalities in about 40% and neural tube defects in about 39% of cases. The mode of delivery for the fetuses with omphalocele of 5 cm and larger should be cesarean section to prevent the risk of rupture, though it depends on the presence or absence of associated abnormalities. When associated with other abnormalities, the mortality may raise to as much as 80%, and even higher with chromosomal abnormalities. But prognosis is excellent for isolated bowel-containing omphalocele. With liver containing omphaloceles the surgical risk and the postsurgical morbidity is high.[21]

Gastrochisis

This is a rare abnormality with a paraumbilical defect in the anterior abdominal wall with herniation of the bowel loops and these bowel loops are floating freely in the amniotic fluid. Incidence is documented as 1:10,000 to 1:15,000 live births. Very rarely stomach or urogenital organs may herniate from this defect. The defect arises because of early regression of right umbilical vein or any other vascular accident during embryogenesis. Exposure of the viscera and the bowel loops to the amniotic fluid leads to chemically induced inflammation and perforation of the bowel loops. It is considered a sporadic event with multifactorial etiology. It has been found to be more common in very young mothers, maternal smoking and maternal consumption of vasoactive drugs.

Ultrasound Diagnosis

Breach in the anterior abdominal wall with free floating bowel loops in the amniotic fluid is the diagnostic criteria **(Figures 22A and B)**. The neck of the defect is usually small, often <2 cm and therefore there is a high chance of compression of the mesenteric pedicle. This may lead to infarction of the bowel loops. Torsion of the bowel loops may also occur. Thickening and edema of the bowel walls, sometimes associated with dilatation is seen in the 3rd trimester. This may indicate obstruction and may progress into infarction and rupture of the bowel loops. A rare mention is also seen about vanishing bowel loops, this is because of infarction of the bowel loops due to severe obstruction of the bowel loops. Umbilical cord insertion is always seen on the side of the defect **(Figure 22C)**.

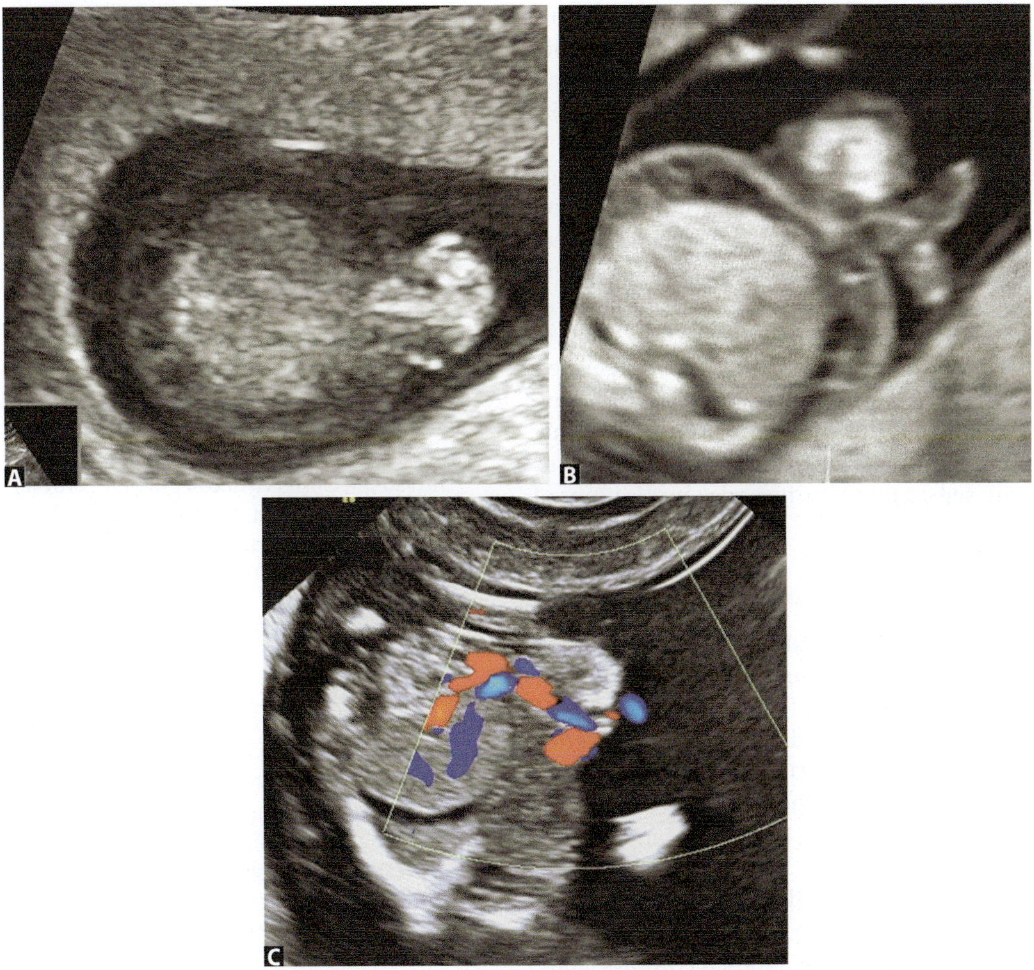

Figure 22: (A and B) B-mode ultrasound image of the fetal abdomen shows free-floating bowel loops suggestive of gastroschisis. This image though also shows marked edema on the fetal abdomen; (C) Gastroschisis with umbilical cord arising from the side of the defect as seen on the Doppler ultrasound image of the fetus

Differential Diagnosis

As described with omphalocele, even gastroschisis needs to be differentiated from omphalocele and limb-body-wall defect. This abnormality is rarely associated with chromosomal abnormalities and even rarely with congenital amyoplasia.

Associated Abnormalities

Association of chromosomal abnormalities is rate but may be associated with other gastrointestinal pathologies like malrotation, atresia, volvulus or infaction in 20–40% of cases.[23,24] About 77% of fetuses with gastroschisis may have growth retardation and about in 33%, preterm labor is likely.

Obstetric Management and Prognosis

In presence of gastroschisis, assessment of the spine and lower limb movements is very important to exclude congenital amyoplasia. Though serial examinations are essential to observe for bowel dilatation and edema. Though some workers prefer a vaginal delivery, operative delivery in a tertiary center may be safer to reduce the risk of bacterial contamination of the exposed bowel loops.

Surgical correction may be done in a single or two consequent surgeries depending on the level and the amount of bowel herniated. In cases of single step surgery where there is a chance of sudden increase in the intra-abdomimal pressure, silastic bag may be used. Though it is heartening that with single step or two step surgery the post-surgery outcome is good with postoperative mortality of only 15%. The prognosis is especially bad in cases with sepsis, prematurity and complications of mesenteric ischemia.

Body-Stalk Abnormalities

It is a rare abnormalitiy with incidence of about 1:14,000 fetuses. It is a large anterior abdominal wall defect due to failure of formation of body stalk. This leads to absence of umbilical cord and umbilicus and the placenta is fused to the herniated viscera.[25,26]

These findings can be typically appreciated on ultrasound.

It is often associated with scoliosis, kyphosis, neural tube defects, gastrointestinal and genitourinary abnormalities. It is always fatal.

DIAPHRAGMATIC DEFECTS

These are widely discussed in chapter on noncardiac thoracic abnormalities.

REFERENCES

1. Gross RE. The surgery of infancy and childhood. Philadelphia, PA WB Saunders; 1953.
2. Metkus AP, Filly RA, Stringer MD, et al. Sonographic predictors of survival in fetal diaphragmatic hernia. J Pediatr Surg. 1996;31:148-51.
3. Satoh S, Takashima T, Takeuchi H, et al. Antenatal sonographic detection of the proximal oesophageal segment: specific evidence for congenital oesophageal atresia. J Clin Ultrasound. 1995;23:419-23.
4. Stringer MD, Mc Kenna KM, Goldstein RB, et al. Prenatal diagnosis of oesophageal atresia. J Pediatr Surg. 1995;30:1258-63
5. Stoll C, Alembik Y, Dott B, Roth MP. Evaluation of prenatal diagnosis of congenital gastrointestinal atresias. Eur J Epidemiol. 1996;12:611-6.
6. Palidini D, Volpe P. Anomalies of the gastrointestinal tract and abdominal wall in Ultrasound of congenital fetal anomalies. Informa Health Care; 2007.pp. 207-30.
7. Geary MP, Chitty LS, Morsison JJ, et al. Perinatal outcome and prognostic factors in prenatally diagnosed congenital diaphragmatic hernia. Ultrasound Obstet Gynecol. 1998;12(2):107-11.
8. Escobar MA, Ladd AP, Grosveld JL, et al. Duodenal atresia and stenosis: long-term follow-up over 30 years. J Pediatr Surg. 2004;39:867-71.
9. Heling KS, Wauer RR, Hammer H, et al. Reliablity of the lung-to-head ratio in predicting outcome and neonatal ventilation parameters in fetuses with congenital diaphragmatic hernia. Ultrasound Obstet Gynecol. 2005;25(2):112-8.
10. Paralekar S. Sonography of normal fetal bowel. J Ultrasound Med. 1991;10:211-3.
11. Deprest J, Jani J, Gratacos E, et al. FETO task group. Fetal intervention for congenital diaphragmatic hernia: the European experience. Semin Perinatol. 2005;29(2):94-103.
12. Heling KS, Wauer RR, Hammer H, et al. Reliability of lung-to-head ratio in predicting outcome and neonatal ventilation parameters in fetuses with congenital diaphragmatic hernia. Ultrasound Obstet Gynecol. 2005;25(2):112-8.
13. Harrison MR, Keller RL, Hawgood SB, et al. A randomized trial of fetal endoscopic tracheal occlusion for severe fetal congenital diaphragmatic hernia. N Engl J Med. 2003;349(20):1916-24.
14. Shulman A, Mazkereth R, Zalel Y, et al. Prenatal identification of oesophageal atresia: the role of ultrasonography for evaluation of functional anatomy. Prenatal Diagn. 2002;22(8):669-74.
15. Cham KL, Tang MHY, Tse HY, Tang RYK, Tam PKH. Meconium peritonitis: prenatal

diagnosis, postnatal management and outcome. Prenat Diagn. 2005;25:676-82.

16. Chen CP, Cheng SJ, Chang TY. Prenatal diagnosis of choledochal cyst using ultrasound and magnetic resonance imaging. Ultrasound Obstet Gynecol. 2004;23(1):93-4.
17. Macken MB, Wright JR, Lau H, et al. Prenatal sonographic detection of congenital hepatic cyst in third trimester after normal second-trimester sonographic examination. J Clin Ultrasound. 2000;28(6):307-10.
18. Roberts AM, Mitchell JM, Pattison NS. Fetal liver length in normal and isoimmunised pregnancies. Am J Obstet Gynecol. 1989;161: 42-6.
19. Laberge JM, Patenaude Y, Desilets V, et al. Large hepatic mesenchymal hamartoma leading to mid-trimester fetal demise. Fetal Diagn Ther. 2005;20(2):141-5.
20. Queisser-Luft A, Stopfkuchen H, Stolz G, et al. Prenatal diagnosis of major malformations: Quality control of routine ultrasound examinations based on five-year study of 20,248 newborn fetuses and infants. Prenatal Diagn. 1998;18(6):567-76.
21. Martin RW. Screening for fetal abdominal wall defects. Obstet Gynecol Clin North Am. 1998;25(3):517-26.
22. Brantberg A, Blass HGK, Haugen SE, Eiknes SH. Characteristics and outcome of 90 cases of fetal omphalocoele. Ultrasound Obstet Gynecol. 2005;26:527-37.
23. Grandjean H, Larroque D, Levi S. The performance of routine ultrasonographic screening of pregnancies in the eurofetus study. Am J Obstet Gynecol. 1999;181(2):446-54.
24. Luck CA. Value of routine ultrasound scanning at 19 weeks: a four year study of 8849 deliveries. BMJ. 1992;304(6840):1474-8.
25. Kurkchubasche AG. The fetus with an abdominal wall defect. Med Health RI. 2000;84(5):159-61.
26. Oguniemy D. Gastroschisis complicated by midgut atresia, absorption of bowel and closure of abdominal wall defect. Fetal Diagn Ther. 2001;16(4):227-30.

9

CHAPTER

Fetal Urinary Tract Anomalies

S Boopathy Vijayaraghavan, Sathiya Senthil

Congenital abnormalities of urinary tract are quite common with an incidence of 1 to 4 in 1000 pregnancies.[1] Prenatal sonographic diagnosis of fetal urinary tract malformation has proved to be useful in the prevention of serious renal damage in children and young adults. The diagnostic accuracy of sonography in prenatal diagnosis of urinary tract malformation is constantly improving. Prenatal diagnosis of urinary tract anomalies requires a systematic ultrasound assessment of fetal kidneys, urinary bladder, amniotic fluid volume and associated anomalies. Urinary tract anomalies may form part of some chromosomal anomalies, syndromes or associations, some of which can be recurrent or inherited. Hence, when urinary tract anomalies are seen in a fetus, associated anomalies have to be searched for in detail and a detailed family history has to be taken. Renal scan is recommended for parents and siblings of fetuses suspected to have certain renal abnormalities (polycystic kidney disease, bilateral renal agenesis/dysgenesis) because it may help to diagnose the type of kidney disease in the fetus.

ULTRASOUND SCANNING TECHNIQUE OF FETAL URINARY TRACT

The fetal kidneys can be seen satisfactorily on sonography from late first trimester (12 weeks onwards). The Endovaginal Sonography (EVS) is complementary in first trimester. The kidneys are seen best in coronal scan of the fetal abdomen. They are seen as oval echogenic structures on either side of spine **(Figure 1)**. In second and third trimester, the ultrasound assessment of kidneys is made on a minimum of two scan planes—axial and longitudinal. A third coronal plane may be necessary in certain situations. The highest frequency transducer that allows adequate penetration of the maternal abdomen should be used. On axial scan, the kidneys are seen as round echopoor structures on either side of fetal spine with a horizontally oriented slit like fluid-filled renal pelvis. On longitudinal scan, the kidney appears oval with the adrenal gland located cranially. On coronal scan, the kidneys appear as bean-shaped structures on either side of the spine. In second trimester, it appears echopoor **(Figure 2)**. In the third

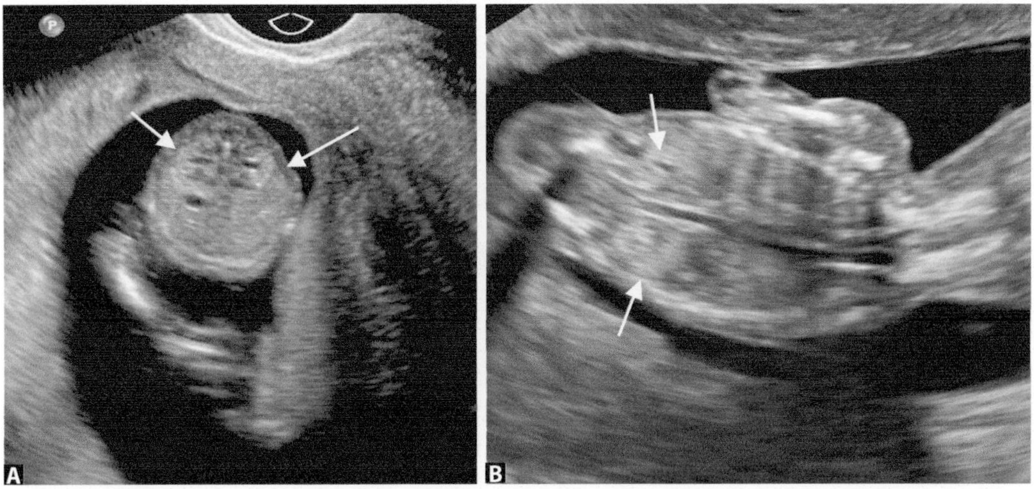

Figure 1: Normal appearance of the kidneys in first trimester: (A) Axial; (B) coronal planes of the fetal abdomen showing the echogenic kidneys (arrows)

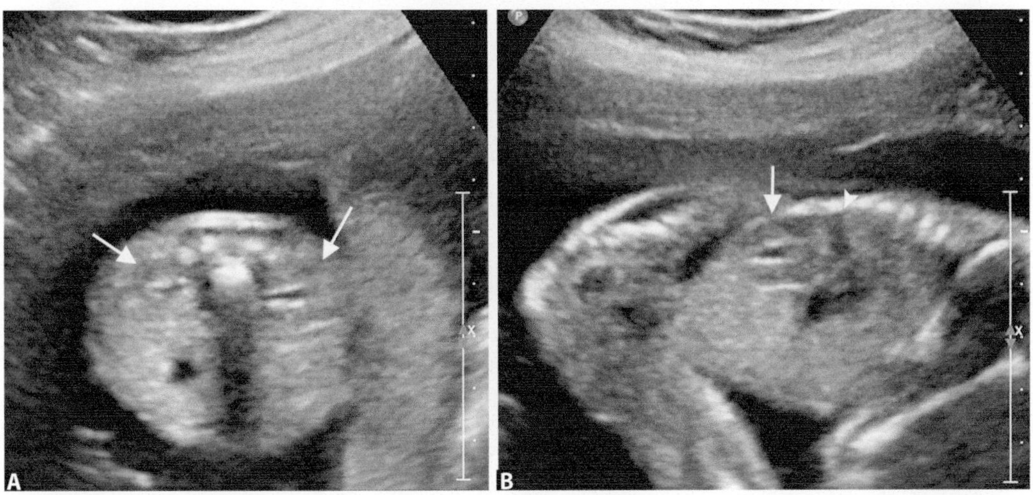

Figures 2: Normal appearance of kidneys in second trimester: (A) Axial scan from posterior aspect shows the round echo-poor kidneys (arrows) on either side of the spine with slit like fluid-filled renal pelvis in the center; (B) Longitudinal scan shows the oval kidney (arrow) with the echo-poor adrenal (arrowhead) above it

trimester, the corticomedullary differentiation (CMD) is distinctly is made out. The medullary pyramids are seen as triangular echopoor areas towards the inner aspect of the kidney. Towards term, the medullary pyramids are prominent **(Figure 3)** and should not be mistaken for dilated calyces. They can be differentiated on coronal scan, where the dilated calyces will communicate with medially placed renal pelvis while the renal pyramids will not. In selected situations, high frequency probe can be used to scan the kidneys to look for parenchymal abnormalities like echogenicity, cysts and corticomedullary differentiation. Urinary bladder is seen as an echopoor cystic structure in axial scan of the fetal pelvis **(Figure 4)**. In longitudinal and coronal scan, it appears fusiform.

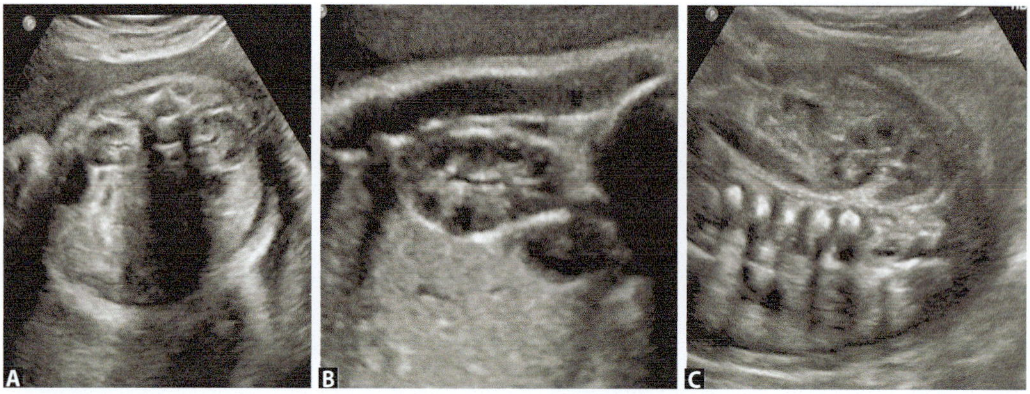

Figure 3: Normal appearance of kidneys in third trimester: (A) Axial scan; (B) Longitudinal scan shows good corticomedullary differentiation (CMD) with the echopoor triangular pyramids on the inner side of the kidney; and (C) Coronal scan showing the bean-shaped kidney

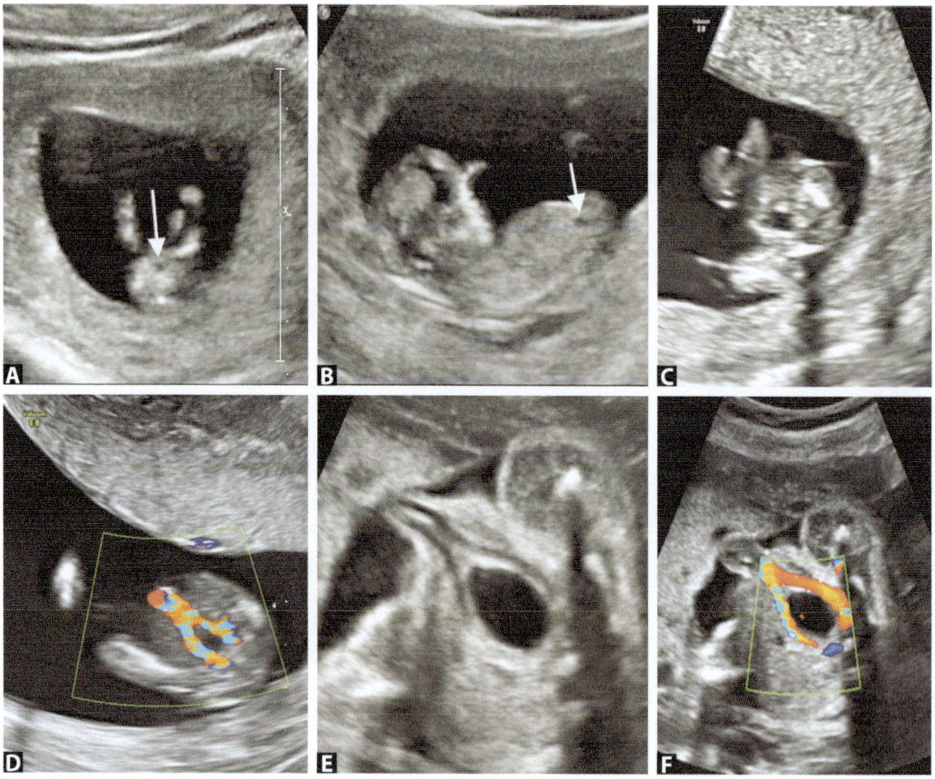

Figure 4: Normal appearance of the urinary bladder at 11 weeks: (A) Axial; (B) Longitudinal scan of the fetus showing the tiny urinary bladder (arrow); At 13 to 14 weeks—(C) Axial scan; (D) Oblique coronal scan with color Doppler showing the umbilical arteries skirting around the urinary bladder; and (E and F) Similar images in second trimester

When the color box is turned on, the two umbilical arteries are seen skirting the urinary bladder **(Figures 4E and F)**. It exhibits alternate cycles of filling and emptying due to fetal micturition. Hence if fetal urinary bladder is not seen, scan has to be repeated to confirm persistent nonvisualization. In urinary bladder outflow obstruction, the urinary bladder remains overdistended over time. The fetal urinary bladder can be visualized consistently from 12 weeks of gestation **(Figures 4A and B)**. In second trimester endovaginal sonography can be done for better visualization of the kidneys and urinary bladder if the fetus is in breech presentation. In certain situations, fetal perineal sonography[2] and sonographic fetal micturating cystourethrogram (SFMCUG)[3] have to be performed. A midline sagittal section of the fetal pelvis, perineum and external genitalia is obtained **(Figure 5)** and the same section is observed continuously for the occurrence of fetal micturition. During micturition, the urinary bladder is seen to contract, the urethra distends slightly with fluid and a urinary stream from the external urethral meatus is observed. The urinary stream can be seen on both gray scale and color Doppler sonography **(Figure 6)**. When micturition is observed, it is stored as a cine loop. This cine loop can then be reviewed either as cine at varying speed or as multiple freeze frames. The same section is also useful to look for ectopic ureteric opening.

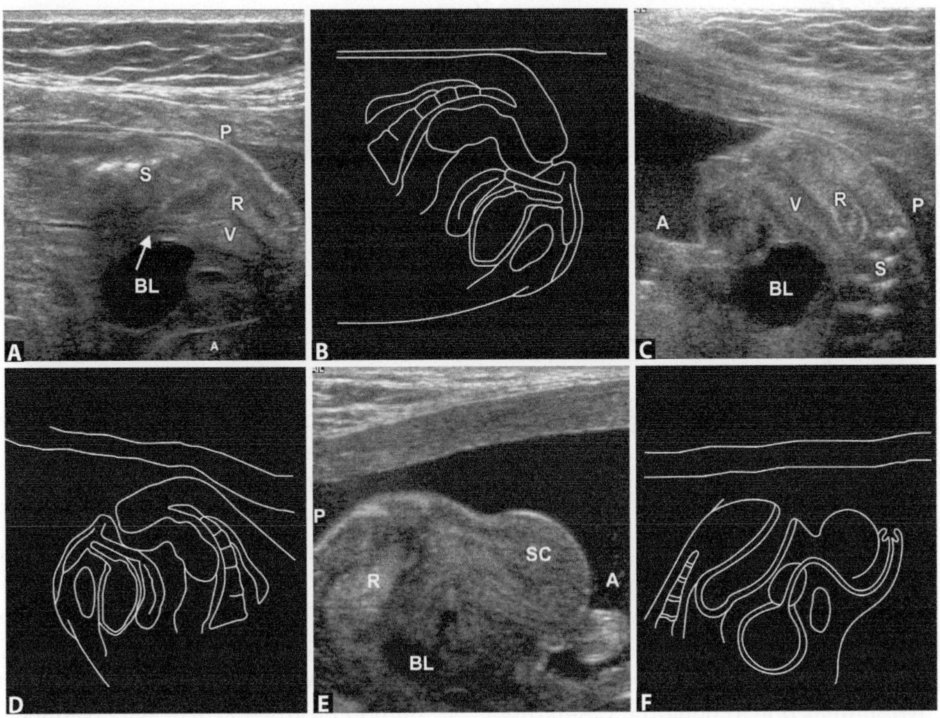

Figure 5: Fetal perineal scan in a female fetus from posterocaudal approach (A and B) and anterocaudal approach (C and D) showing the urinary bladder (BL) and urethra anteriorly, vagina (V) and uterus (arrow) in the middle and rectum (R) posteriorly. A indicates anterior, P—posterior and S—sacrum. (E and F) Fetal perineal scan in a male fetus showing the urinary bladder (BL) and urethra anteriorly and rectum (R) posteriorly. A indicates anterior, P—posterior and SC—scrotum

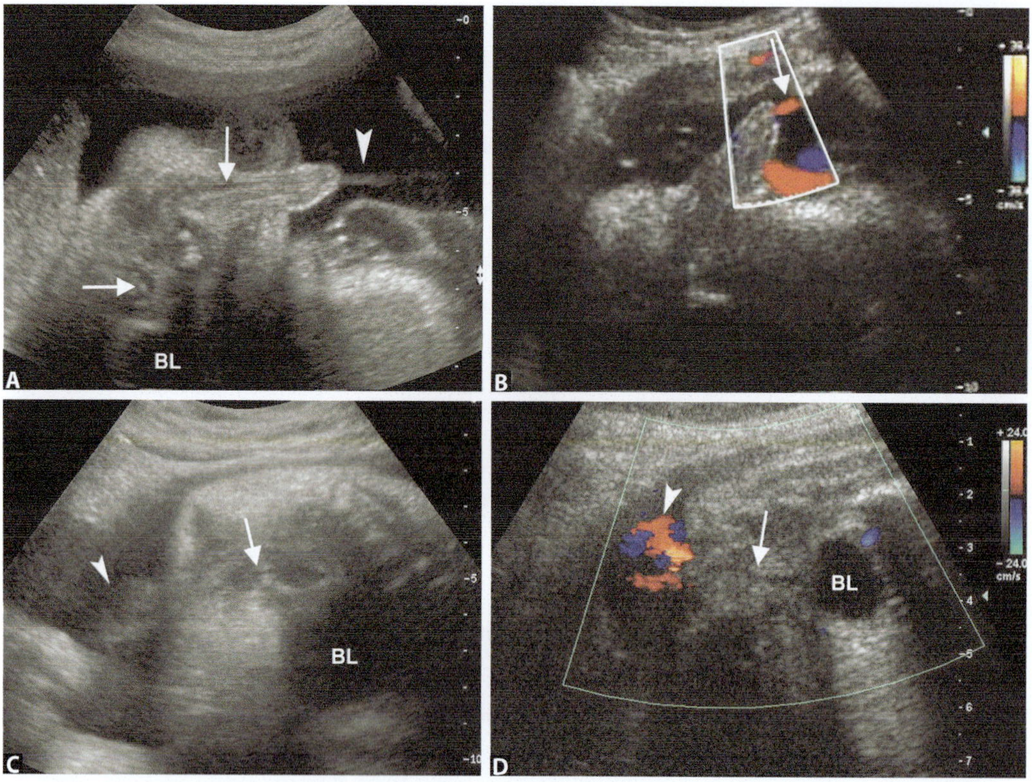

Figure 6: Fetal sonographic micturating cystourethrogram (FSMCUG): (A) Midline sagittal gray scale image through the fetal pelvis, perineum and the penis during micturition showing the urinary bladder (BL) slightly fluid distended posterior and anterior urethra (arrows) and the urinary stream from the tip of the penis (arrowhead) in a fetus with normal urethra; (B) Color Doppler image of the same fetus showing the urinary stream from the tip of the penis; (C) Gray scale; and (D) Color Doppler images of micturition in a female fetus showing the urinary bladder (BL) urethra (arrow) and the urinary stream (arrowhead)

AMNIOTIC FLUID AND URINARY TRACT ANOMALY

The fetal urine is the major source of amniotic fluid volume after 16 to 18 weeks. Hence, there is a close association between the urinary tract pathology and amniotic fluid volume. In Barter's syndrome, fetal anemia and recipient in twin-to-twin transfusion syndrome, there is polyhydramnios due to polyuria. When there is decreased urine output due to urinary tract anomaly or fetal growth restriction (FGR), it will result in oligohydramnios. Decrease in urine output is seen in either urinary bladder outflow obstruction or bilateral renal disease or obstruction. Hence when there is oligohydramnios, the following protocol has to be followed.

1. Premature rupture of membranes (PROM) as the cause of oligohydramnios should be ruled out.
2. Urinary bladder should be looked for. It may be seen and may appear normal. It may appear over distended in urinary bladder outflow obstruction. If urinary bladder is not seen, then the scan has to be repeated at short intervals to see if it is not seen persistently.
3. If urinary bladder is not persistently seen, then the renal fossa should be looked for to rule out diseased kidneys or renal agenesis.

4. If urinary bladder and kidneys are normal then the placenta has to be assessed for hypermaturity. Color Doppler assessment of umbilical artery has to be done to rule in or out placental dysfunction with/without fetal growth restriction.

URINARY TRACT DILATATION

Urinary tract dilatation (UTD) is one of the most common anomalies that can be picked up prenatally. It occurs in 1–2% of all pregnancies.[4] Its prenatal detection helps to manage the condition prior to the development of complications such as urinary tract infection (UTI), calculus formation or renal dysfunction postnatally. In most of the cases (50 to 70%), the urinary tract dilatation is transient or physiologic without any clinical significance. In the rest, it may be due to obstructive pathology like pelviureteric junction obstruction (10 to 30%), primary obstructive megaureter (5 to 15%), posterior urethral valves (1 to 5%) or vesicoureteric reflux (10 to 40%).[5] The less common causes can be ectopic ureter, duplex collecting system, and urethral atresia or prune belly syndrome. The etiology may not be defined before birth in all cases and is diagnosed postnatally with imaging which includes ultrasound and micturating cystourethrogram (MCUG). There are considerable variations in the follow-up evaluation of fetuses and postnatal follow-up of children with urinary tract dilatation. There is no uniformity on how to define, classify and grade urinary tract dilatation during prenatal and postnatal periods. Different terminologies like hydronephrosis, pyelectasis, and renal pelvis dilatation with overlapping meanings are used to describe urinary tract dilatation leading to misinterpretation between the imagers and clinicians. Urinary tract dilatation is a dynamic process fluctuating over time and with varying conditions like degree of distension of urinary bladder prenatally and hydration and patient position postnatally. Hence, urinary tract dilatation can present as a spectrum of severity—for example, not all cases of posterior urethral valves present with severe urinary tract dilatation as discussed and illustrated later.

In 2014, a multidisciplinary consensus on the classification of prenatal and postnatal urinary tract dilatation has been published,[4] where a statement of unified description of urinary tract dilatation with consistent terminology and standardized scheme for the perinatal evaluation of these patients has been put forth. This system is designed to be used in cases of isolated urinary tract dilatation and not to be applied to unique situations or anomalous kidneys. The statement recommends the consistent use of the term "urinary tract dilatation". The ideal technique for anteroposterior renal pelvic diameter (APRPD) measurement is based on images of the kidney obtained with the fetus in an anterior-posterior plane.[4] For optimal visualization of the fetal kidneys, and measurement of the AP diameter of renal pelvis dilatation, the spine should be demonstrated at the 12 or 6 o'clock positions. In addition, the measurement should be taken at the maximal diameter of intrarenal pelvis dilatation **(Figure 7)** rather than that of the extrarenal pelvis dilatation. Additional sonographic features to be evaluated are: (1) calyceal dilatation; (2) Parenchymal thickness by subjective assessment; (3) parenchymal appearance—(a) echogenicity assessed subjectively by comparison with liver and spleen (b) presence or absence of cortical cyst (c) corticomedullary differentiation; (4) ureteric dilatation; (5) abnormalities of urinary bladder like wall thickness, over distension, presence of ureterocele or dilated urethra; and (6) oligohydramnios.

The renal pelvis is considered normal if the APRPD is <4 mm at <28 weeks gestation, <7 mm at ≥28 weeks and <10 mm postnatally without calyceal dilatation, normal parenchyma, nonvisualized ureter and normal urinary bladder. Above these threshold measurements, it is diagnosed as

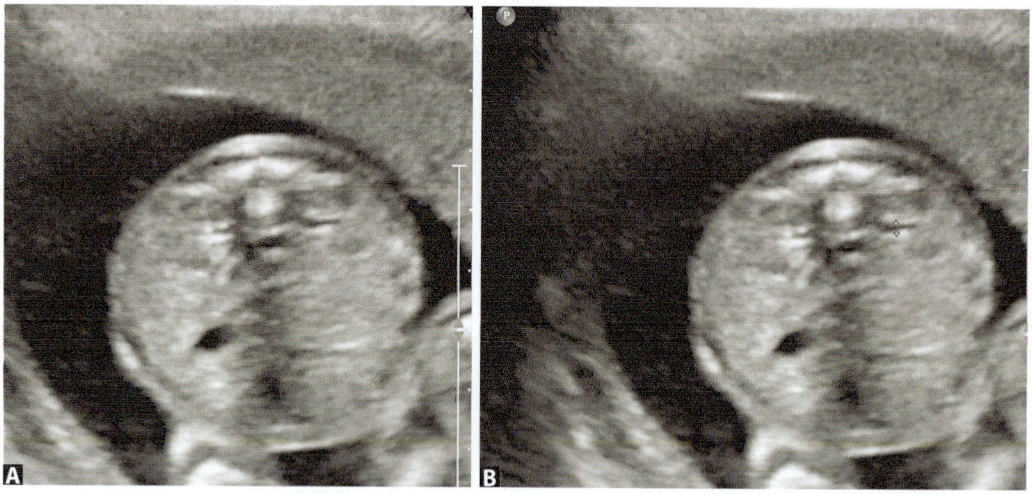

Figure 7: Technique of measurement of anteroposterior renal pelvic diameter (APRPD): Axial scan of fetal abdomen demonstrates the fetal spine at 12 o'clock position (A) and placement of calipers for the measurement (B)

urinary tract dilatation (UTD). In antenatal period, the UTD is classified into two groups—a low-risk group of UTD A1 with low risk for postnatal uropathy and an increased risk group of UTD A2–3 with increased risk for postnatal uropathy.[4] In fetuses of UTD A1, the APRPD is 4 to <7 mm at <28 weeks **(Figures 8A and B)** and 7 to <10 mm at ≥28 weeks **(Figures 8C and D)** with normal renal parenchyma, nonvisualized or undilated ureter, normal urinary bladder with normal amniotic fluid volume. They may have central calyceal dilatation. In fetuses with UTD A2–3, the APRPD is ≥7 mm at <28 weeks **(Figures 9A and B)** and ≥10 mm at ≥28 weeks **(Figures 9C and D)** or any one of the following findings: dilatation of peripheral calyces **(Figures 9E and F)**, abnormal parenchymal thickness or appearance **(Figures 9G and H)**, dilated ureter **(Figure 9I)** an abnormal urinary bladder or oligohydramnios.

Based on the UTD classification system, a follow-up management scheme has been proposed. For UTD A1 diagnosed before 32 weeks, a follow-up prenatal ultrasound is recommended at ≥32 weeks. If the ultrasound at ≥32 weeks reveals resolution of the UTD with normal renal parenchyma, bladder and ureters, no further prenatal or postnatal follow up is necessary. If there is persistent UTD A1 or UTD A2–3, evaluation after birth is recommended. Postnatal evaluation should include two ultrasound evaluations: the first at >48 hours but less than 1 month after birth; and the second 1–6 months later. In fetuses considered at increased risk for postnatal uropathy (UTD A2–3), a follow-up prenatal ultrasound is recommended within 4–6 weeks of the initial diagnosis of urinary tract dilatation. Where there is substantial risk for surgery or renal dysfunction, prenatal consultation with a specialist is recommended. After birth, a follow-up ultrasound is recommended at >48 hours of life to avoid a false negative appearance due to neonatal dehydration. Follow up should be performed earlier for obstructive uropathies, such as suspected posterior urethral valve (as suggested by the finding of a thick-walled bladder with persistent dilatation and a fusiform appearance and/or posterior urethral dilatation on prenatal ultrasound) or for bilateral conditions. Worsening findings on serial prenatal or postnatal ultrasound are associated with increased risk for genitourinary pathology. There is no significant difference

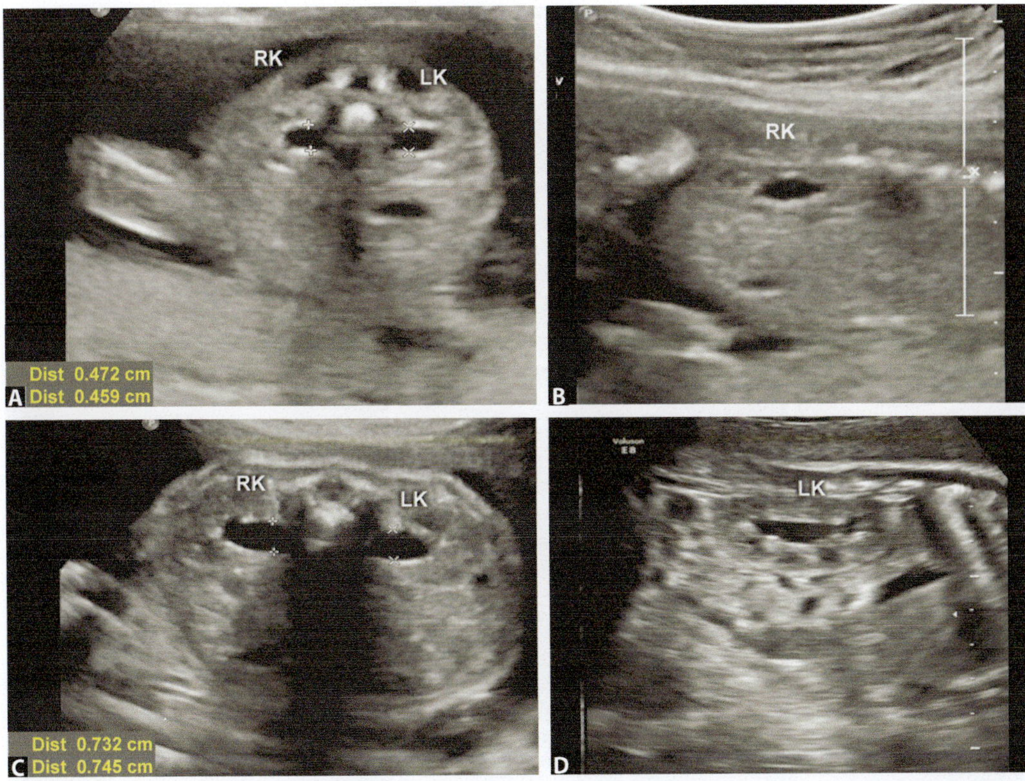

Figure 8: Ultrasound appearance of UTD A1—Fetal kidneys at 21 weeks of gestation: (A) Transverse scan showing anteroposterior renal pelvic diameter (APRPD) measuring less than 7 mm which is within the UTD A1 range; (B) Sagittal scan demonstrates normal parenchyma and no peripheral calyceal dilatation; (C and D) Fetal kidneys at 35 weeks: (C) Transverse scan shows APRPD of less than 10 mm which is within the UTD A1 range for this gestational age; (D) Sagittal scan demonstrates normal parenchyma and no peripheral calyceal dilatation

in risk for postnatal uropathy with respect to gender of the fetus or unilateral versus bilateral urinary tract dilatation. UTD is most often transient and associated with an increased risk of Trisomy 21 anomaly warranting a detailed ultrasound and correlation with aneuploidy screening protocols.[6-10]

CYSTIC RENAL DISEASE

Two main sonographic features lead to the suspicion of renal cystic disease in a fetus: cysts and renal hyperechogenicity.[11-13] Cysts can occur anywhere in the kidney and can occur in one or both kidneys. Renal hyperechogenicities can be visualized in the entire kidney, only the cortex, or only the medulla. There are no objective criteria for comparison of echogenicity up to 32 weeks. At later gestational ages, hyperechogenicity is confirmed when the renal cortex appears hyperechoic compared to liver and spleen.[13,14]

In their article, Imaging and classification of congenital cystic renal diseases,[15] the authors describe a decision tree approach once renal cystic disease is suspected. The basis of approach is a detailed sonographic analysis in addition to assessment of clinical data and the familial history. A detailed ultrasound examination includes renal size, defining the echogenicity of the cortex (hypoechoic, isoechoic or hyperechoic) and

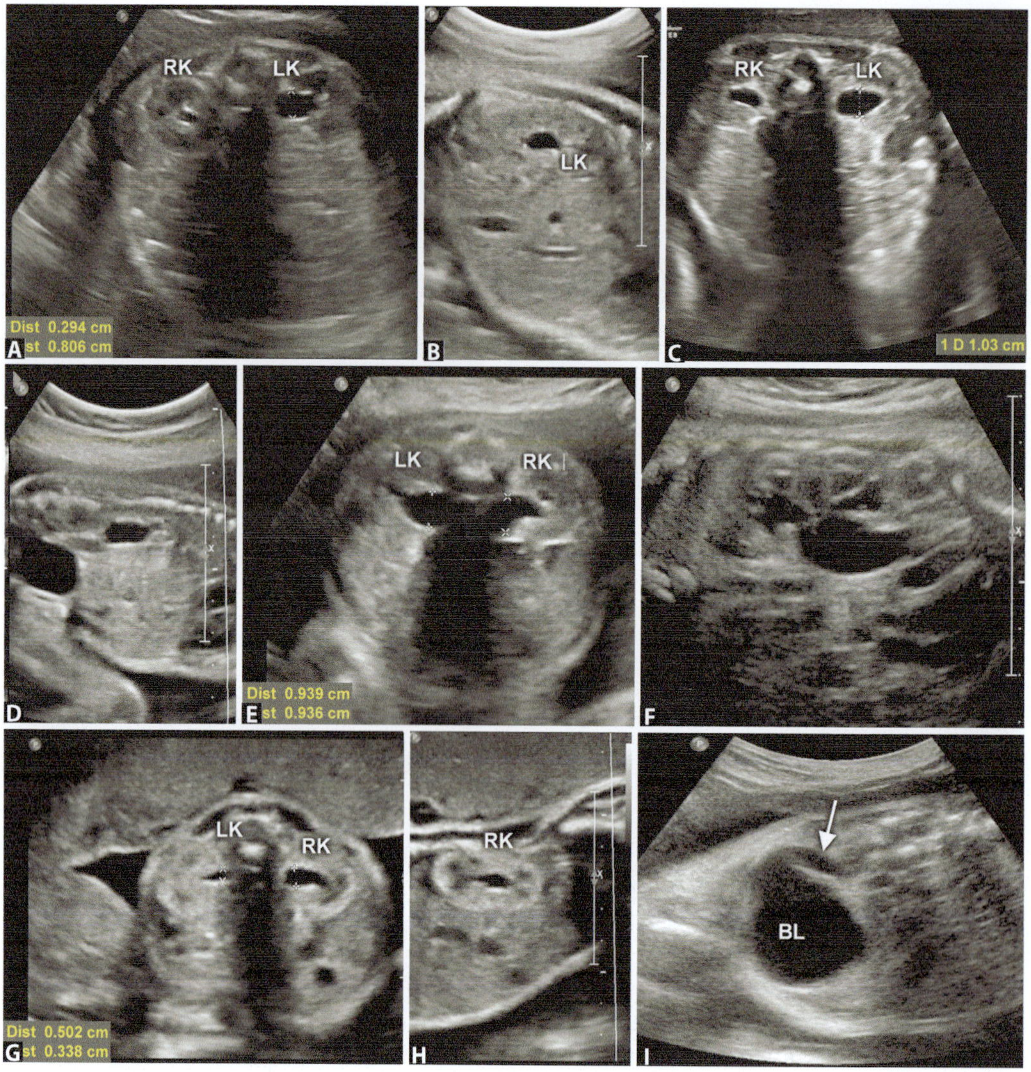

Figure 9: Ultrasound appearance of UTD A2–3: (A and B) Fetal kidneys at 23 weeks gestation:(A) Transverse plane demonstrates an APRPD of more than 7 mm in left kidney (LK) that is in the UTDA2-3 range (B) Sagittal scan showing normal parenchyma. (C and D) Fetal kidneys at 33 weeks: (C)Transverse scan shows anteroposterior renal pelvic diameter (APRPD) of more than 10 mm which is in range of UTDA2-3 range; (D) Sagittal scan shows normal parenchyma; (E and F) Fetus of 37 weeks: (E) Axial scan shows APRPD of less than 10 mm but (F) Coronal scan showing peripheral calyceal dilatation putting this in UTDA-2–3 group. (G and H) Fetus at 25 weeks showing APRPD of less than 7 mm but demonstrates abnormal echogenic parenchyma leading to classification of UTDA 2–3 group; (I) oblique scan demonstrates dilated ureter leading to classification of UTDA 2–3 group

medulla (hypoechoic, hyperechoic) assessing the corticomedullary differentiation (CMD) (preserved, absent, reversed), evaluating cysts (number, size, location), calcifications and assessing the pelvicalyceal system. Whenever cystic kidneys are suspected, it is useful to perform a sonographic examination of the parents to check for unknown familial disease.

Decision Tree Approach to Renal Cystic Disease (Figure 10)[15]

- The first step is to rule out dysplasia associated with obstructive uropathy in which there is dilatation of the collecting system. The common cause of hyperechoic cortex with/without cysts is obstructive dysplasia. It can be unilateral or bilateral. The kidneys can be of variable sizes with hyperechoic normal or thinned irregular cortex, absent CMD and with/without cysts **(Figure 11)**.
- The second diagnosis to be considered is multicystic dysplasia of kidneys. There are multiple cysts of variable size without connections between them and with no or little parenchyma **(Figure 12)**. They can be unilateral or bilateral **(Figure 13)**,

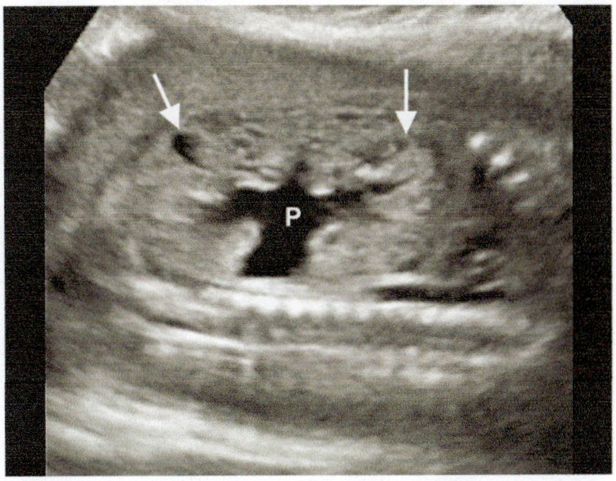

Figure 11: Renal dysplasia with obstruction: Longitudinal scan of the kidney shows echogenic parenchyma without CMD and with small cysts (arrows). The collecting system (P) is dilated

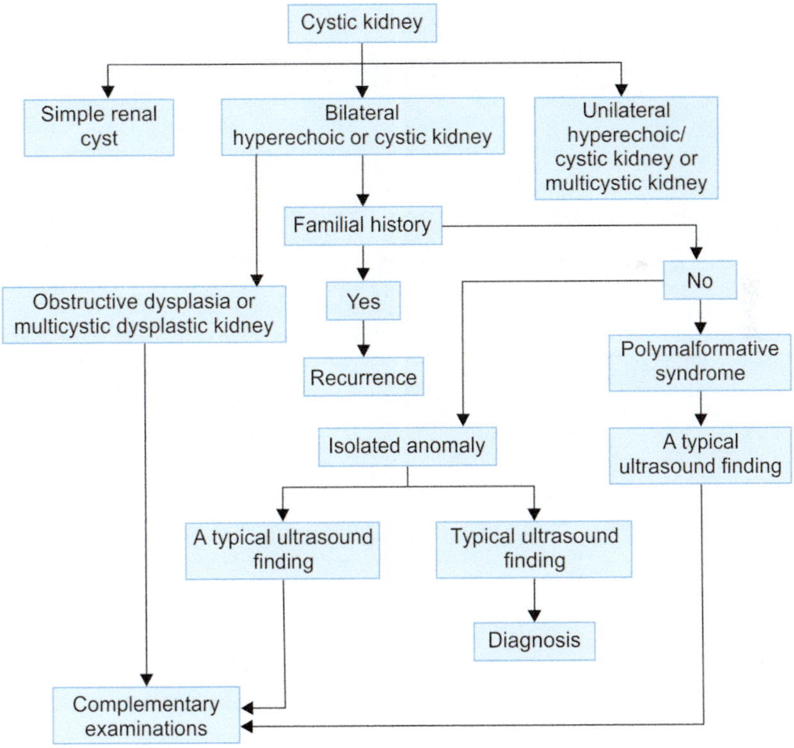

Figure 10: Decision tree approach to cystic renal disease

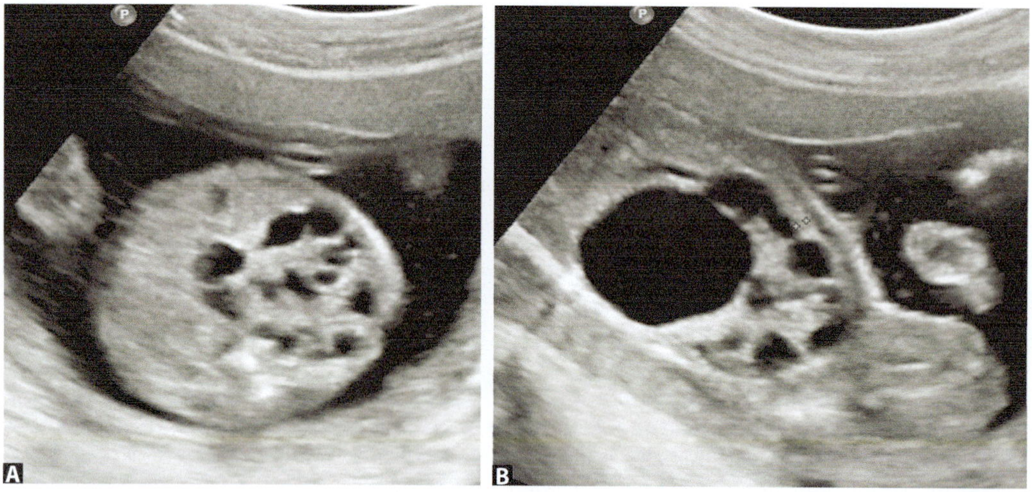

Figure 12: Multicystic dysplasia: (A) Axial and (B) Longitudinal scan of the renal fossa showing multiple cysts of varying size without connection between them and without normal parenchyma

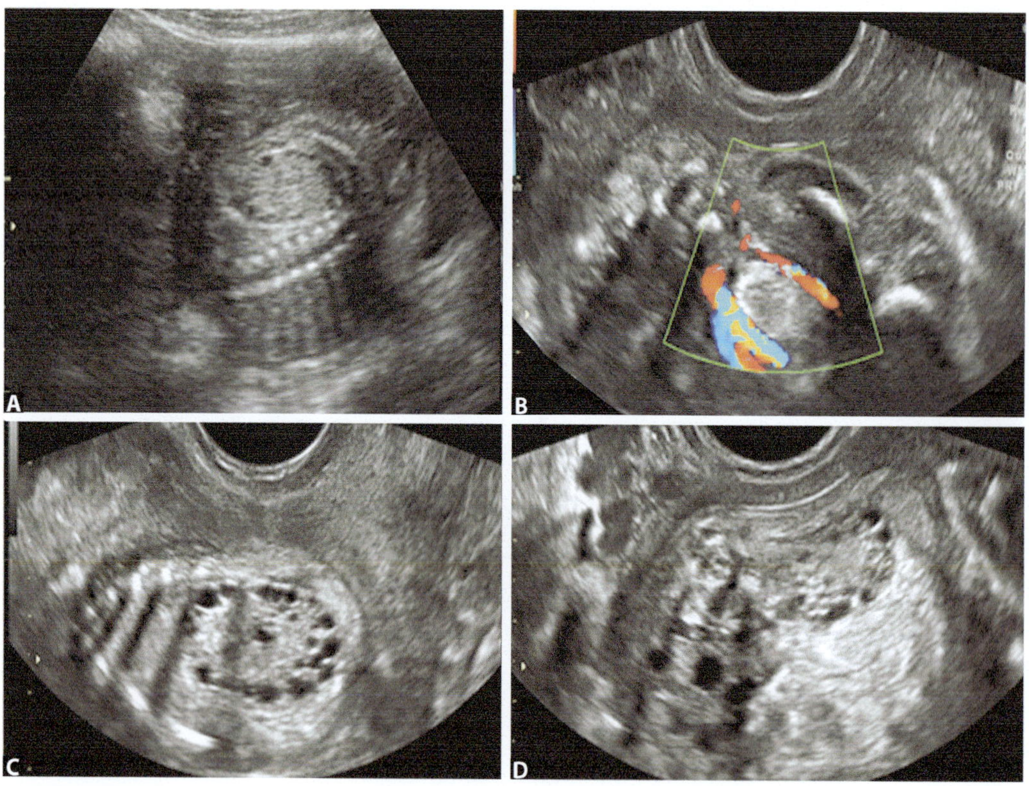

Figure 13: Bilateral multicystic dysplasia: (A) Transabdominal sonography of a 19 weeks fetus in breech presentation shows anhydramnios with apparently normal kidney; (B) Endovaginal sonography of pelvis showing the nonvisualized urinary bladder between the umbilical arteries; (C) Longitudinal scan of one kidney showing the typical appearance of MCD and (D) axial scan demonstrating MCD of both kidneys, explaining the anhydramnios

involve upper or lower poles of duplex kidney **(Figure 14)**, one moiety of horseshoe kidney **(Figure 15)** or affect an ectopic kidney **(Figure 16)**. It is due to an abnormal development or associated with a significant percentage of cases with early obstruction. It may form part of some syndromes like Branchio-oto-renal syndrome, cerebro-reno-digital syndrome or VACTERL association. It can be associated with genital malformations both in girls (hemiuterus or uterine agenesis) and in boys (absent testis, seminal vesicle agenesis or cyst). The cysts can involute during pregnancy or after birth.[16,17] The appearance of multicystic kidney may show some variations. One pattern shows peripheral small cysts and a large central cyst. This mimics hydronephrosis due to pelviureteric junction obstruction **(Figure 17)**. The differentiating features are: the peripheral cysts not communicating with the central cyst; the varying size of peripheral cysts and absence of renal parenchyma. Multicystic kidney is a nonfunctioning kidney. If it is unilateral and the other kidney and the amniotic fluid volume are normal, the condition is compatible with normal postnatal life. If it is bilateral, there will be anhydramnios and is not compatible with postnatal life.

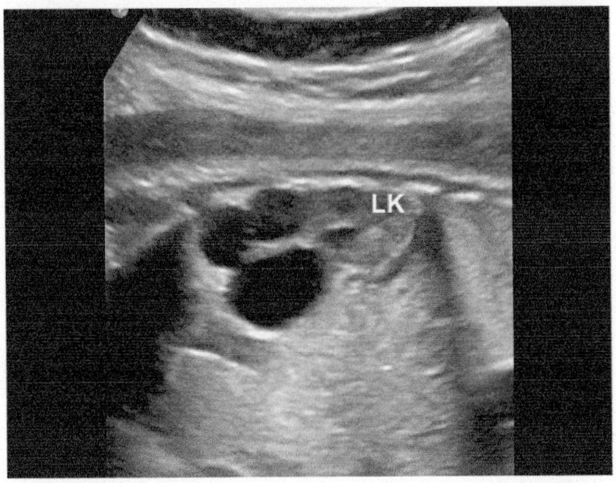

Figure 14: Segmental multicystic dysplasia: Longitudinal scan of the kidney showing the MCD of lower half of the kidney. The upper half (LK) appears normal

- Simple renal cyst is very rare in the fetuses. It is seen as a well-defined unilocular anechoic lesion with thin smooth walls and clear fluid **(Figure 18)**. Hydronephrosis of

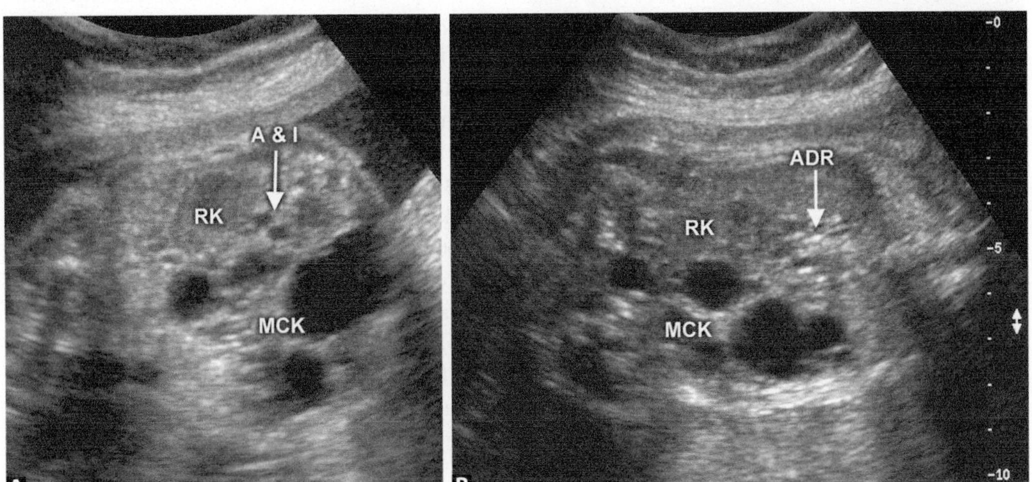

Figure 15: Horseshoe kidney with multicystic dysplasia of one moiety: (A) Axial and (B) Coronal scan of the fetal abdomen demonstrating the Horseshoe kidney with isthmus anterior to the aorta and inferior vena cava (arrow A and I) with multicystic dysplasia (MCK) of the left moiety and isthmus with normal lower placed right kidney (RK) and elongated right adrenal (ADR) above the right kidney

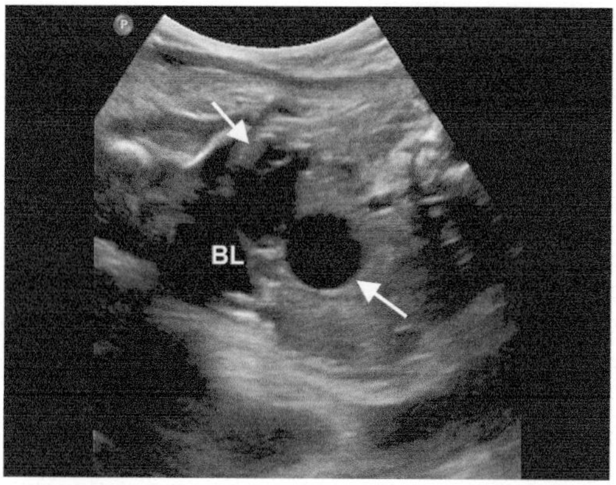

Figure 16: Multicystic dysplasia of ectopic pelvic kidney: Transverse scan of fetal pelvis showing the multicystic dysplasia of ectopic presacral kidney (arrows) posterior to urinary bladder (BL)

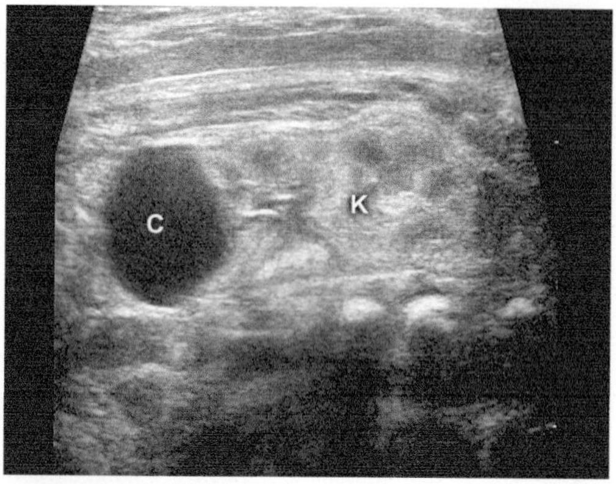

Figure 18: Simple renal cyst (C) seen in a longitudinal scan of the kidney (K) seen as a well defined round anechoic lesion with thin smooth walls and clear fluid in the lower pole

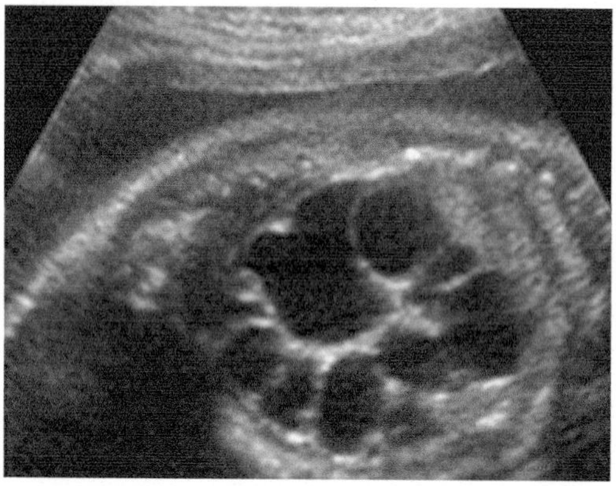

Figure 17: Coronal scan of multicystic dysplastic kidney demonstrating the variant appearance of the central and medial large cyst with peripheral cysts mimicking hydronephrosis due to pelviureteric junction obstruction. Differentiating features are varying size of peripheral cysts, lack of connection with the larger central cyst and absent parenchyma

one of the moieties in duplex kidney is to be ruled out by looking for continuity with ureter on coronal scan which is discussed and illustrted later.

- If the foregoing diagnoses are unlikely, then the inherited renal cystic disease should be considered. Knowledge of familial history is essential. If there is familial history of renal cystic disease, fetus with abnormal kidneys suggests recurrence of the disease. If there is no familial history, the fetuses could be categorized into two groups:
  1. Isolated renal finding.
  2. Those associated with other organ malformations.

Both categories of fetuses can be further divided into those with typical ultrasound patterns suggestive of specific diagnoses and those with atypical ultrasound patterns.

- A typical pattern means all sonographic features such as a typical pattern of cysts (size, location, number), appearance of the parenchyma (echogenicity, CMD), and renal size that leads to a straightforward specific diagnosis (isolated or associated with other malformations) like Autosomal Recessive Polycystic kidney disease (ARPKD). Nonspecific or atypical pattern means that no significant features are present that lead to a specific diagnosis and needs an approach with differential diagnosis tables. In rare cases, supplementary examinations, such as genetic studies and MRI may be necessary to reach the diagnosis.[18,19]
- Typical ultrasound patterns can be seen both as isolated findings and as polymalformative syndromes. Although the ultrasound findings are typical of these conditions, they need a genetic confirmation.

Renal Anomalies with Typical Ultrasound Pattern Seen as Isolated Findings

Autosomal Recessive Polycystic Kidney Disease (ARPKD)

ARPKD is the most common childhood ciliopathy with incidence of 1/20,000 live births. It is caused by mutation in the PKHD 1 gene. The extent of ARPKD can be variable and evolve over time. They are seen as a spectrum, depending on the time of manifestation and severity, as fetal, infantile and juvenile. Fetal type presents in second trimester as oligohydramnios. Both the kidneys are markedly enlarged (>4SD) and echogenic, filling almost the entire abdomen and even bulging out. There is no CMD with/without evident cysts **(Figure 19)**. The hyperechogenicity is due to the multiple interfaces of the dilated renal tubules. High frequency scan will show numerous tiny linear cysts. The urinary bladder will not be seen. The infantile type has similar features but manifests in the third trimester. The kidneys are seen as very large and echogenic with hyperechoic medullary pyramids and oligohydramnios. The rare less severe juvenile type, presents as slightly enlarged kidneys with enlarged echogenic pyramids (reverse CMD) **(Figure 20)**, normal urinary bladder and

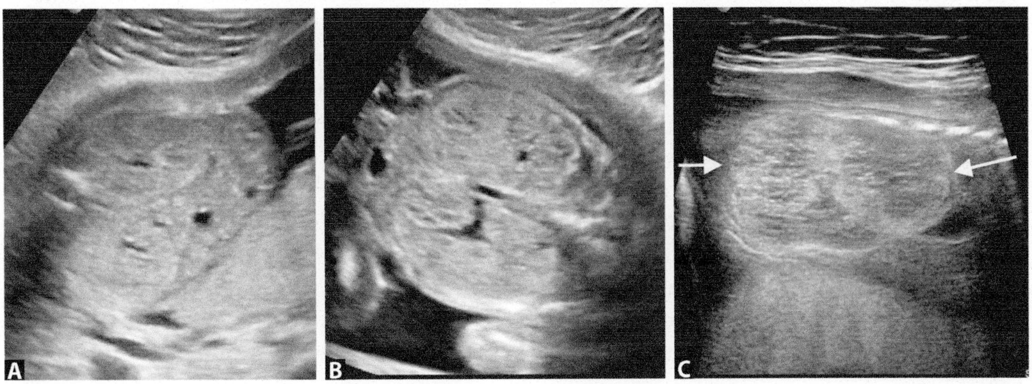

Figure 19: Autosomal recessive polycystic kidney: (A) Axial and (B) Coronal scan of the fetal abdomen demonstrating the markedly enlarged hyperechoic kidneys without CMD. There is oligohydramnios; (C) High frequency scan of the kidney (arrows) shows tiny linear cysts in medulla

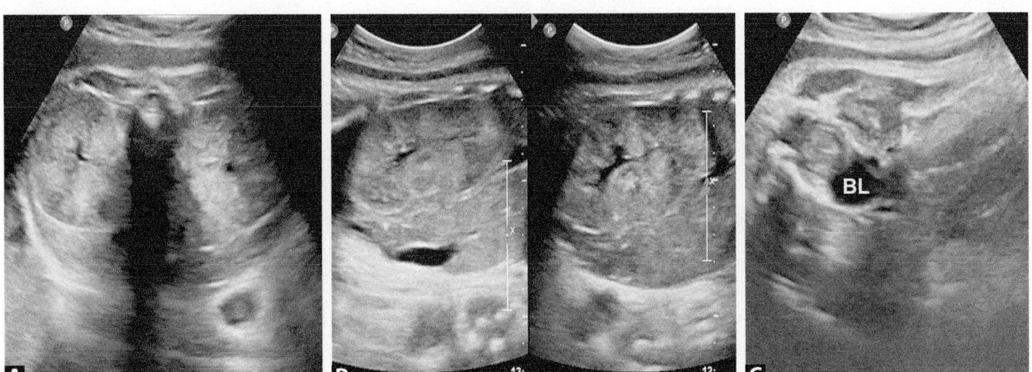

Figure 20: Juvenile autosomal recessive polycystic kidney in fetus of 35 weeks: (A) Axial and (B) Longitudinal scan demonstrating enlarged kidneys with enlarged echogenic pyramids (reverse CMD); (C) shows normal urinary bladder (BL)

normal amniotic fluid volume. The children with this type develop hepatic fibrosis in their later childhood.[15]

Glomerulocystic Kidney Disease (GCKD)

Fetus shows diffusely hyperechoic and enlarged (+2SD) kidneys without CMD but with multiple subcapsular cysts and additional cortical cysts **(Figure 21)**. The cysts develop in utero or postnatally. This condition has autosomal dominant transmission. The same pattern is seen in autosomal dominant polycystic kidney disease (ADPKD). The appearance should lead to scan of parents. The same pattern can be seen in HNF1B/TCF2 gene mutation. Besides producing renal cysts, TCF2 mutations express various other renal anomalies (renal agenesis, hypoplasia, horseshoe kidney, cystic dysplasia) and genital malformation. Because several TCF2 mutations can occur, the ultrasound findings of disease vary. Cysts can develop in the cortex (subcapsular), at the cortico medullary junction, or in the medulla. Detectable cysts can develop in utero or after birth. The cysts can be very large (more than several centimeters). TCF2 mutations can be confirmed only with knowledge of a familial history or results of genetic studies.[20-24]

Autosomal Dominant Polycystic Kidney Disease (ADPKD)

ADPKD affects about 1/1000 people. It is an important differential diagnosis of hyperechoic kidneys with increased CMD due to hyperechoic cortex with cortical cysts **(Figure 22)**. ADPKD affects the kidneys, liver, pancreas and macrovessels. Two mutations have been recognized PKD1 and PKD2.[25,26] PKD1 causes more renal disease. PKD2 causes extrarenal manifestations such as intracranial aneurysm. Only the renal involvement can be detected in utero, as renal cysts. The clue to the diagnosis is a familial history or detection of yet unknown familial disease with renal ultrasound of the parents and grandparents. ADPKD can resemble GCKD appearance.

Nephronophthisis

Nephronophthisis shows the fourth typical pattern where the kidneys are hyperechoic, normal sized or small and without CMD with renal cysts at the corticomedullary junction **(Figure 23)**. It is a group with autosomal

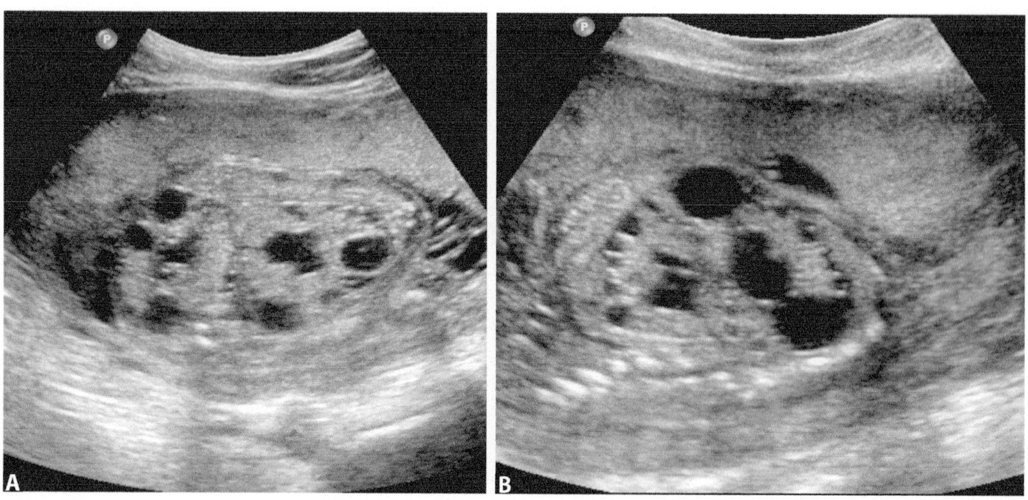

Figure 21: Glomerulocystic kidney disease: (A) Axial and (B) Longitudinal scans revealing enlarged hyperechoic kidneys without CMD with multiple cysts, some of them are subscapular

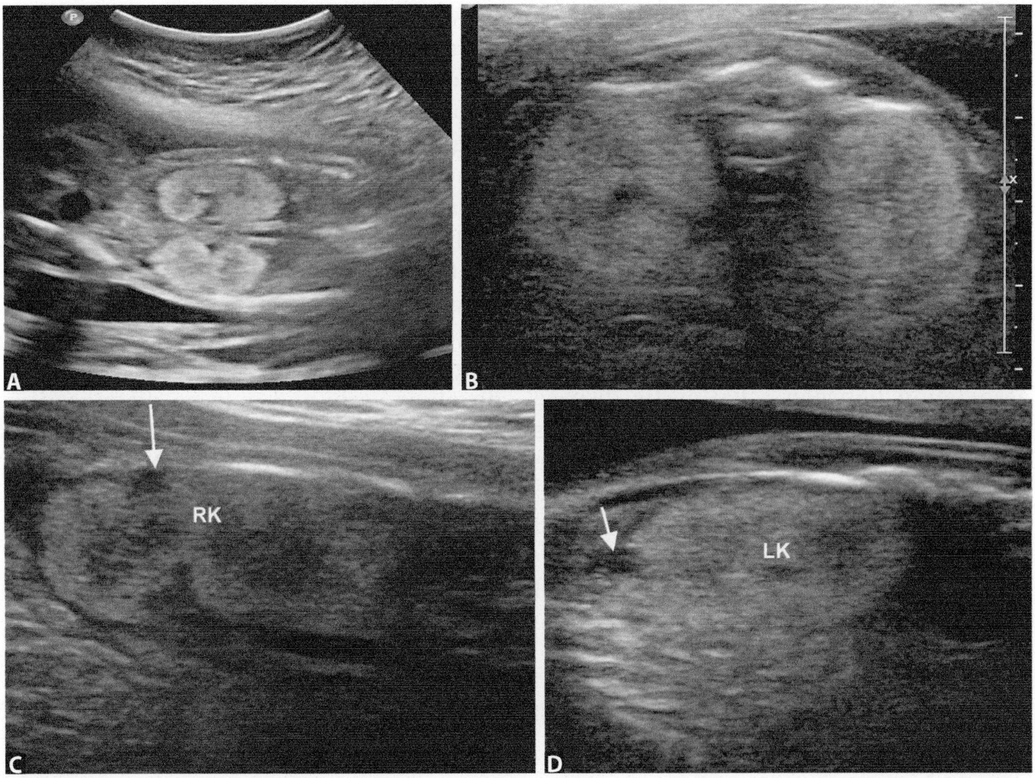

Figure 22: Autosomal dominant polycystic kidney: (A) Coronal scan demonstrating bilateral enlarged hyperechoic kidneys with increased CMD. High frequency axial; (B) and longitudinal (C&D) scan demonstrating the small cortical cysts (arrow) in both kidneys

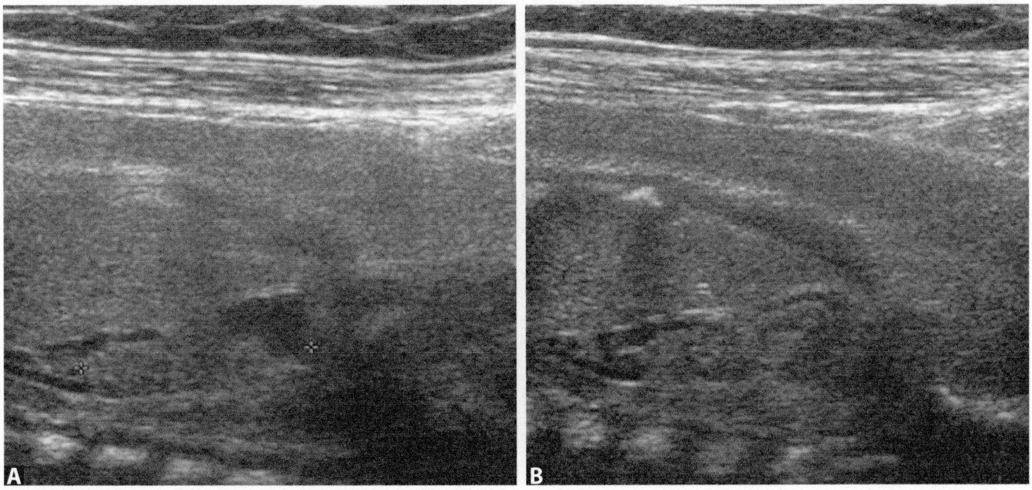

Figure 23: Nephronophthisis: High frequency scan of the kidneys reveal small echogenic kidneys with cysts

recessive inheritance. It can be diagnosed at any age. The same pattern can be seen in various syndromes.[27-29]

Renal Anomalies with Typical Ultrasound Pattern Seen as Polymalformative Syndromes

Renal cystic disease may be seen as part of some syndromes. When there are renal anomalies, complete survey of the fetus has to be performed to detect associated malformation in other organ systems. The association between renal cystic disease and malformations of other systems is found to be characteristic of a syndrome or association. In Bardet-Biedl syndrome (BBS), renal changes of markedly enlarged (>4SD) diffusely hyperechoic kidneys with loss of CMD are associated with postaxial polydactyly, hypogonadism, obesity and retinitis.[18] It is an autosomal recessive genetically heterogenous ciliopathy. The renal changes and polydactyly are seen prenatally **(Figure 24)**. Meckel-Gruber Syndrome is another autosomal recessive syndrome in which the kidneys are markedly enlarged (4SD) with enlarged hypoechoic medulla containing cysts associated with postaxial polydactyly and anomalies of central nervous system, more commonly encephalocele **(Figure 25)**.[30] The Meckel Gruber syndrome develops early and may be diagnosed in first trimester and renal medullary changes are more profound compared to BBS. The combinations of renal, hepatic and pancreatic dysplasia (RHPD) also known as Ivemark II syndrome, is very rare and uniformly fatal. The patterns of renal, hepatic and pancreatic

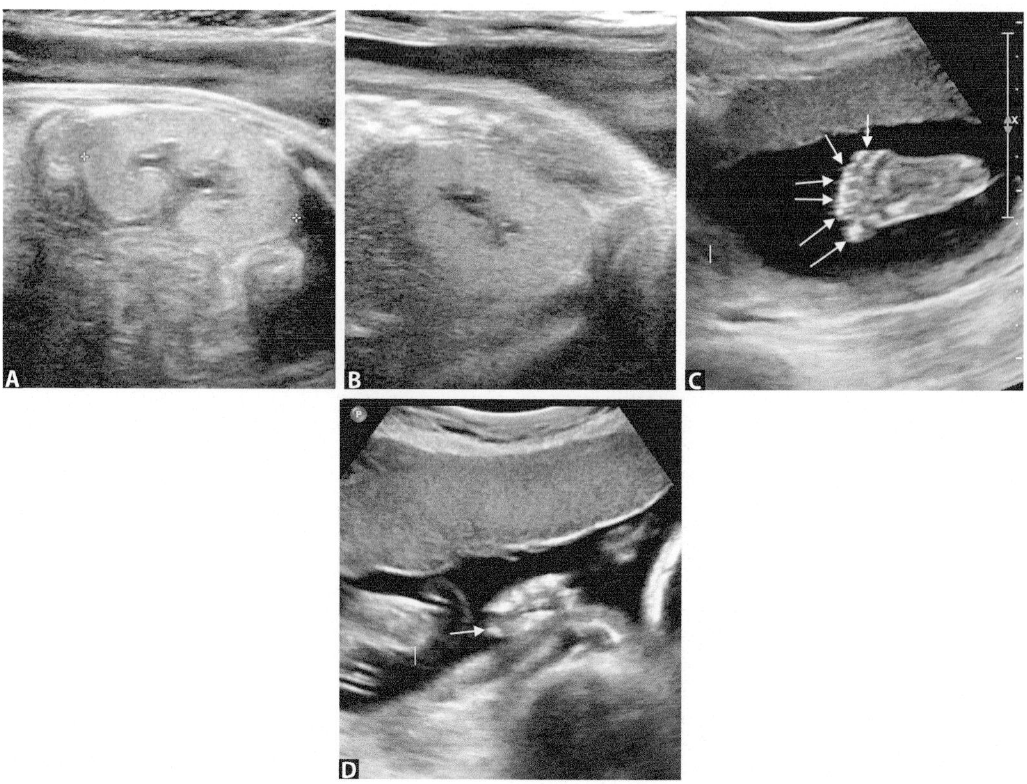

Figure 24: Bardet-Biedl syndrome: High frequency longitudinal scan of the kidneys ((A and B) demonstrating enlarged hyperechoic kidneys without CMD with polydactyly of foot (C) and hand (D)

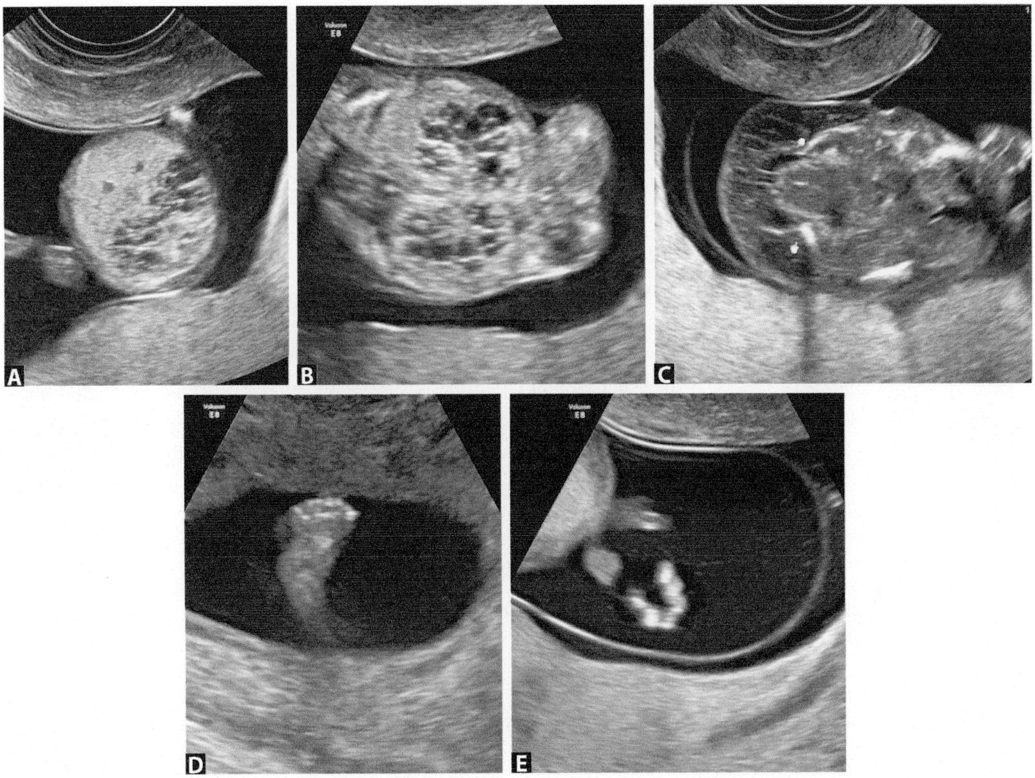

Figure 25: Meckel-Gruber system: (A) Axial and (B) Coronal scan demonstrating the bilateral markedly enlarged kidneys with enlarged hypoechoic medulla containing cysts associated with (C) encephalocele (pointing fingers) and polydactyly of foot (D) and hand (E)

involvement were indistinguishable from those reported in several other syndromes, including Jeune Asphyxiating Thoracic Dystrophy (JATD) and Ellis-Van Creveld syndrome (EVC). In the MIM system, RHPD is described along with autosomal recessive polycystic kidney disease. Renal hepatic pancreatic dysplasia (Ivemark II syndrome) shows renal cystic changes of glomerulocystic or medullary dysplasia type, hepatic dysplasia in the form of dilated bile ducts and pancreatic cysts **(Figure 26)**.[31]

Renal Anomalies with Atypical Ultrasound Pattern

1. Simple renal cyst.
2. Bilateral echogenic kidneys.

The incidence of this finding on prenatal sonography is increasing and becoming a challenge in differential diagnosis. The conditions which can present with this feature are as follows:

A. Renal cystic disease which has been discussed earlier.
B. Cytomegalovirus (CMV) infection: In CMV infection, the kidneys are either normal in size or slightly enlarged and echogenic. The corticomedullary differentiation is present **(Figure 27)**. The urinary bladder and amniotic fluid volume are normal. There may be other markers of CMV infection.[15,16]
C. Nephrotic syndrome—Finnish type
D. Medullary nephrocalcinosis **(Figure 28)**
E. Some trisomies.
F. Transient finding in normal fetuses: Echogenic kidneys of normal size, normal urinary bladder and normal amniotic fluid volume have good outcome and are usually normal.[15]

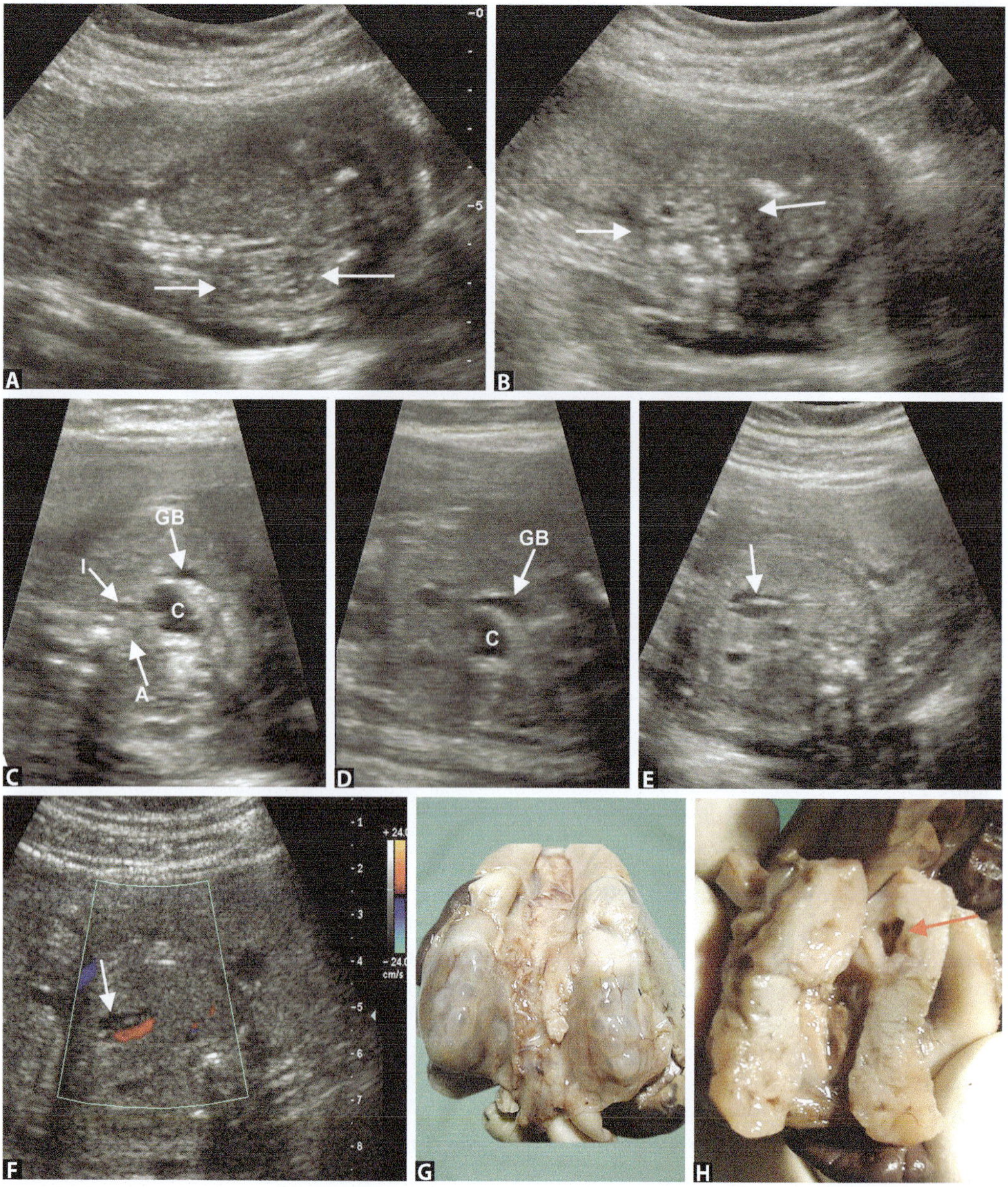

Figure 26: Renal hepatic pancreatic dysplasia: Longitudinal scan of the kidneys (arrows) showing multiple cysts in them (A) Left kidney; (B) Right kidney. Transverse; (C) and longitudinal; (D) scans of upper abdomen showing the pancreatic cyst (C) A—Aorta; GB—Gallbladder and I—Inferior vena cava; (E) Transverse scan of liver showing dilated right and left hepatic ducts (arrow) anterior to right and left branches of the portal vein; (F) Color Doppler scan of same section confirms blood flow in portal vein; (G) Autopsy picture of bilateral multicystic kidneys; (H) Autopsy picture of cut section of pancreas showing the irregular cyst in head of the pancreas

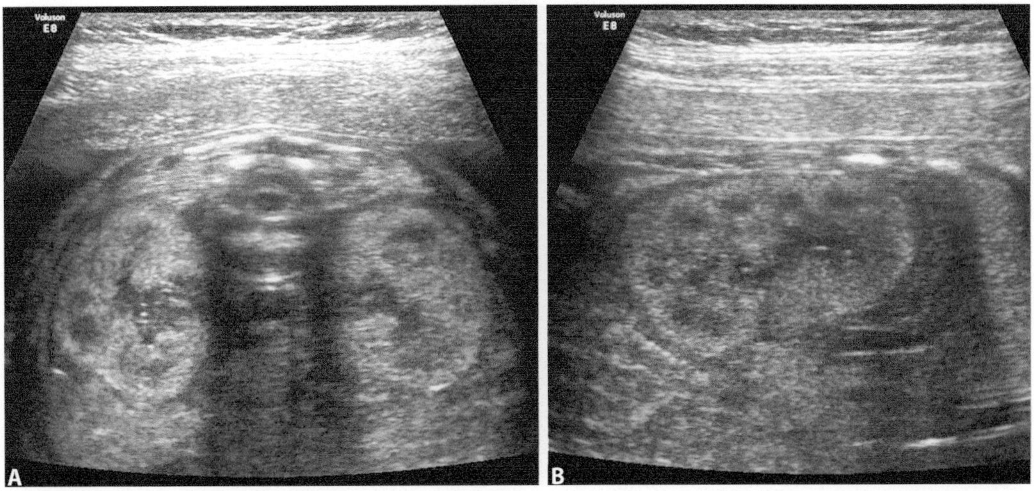

Figure 27: Cystomegalovirus (CMV) infection: High frequency (A) Axial and (B) longitudinal scan, demonstrating slightly enlarged echogenic kidneys with preserved CMD

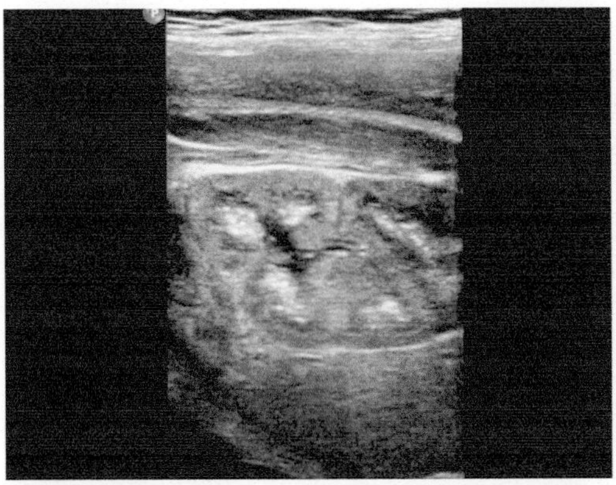

Figure 28: Medullary nephrocalcinosis: Longitudinal high frequency scan of the kidney shows bunches of small calcifications in the medullary pyramids

NONVISUALIZED KIDNEY

Unilateral Nonvisualized Kidney

On axial scan, one kidney may not be seen. A coronal or sagittal scan will confirm the same by showing elongated adrenal gland replacing the kidney (lying down adrenal sign). Rest of the fetal abdomen should be evaluated to look for an ectopic kidney. Unilateral nonvisualized kidney may be due to:

1. *Unilateral renal agenesis:* Unilateral renal agenesis is due to failure of development of ureteric bud. It is three to four times more common than bilateral renal agenesis (1 in 1000 newborn). The kidney is absent and an ectopic kidney is not seen **(Figure 29)**. The contralateral kidney can be enlarged due to compensatory hypertrophy and there is higher incidence of renal abnormalities like vesicoureteral reflux. Unilateral renal agenesis can be the main sign of many nonchromosomal syndromes the risk being 20 to 25%. The most common are Fraser syndrome and VACTERL association. The risk of chromosomal anomaly is low (<1%).[1]
2. *Unilateral ectopic kidney:* The incidence of renal ectopia varies between 1:500 and 1:1200. The kidney may be ectopic, low lumbar or presacral **(Figure 30)** in position. There is possibility of crossed renal ectopia with/without fusion where the ectopic kidney is located on the opposite side of the abdomen relative to its ureteral insertion into the bladder **(Figure 31)**. Crossed fused ectopia can have obstructive features. Ectopic kidney is identified by the morphology and the fluid-filled renal pelvis in the center.

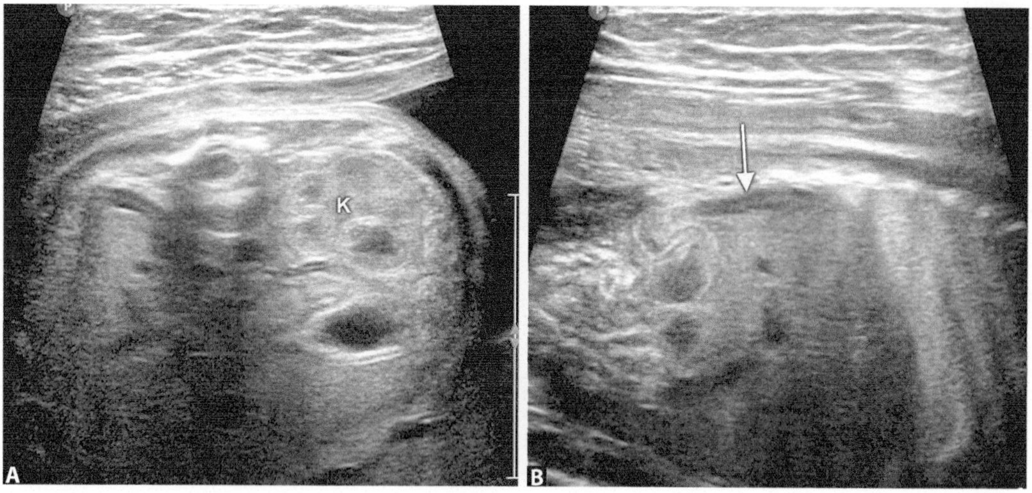

Figure 29: Unilateral renal agenesis: (A) Axial scan revealing the normal kidney (K) on one side and nonvisualized kidney on opposite side; (B) Longitudinal scan demonstrating the elongated adrenal (arrow) of lying down adrenal sign

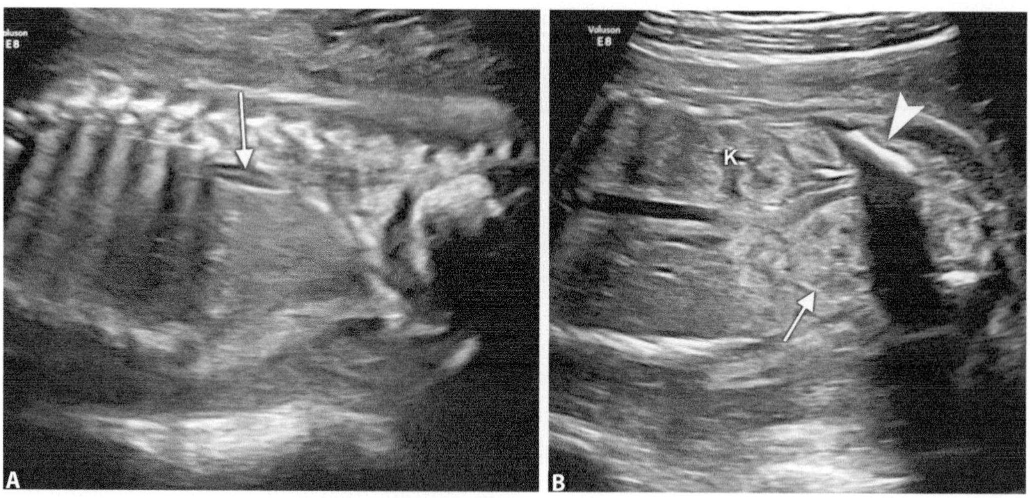

Figure 30: Ectopic presacral kidney: (A) Longitudinal scan of renal area showing the lying down adrenal sign(arrow); (B) Coronal scan of the fetal abdomen and pelvis behind the urinary bladder demonstrates the normally located kidney (K) and ectopic kidney in the pelvis (arrow). Arrowhead indicates iliac bone

Bilateral Nonvisualized Kidneys

When both kidneys are not seen in the renal fossa, it may be due to bilateral renal agenesis and bilateral ectopic kidneys.

1. Bilateral renal agenesis (BRA): It is a lethal congenital anomaly with an incidence of 1 in 4000 births. The ureteric bud fails to develop, nephrons do not form, and no urine is produced. The sonographic signs are anhydramnios and nonvisualization of kidneys and bladder **(Figure 32A)**. The lying down adrenal sign helps to confirm that the kidneys have not developed in the flank. The bowel or adrenal glands can be mistaken for kidneys. The image quality will be poor due to oligohydramnios.

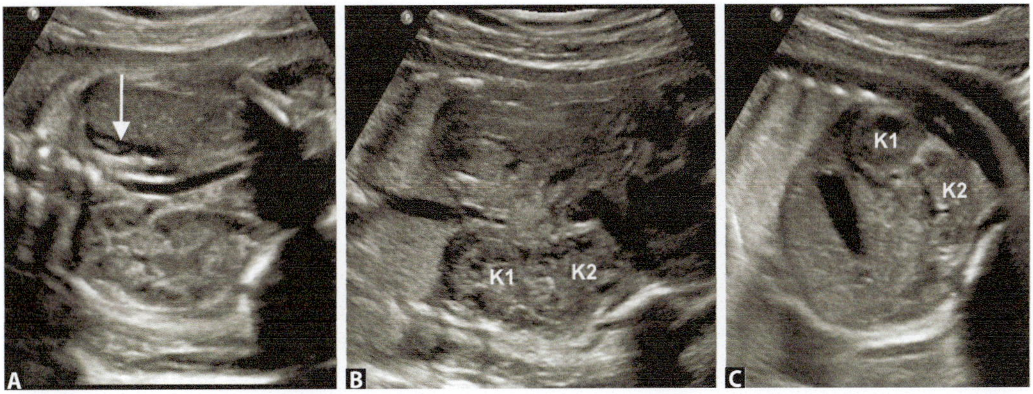

Figure 31: Crossed renal ectopia: Coronal scans of fetal abdomen showing the lying down adrenal sign (arrow) on one side (A); and both kidneys (K1 and K2) on the other side with fusion (B); (C) Oblique scan in another fetus shows crossed renal ectopia without fusion

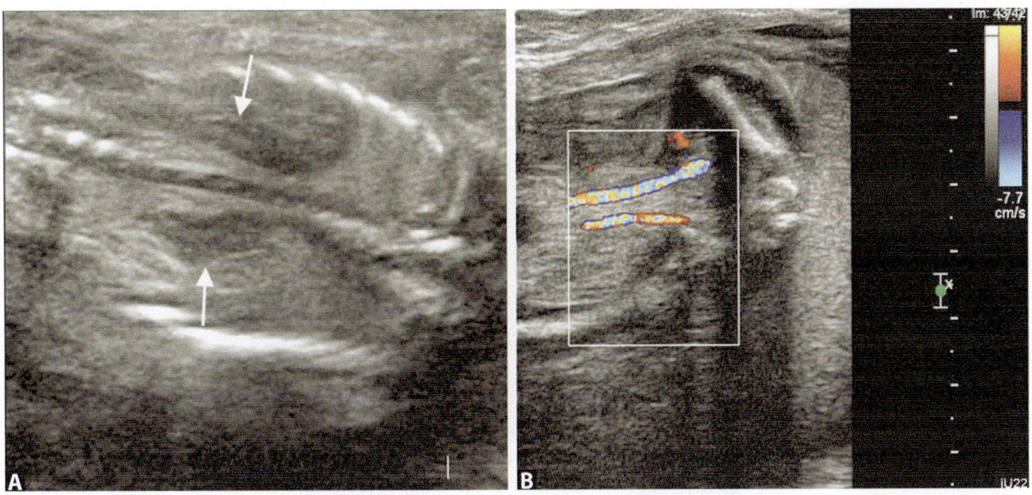

Figure 32: Bilateral renal agenesis: (A) Coronal scan of the fetal trunk demonstrates anhydramnios and bilateral lying down adrenal sign (arrows); (B) CDS of pelvis revealing the nonvisualized urinary bladder between the two umbilical arteries diagnostic of bilateral renal agenesis

High resolution scan using linear probe can be used to visualize the renal fossa better. If the fetus is in breech presentation, transvaginal scan can be used to visualize the renal fossa. Color Doppler study can be used to diagnose absent renal arteries and to confirm that the urinary bladder is not seen between the two umbilical arteries **(Figure 32B)**. If there is single umbilical artery along with bilateral renal agenesis and it is arising from abdominal aorta instead of iliac artery, it is aberrant vitelline artery. In such a situation sirenomelia has to be ruled out.[32] BRA may be a component of caudal regression syndrome.[1]

2. Bilateral ectopic kidneys: When both kidneys are not seen in the renal fossa but the bladder is seen, then the kidneys may be located ectopically in the pelvis close to bladder or iliac wing **(Figure 33)**. It may not be possible always to see the two ectopic kidneys separately, to differentiate

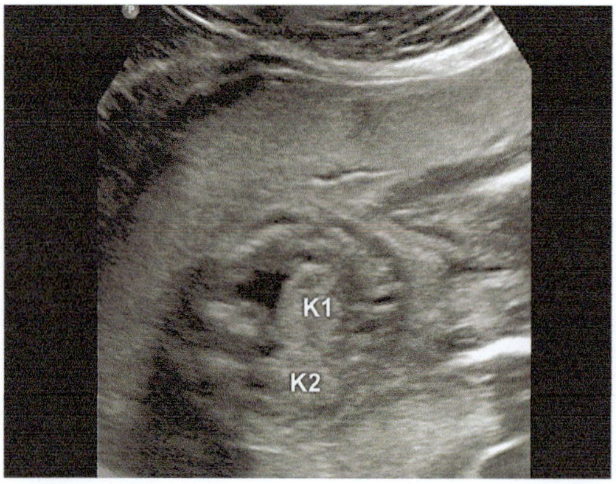

Figure 33: Bilateral ectopic kidneys: Oblique scan of fetal pelvis demonstrating both kidneys (K1 and K2) located ectopically in the pelvis

from unilateral ectopic kidney on one side and unilateral renal agenesis on the other side. The amniotic fluid volume is normal in bilateral ectopic kidneys or when at least one kidney is present.

UNILATERAL SMALLER KIDNEY

Unilateral smaller kidney may be due to horseshoe kidney, congenital hypoplasia or vesicoureteric reflux. Horseshoe kidney occurs in 1 in 400 to 500 births. The inferior poles of the kidneys are fused. It is considered when one kidney is smaller **(Figure 34A)** or when the orientation of the renal pelvis

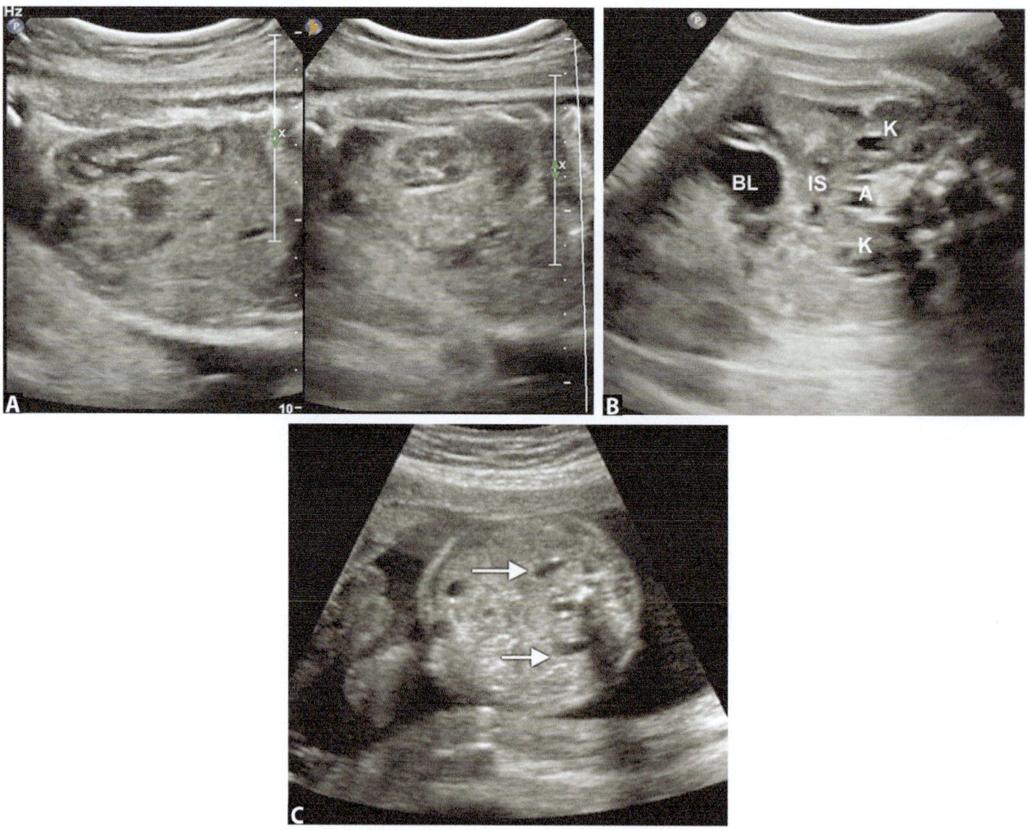

Figure 34: Horseshoe kidney: (A) Longitudinal scans of the kidneys reveals a smaller kidney on one side; (B) Oblique coronal scan demonstrates the isthmus (IS) anterior to aorta (A) connecting the two kidneys (K). BL—urinary bladder; (C) Axial scan of another fetus with horseshoe kidney shows the anteroposterior orientation of the renal pelvis of both kidneys (arrows)

is anteroposterior instead of the normal horizontally placed pelvis **(Figure 34C)**. Transverse and coronal scan will demonstrate the bridge of renal tissue (isthmus) connecting the lower poles of both kidneys **(Figure 34B)**.

HYDRONEPHROSIS

Pelviureteric junction (PUJ) obstruction: Most cases of PUJ obstruction are functional rather than fixed anatomic lesions. It is more common in males and is more often unilateral. There is dilatation of calyces and pelvis. On coronal scan, the peripheral dilated calyces communicate with the medial larger renal pelvis. The ureter and bladder are not dilated **(Figure 35A)**. The prognosis is dependent on parenchymal thickness **(Figure 35B)**, hyperechogenic parenchyma with/without cysts **(Figure 35C)**, anteroposterior diameter of renal pelvis **(Figure 35D)** and whether the renal pelvis is intrarenal or extrarenal. In intrarenal pelvis **(Figure 36)**, the parenchymal atrophy is seen early as the pressure is extended to the parenchyma, while in extrarenal pelvis, the renal pelvis can reach enormous proportion with good preservation of the parenchyma **(Figure 37)**. When the pelviureteric junction obstruction is bilateral **(Figure 38)**, the prognosis depends upon the severity, duration of obstruction and on amniotic fluid volume.

Hydroureteronephrosis

There is dilatation of calyces, pelvis and ureter. It may be unilateral and bilateral. The level of obstruction varies.

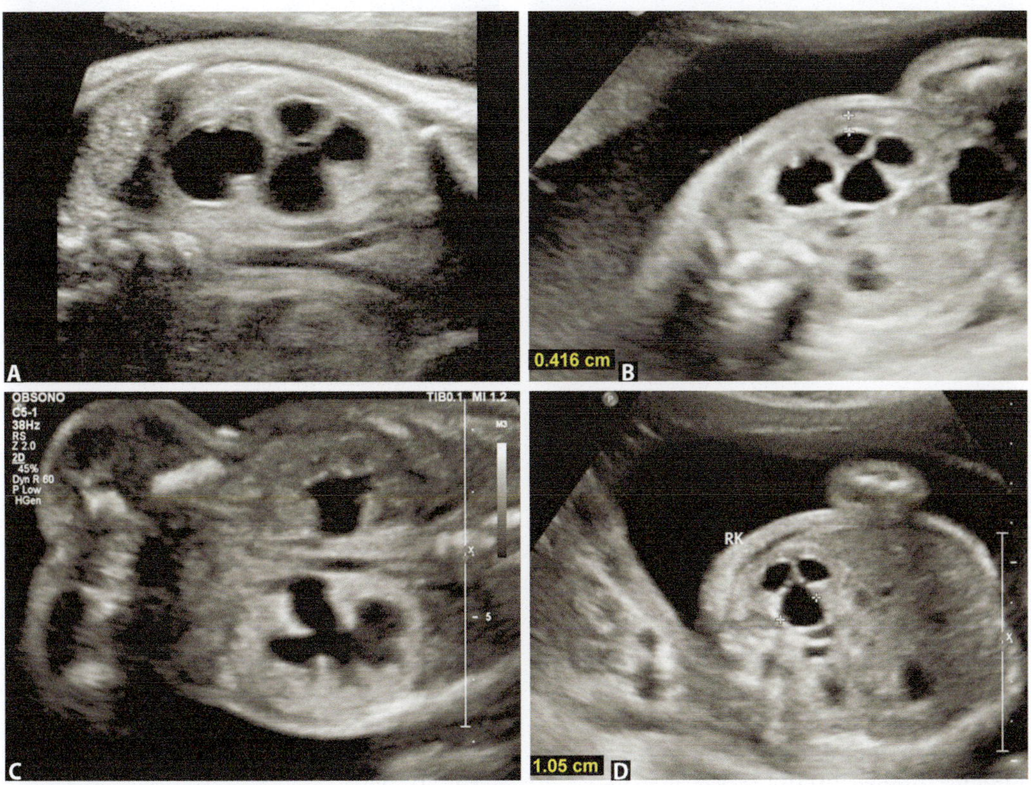

Figure 35: Pelviureteric junction (PUJ) obstruction: (A) Coronal scan of the kidney shows the peripheral symmetrically dilated calyces communicating with the dilated pelvis. The ureter is not dilated. Images showing thin parenchyma; (B) Echogenic parenchyma; (C) and measurement of APD (D) in PUJ obstruction

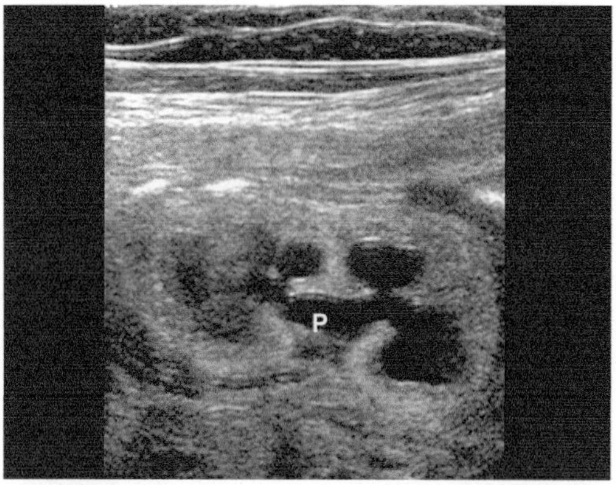

Figure 36: Coronal scan of a kidney with pelviureteric junction obstruction demonstrating a slightly dilated intrarenal pelvis (P) with echogenic parenchyma indicating dysplasia

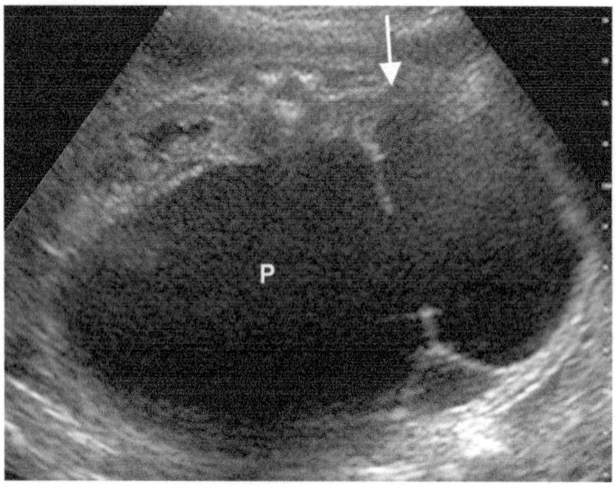

Figure 37: Axial scan demonstrating a grossly dilated extrarenal pelvis (P) filling most of the abdomen with well-preserved renal parenchyma (arrow)

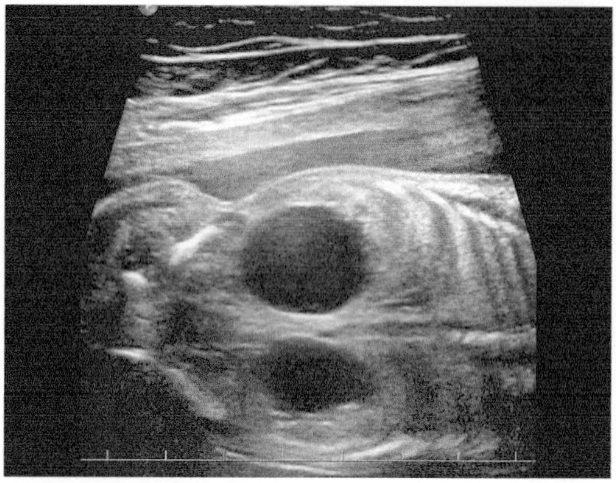

Figure 38: Coronal scan of fetal abdomen demonstrating bilateral pelviureteric junction obstruction

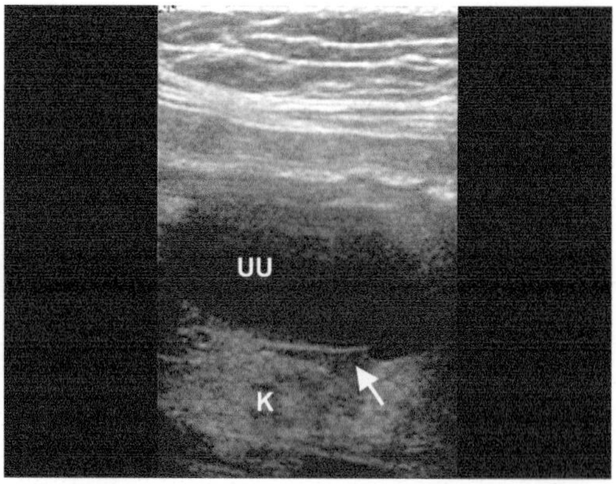

Figure 39: Ureteric Valve: Longitudinal scan showing the cystic dilatation of the upper ureter (UU) continuous with the slightly dilated renal pelvis (arrow). K; indicates the kidney

Unilateral Hydroureteronephrosis

Mid ureteric obstruction is due to ureteric valve. It is seen as a cystic dilatation of the proximal ureter with hydronephrosis. The renal pelvis is connected to the cystically dilated upper ureter **(Figure 39)**. This has to be differentiated from retroperitoneal lymph cyst which is multiseptated and displaces the kidney without hydronephrosis. When the ureteric dilatation is seen up to urinary bladder **(Figure 40)** the causes may be:

1. Primary obstructive mega ureter.
2. Vesicoureteric reflux.
3. Ureterocele.
4. Ectopic ureteric opening.

In the fetus, the primary obstructive mega ureter and vesicoureteric reflux cannot be usually differentiated. Occasionally in vesicoureteric reflux, the kidney is smaller and the collecting system shows intermittent dilatation, varying grades of dilatation over time or ureteric hyperperistalsis **(Figure 41)**. Vesicoureteric reflux can be associated with duplex collecting system with hydroureteronephrosis of lower moiety. Ureterocele is seen as a thin-walled cystic structure within the urinary bladder

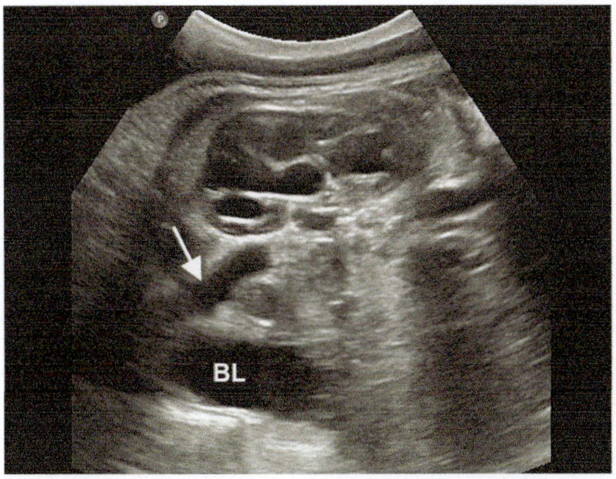

Figure 40: Hydroureteronephrosis: Oblique coronal scan demonstrating hydronephrosis of the kidney and dilated ureter (arrow) up to urinary bladder (BL)

(Figure 42). It is seen well when the bladder is partially full and can be overlooked when the bladder is empty or well distended. It is more often associated with duplex collecting system with hydroureteronephrosis of the upper moiety. Ureterocele collapses and distends over time and hence it may not be obvious all the time.

Ectopic Ureteric opening

The incidence of ureteric anomalies at autopsy is 2-3%. Ureteric ectopia is more common in females (70-90%) and is usually associated with duplication (80-90%).[33,34] In both sexes, the most common site of an

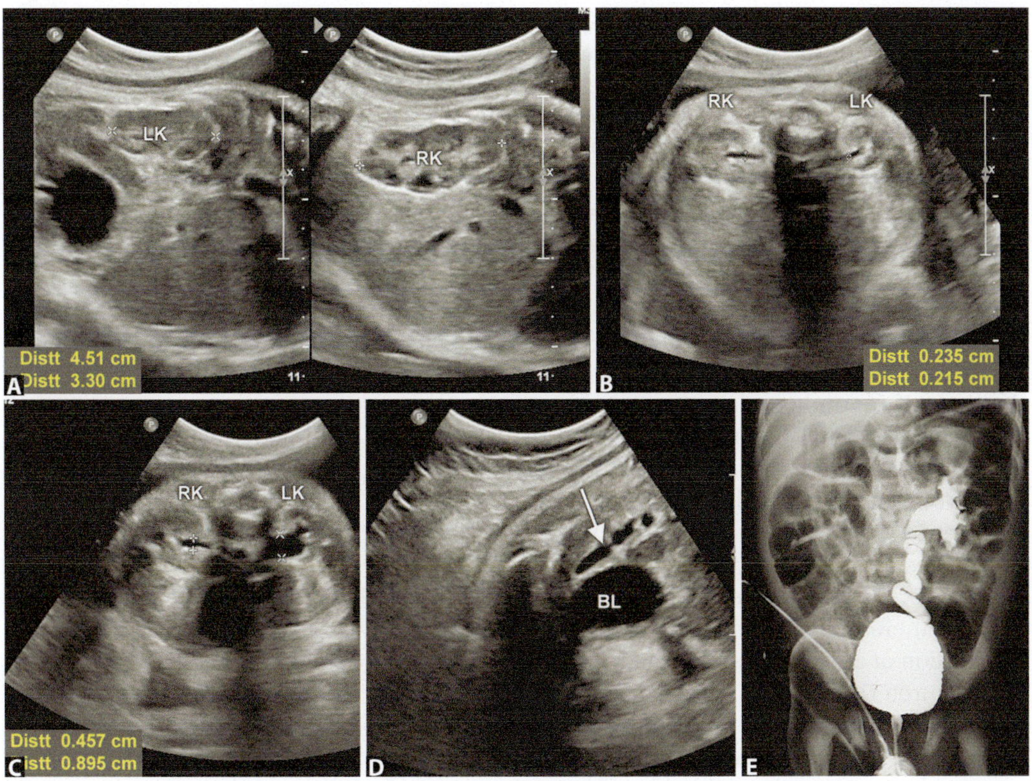

Figure 41: Vesicoureteric reflux: (A) Longitudinal scans showing the smaller left kidney (LK) compared to normal right kidney (RK). Axial scan at two different times shows normal left renal pelvis in (B) and dilated left renal pelvis in (C); (D) Oblique scan shows dilated left ureter (arrow). It showed hyperperistalsis; (E) Postnatal MCU shows the grade III vesicoureteric reflux on left side

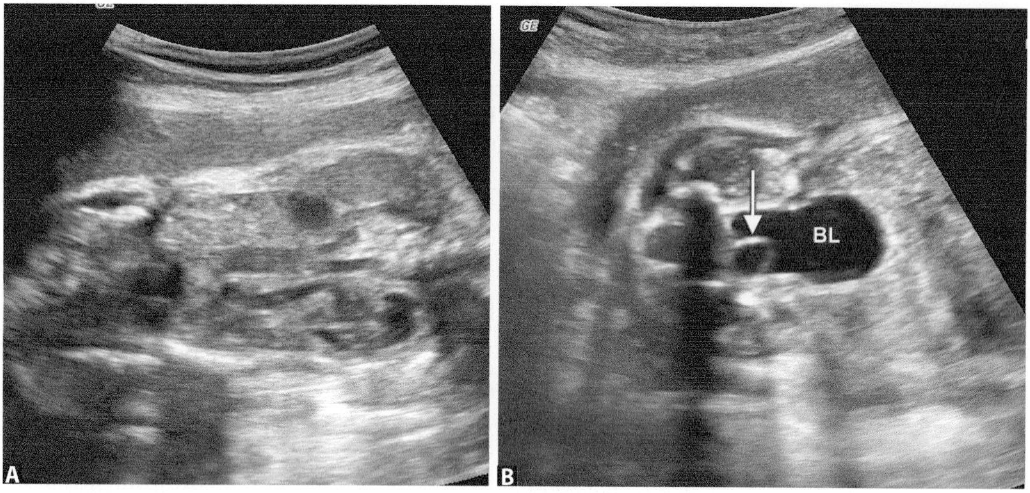

Figure 42: Ureterocele: (A) Coronal scan reveals hydroureteronephrosis; (B) Coronal scan of fetal pelvis demonstrates the ureterocele (arrow) within the urinary bladder (BL)

ectopic opening of the ureter is into the urethra. Other sites are the seminal vesicle, ejaculatory duct and vas deferens in males and the vagina and uterus in females. During normal development, the ureteric buds are incorporated into the urogenital sinus. This is followed by caudal movement of the mesonephric duct and cranial migration of the ureter, with the mesodermal tissue between them differentiating into the bladder neck and trigone. In ureteric ectopia, separation of the two orifices and cranial migration of the ureter do not occur. If it is bilateral, because of lack of appropriate stimuli, there is deficient development of the bladder neck and trigone.[35,36] Associated anomalies in males are agenesis or dysplasia of the kidney and agenesis or cysts of the seminal vesicles. In females, there can be uterine anomalies and duplication or atresia of the vagina. In case of ectopic ureteric opening, the dilated ureter is seen to extend low in the pelvis beyond the urinary bladder, indicating an ectopic opening below the urinary bladder **(Figure 43A)** which is seen better on fetal perineal sonography **(Figures 43B and C)**. On fetal perineal sonography real-time visualization of the continuity of ureteric peristalsis as a distension of the urethra, although rare, can confirm an ectopic ureteric opening into the urethra.[2] It is associated with duplex collecting system with hydroureteronephrosis of the upper moiety.

In hydronephrosis, the appearance of renal parenchyma is useful in predicting the prognosis of the function of that kidney. The echogenic parenchyma indicates dysplasia. There may be peripheral tiny cysts in obstructive dysplasia of the kidney.

Duplex Collecting System of Kidneys

Duplication of the collecting system results from division of the metanephric diverticulum or ureteric bud. They can be seen prenatally if one or both of the moieties are dilated. The two ureters may join together anywhere along their course or they may open separately into the urinary bladder or at ectopic location. The dilatation of the upper moiety is due to ureterocele **(Figure 44)** or ectopic ureteric opening **(Figure 45)** and dilatation of lower moiety is due to pelviureteric junction obstruction **(Figure 46)** or vesicoureteric reflux.

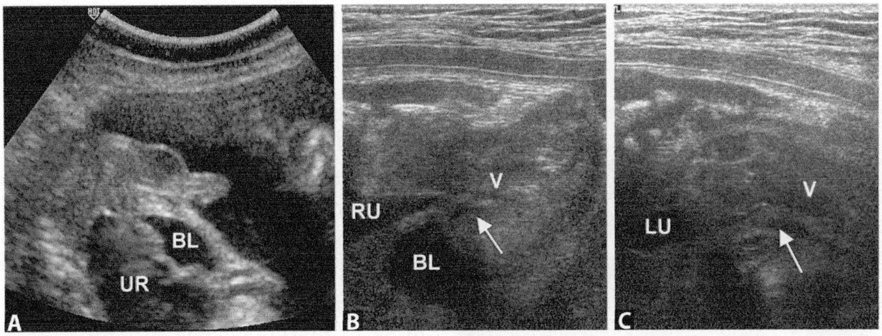

Figure 43: Ectopic ureteric opening:(A) Sagittal scan of fetal pelvis demonstrating the grossly dilated ureter (UR) extending beyond the urinary bladder (BL). Parasagittal perineal scan of the fetus with bilateral ectopic ureteric opening showing distal ends of the right ureter (UR) in A and the left ureter (UR) in B, extending beyond the urinary bladder (BL) and opening into urethra (arrow). V indicates vagina

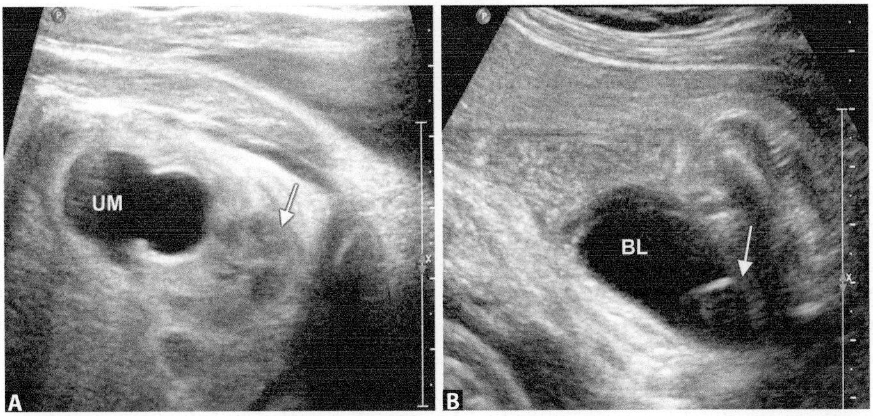

Figure 44: Duplex collecting system: (A) Longitudinal scan of the kidney shows duplex collecting system with hydronephrosis of upper moiety (UM) due to (B) ureterocele (arrow) in urinary bladder (BL)

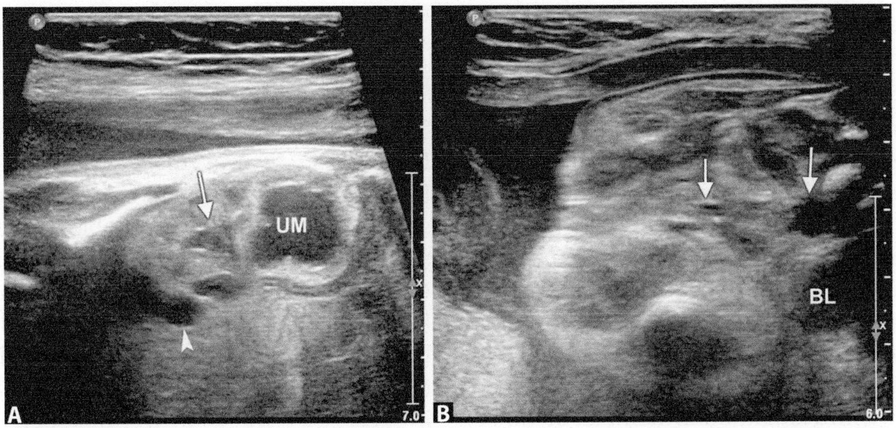

Figure 45: Duplex collecting system: (A) Longitudinal scan of the kidney shows duplex collecting system with hydroureteronephrosis of upper moiety (UM) and normal lower moiety (arrow). Arrowhead points the dilated ureter; (B) Fetal parasagittal perineal scan demonstrates the dilated upper moiety ureter (arrow) opening into the vagina

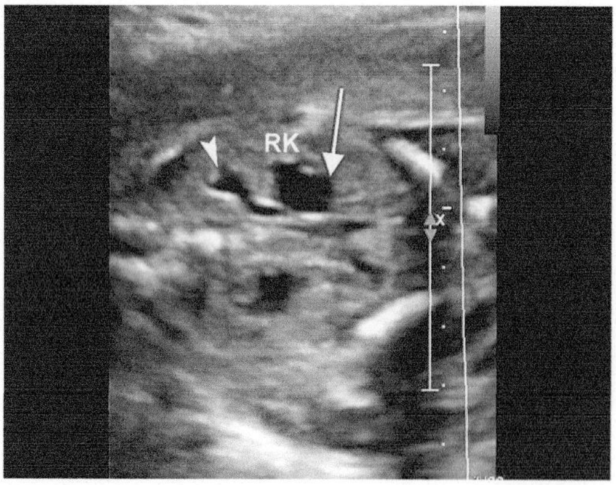

Figure 46: Duplex collecting system: Coronal scan of the right kidney demonstrates duplex collecting system with normal upper moiety (arrowhead). There is hydronephrosis of the lower moiety (arrow)

BILATERAL HYDROURETERONEPHROSIS

When bilateral hydroureteronephrosis is seen, the cause is either bilateral occurrence of conditions described for unilateral hydroureteronephrosis, where the urinary bladder can be normal, or urinary bladder outflow obstruction. In urinary bladder outflow obstruction, the urinary bladder is over distended with thick walls. The walls may be trabeculated, which is discussed and illustrted later.

MEGACYSTIS OR DILATED URINARY BLADDER

A dilated urinary bladder may be due to obstructive or nonobstructive conditions.[37] There is a definite measurement cut off in the first trimester to define dilated bladder. Beyond first trimester, there is no measurement cut off to define them. Megacystis is diagnosed if longitudinal diameter of urinary bladder is 7 mm or more in first trimester (11–14 weeks) **(Figures 47A and B)**. In 11–14 weeks fetuses with a longitudinal diameter of urinary bladder between 7 and 15 mm, 23% of them have a chromosomal anomaly which has to be ruled out. If the karyotyping is normal, the condition resolves in 90% of the fetuses. In the fetuses with longitudinal bladder diameter of more than 15 mm, risk of aneuploidy is only 10%. Fetuses in this group invariably progress to obstructive uropathy.[9] The urinary bladder is normally distensible with cycles of micturition. So it will be seen in varying degrees of distension during the time of scan. Assessment of dilatation of urinary bladder after 14 to 15 weeks is subjective and hence correlation with associated findings such as thickness and echogenicity or trabeculation of its walls **(Figures 47C and D)**, or presence of hydronephrosis indicating obstruction is necessary.[9] Rarely there may be patent urachus extending from the urinary bladder to umbilicus. There may be allantoic cyst in the umbilical cord.

Urethral Atresia

The onset of obstruction is early. So the dilatation of urinary bladder is gross, almost filling the abdomen and may protrude anteriorly. Usually, there is bilateral hydronephrosis with/without parenchymal dysplasia. The urethra is not dilated. The amniotic fluid volume may be normal before 18 weeks but there will be marked oligohydramnios or anhydramnios beyond this gestation **(Figure 48)**.

Posterior Urethral Valves

These are valves in posterior urethra in male fetuses causing varying degree of urinary bladder outflow obstruction. The prenatal sonographic findings are variable in degree of severity and time of manifestation from first to third trimester. The common presentation is with oligohydramnios. There is bilateral hydroureteronephrosis of varying degree **(Figures 49 and 50)**. The urinary bladder is over distended with thick echogenic walls. The posterior urethra is dilated with a key-hole appearance on coronal scan

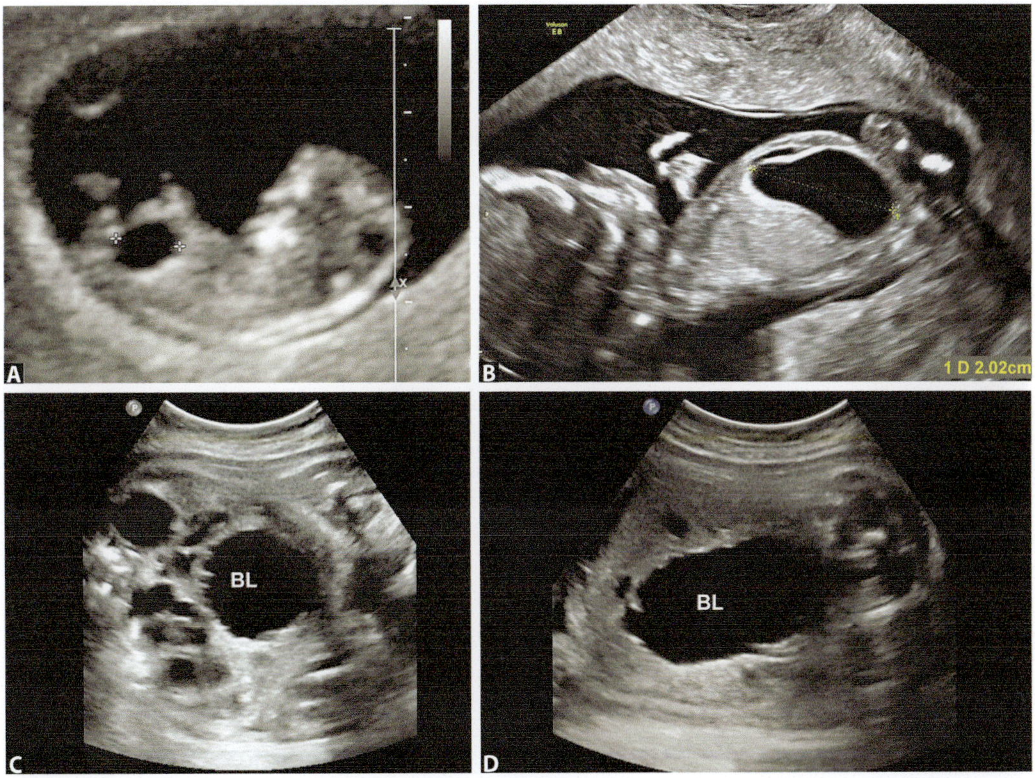

Figure 47: Megacystis: 1st trimester—Longitudinal scan of the fetus shows megacystis with (A) longitudinal diameter of the bladder between 7 to 15 mm, a marker for aneuploidy and (B) above 15 mm indicating obstruction. 2nd and 3rd trimester; (C) Axial; and (D) Coronal scan of pelvis showing over distended and trabeculated urinary bladder (BL) indicating urinary bladder outflow obstruction

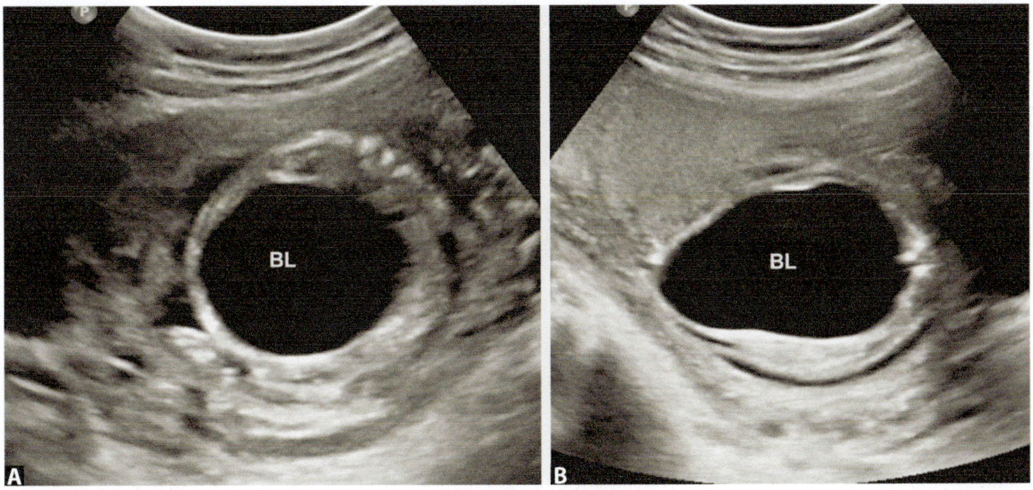

Figure 48: Urethral atresia: Axial (A) and coronal (B) scan of fetal pelvis reveals the markedly over distended urinary bladder (BL) with anhydramnios

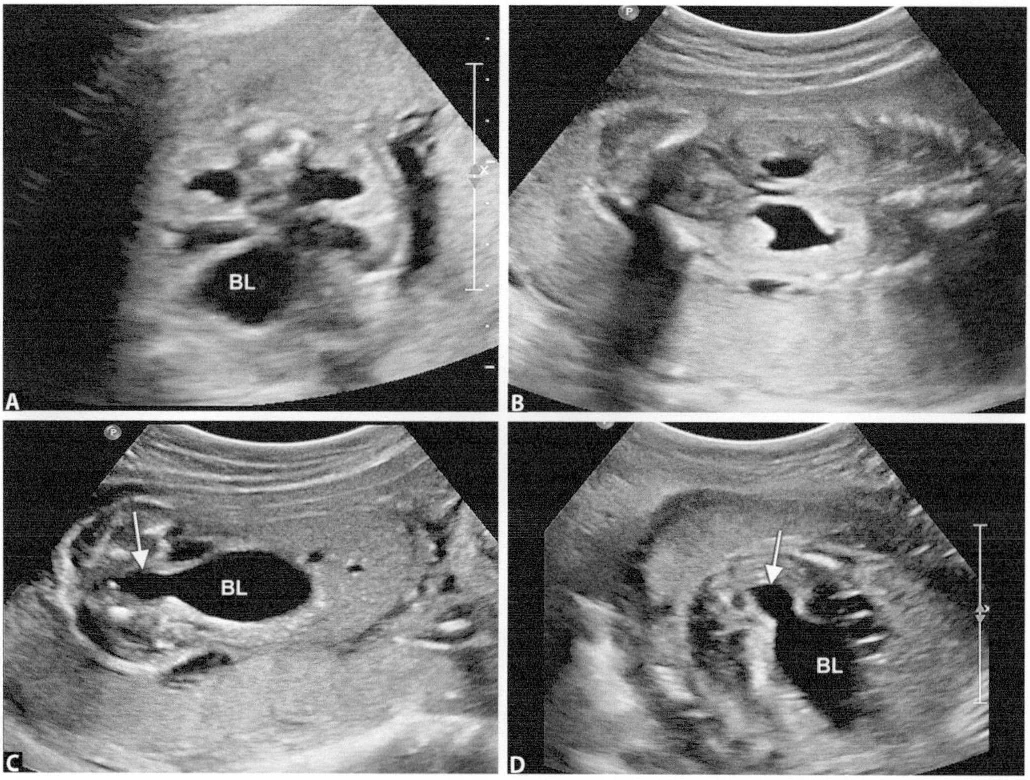

Figure 49: Posterior urethral valves: (A) Axial and (B) coronal scans showing bilateral hydronephrosis and dilated urinary bladder (BL); (C) coronal scan of the fetal pelvis shows the characteristic key hole appearance of dilated urinary bladder (BL) and the posterior urethra (arrow); (D) Sagittal scan of fetal pelvis and perineum demonstrates the cephalocaudal orientation of the dilated posterior urethra (arrow) stopping at root of penis

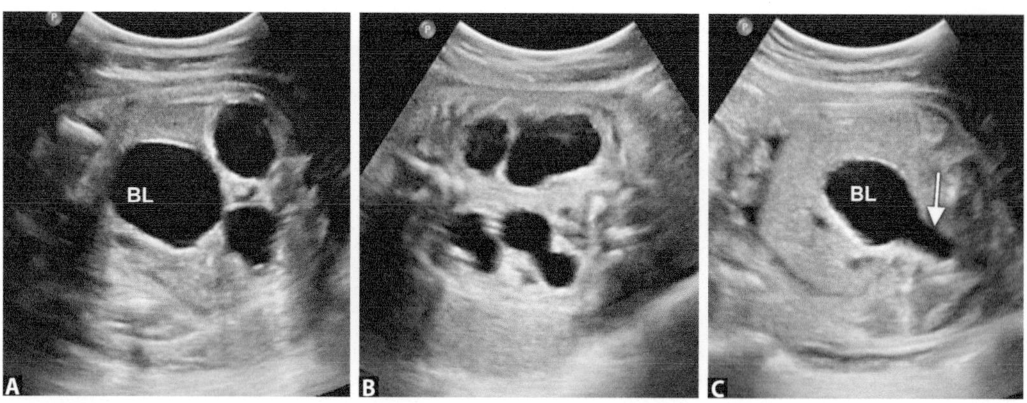

Figure 50: Posterior urethral valve: (A) Axial scan showing the gross bilateral hydronephrosis and dilated urinary bladder (BL); (B) Coronal scan of the kidneys showing bilateral gross hydronephrosis with thin echogenic parenchyma; (C) Coronal scan revealing the dilated urinary bladder (BL) and posterior urethra (arrow)

(Figure 49). In severe form, the renal parenchyma is echogenic with/without small peripheral cysts indicating dysplasia **(Figure 50)**. There may be perinephric urinoma due to rupture of a calyx **(Figure 51)** or urinary ascites due to a breach in urinary bladder **(Figure 52)**. The signs of bad prognosis are oligohydramnios, early manifestation, dysplastic parenchyma, perinephric urinoma and ascites. Sometimes, the posterior urethra is not dilated in resting state. It dilates only during fetal micturition. Hence when suspected a sonographic fetal micturating cystourethrogram (SFMCUG) is to be done. When fetus micturates, the posterior urethra dilates in posterior urethral valves **(Figure 53)**.[3]

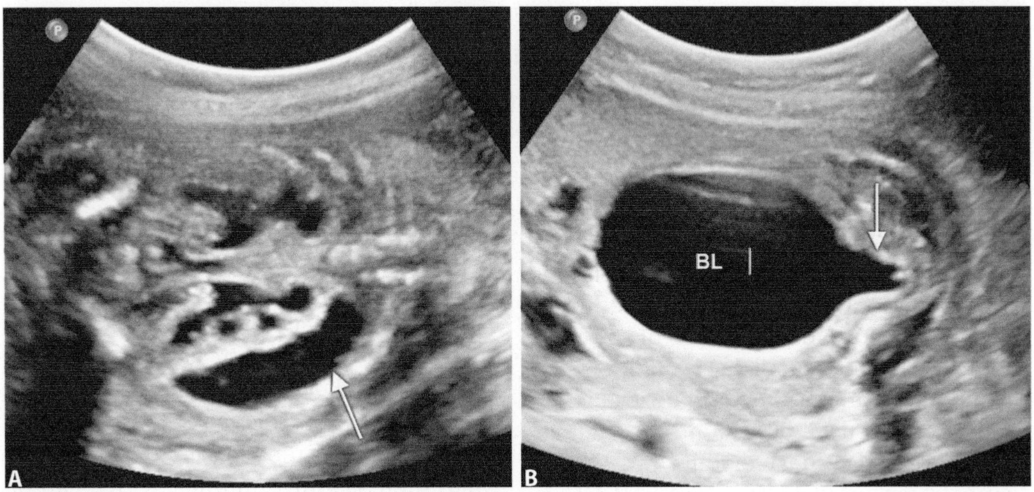

Figure 51: Urinoma: (A) Coronal scan of the kidneys shows bilateral hydronephrosis with a large perinephric urinoma on one side (arrows); (B) Coronal scan of dilated urinary bladder (BL) and posterior urethra (arrow head)

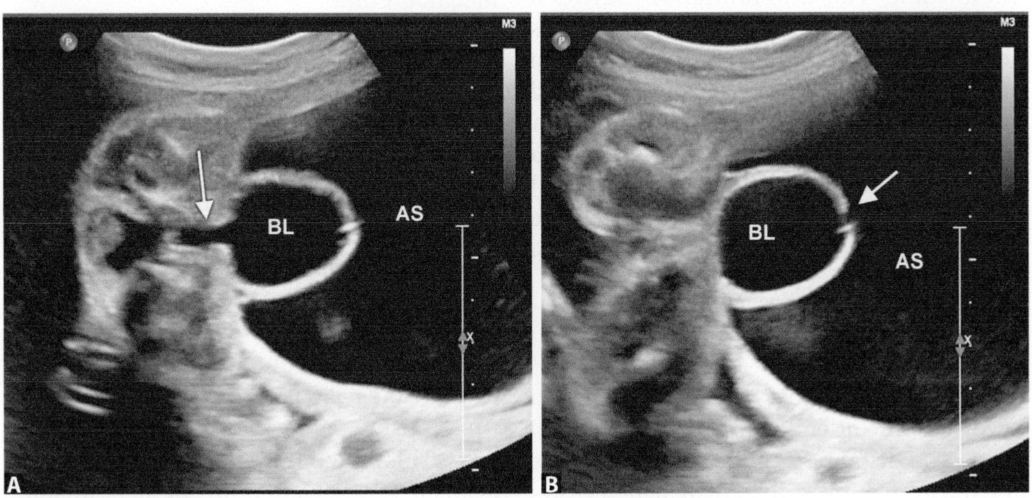

Figure 52: Urinary ascites: Coronal scan of fetal pelvis demonstrating dilated urinary bladder (BL), ascites and dilated posterior urethra (arrow) in (A) and breach in urinary bladder (arrow) in B

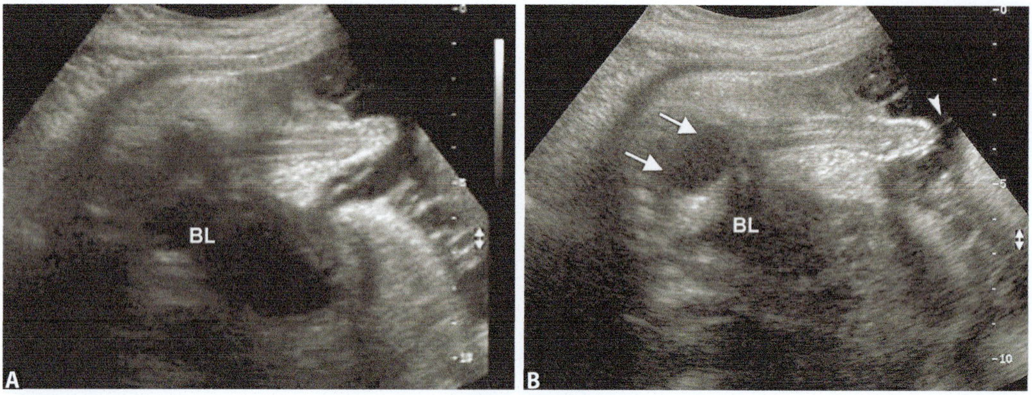

Figure 53: PUV: Fetal SMCUG—Sagittal scan of fetal perineum and pelvis revealing nondilated posterior urethra in resting state (A) and dilated posterior urethra (arrows) during fetal micturition (B). Arrow head demonstrates the stream of urine from tip of penis

Anterior Urethral Valves

This is a very rare condition, where there is obstruction to anterior or penile urethra in male fetuses. It is not clear if the obstruction is due to valves or a small diverticulum which fills up during micturition and obstructs the urethra. On prenatal ultrasound the findings of kidneys and urinary bladder are similar to posterior urethral valves. SFMCUG is necessary for the diagnosis as the anterior urethra is seen to distend only during fetal micturition. The differentiation between posterior and anterior urethral valves is possible only on mid sagittal scan of fetal pelvis showing the urinary bladder and urethra during fetal micturition. In posterior urethral valves, the dilated posterior urethra is cephalo-caudal in orientation **(Figure 53)** whereas in anterior urethral valve the dilatation extends to the horizontal portion up to mid shaft of penis **(Figure 54)**.

Anterior Urethral Atresia

Embryologically, most of the male urethra develops from the endoderm of the urogenital sinus. The distal part of the male urethra is derived from the glandular plate which grows inwards from the tip of the glans penis to meet the urethra derived from the urogenital sinus. Then it canalizes. When there is failure of canalization of the distal ectodermal origin of the urethra it results in anterior urethral atresia. The prenatal onset and sonographic features are similar to urethral atresia except that the fluid distended urethra is seen up to the tip of penis **(Figure 55)**. This can be mistaken for a vessel in a loop of umbilical cord, particularly when there is anhydramnios, which can be ruled out by Color Doppler study.

Megalourethra

Megalourethra is a rare form of functional lower obstructive uropathy characterized by a congenital deficiency of the mesodermal tissues of the phallus leading to a fusiform, or scaphoid dilatation of penile urethra.[38] There is no obstruction to the flow of urine. It may be isolated or associated with proximal urinary tract dilatation and oligohydramnios. In megalourethra, urinary tract dilatation develops as a result of urinary stasis in the dilated penile urethra, which lacks adequate support and balloons during fetal micturition, thus causing passive obstruction of urinary flow. This functional obstruction may also act as a valve like flap mechanism in some cases, producing intermittent mechanical obstruction to the urine stream through the

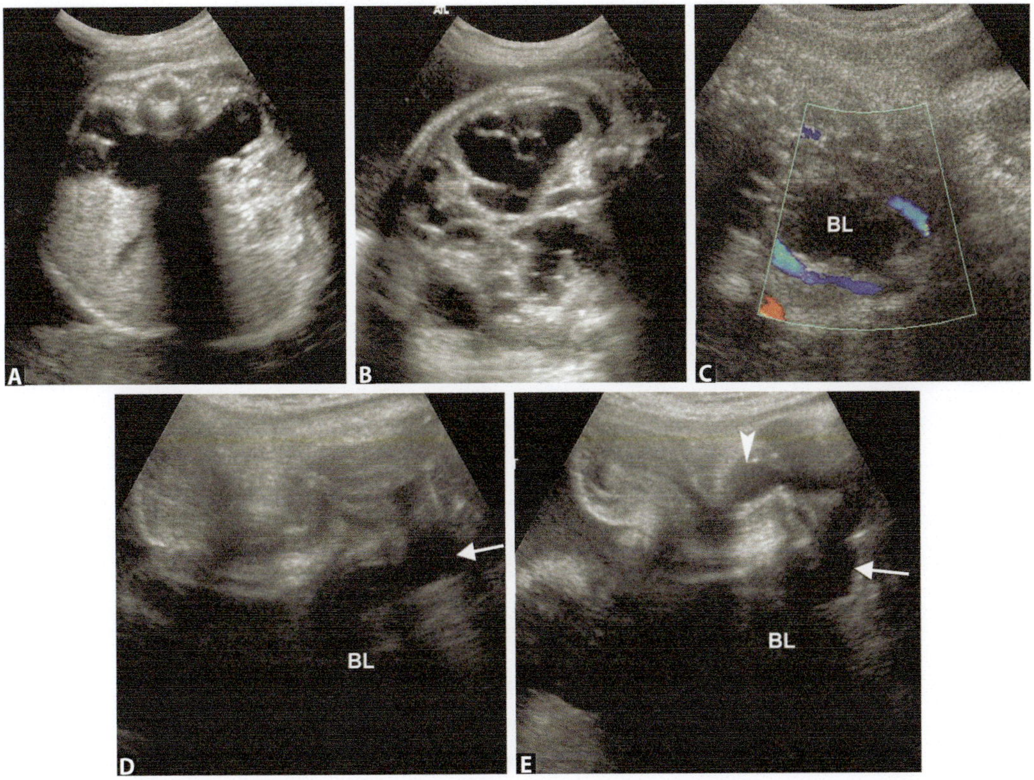

Figure 54: Anterior urethral valves: (A) Axial scan shows bilateral hydronephrosis; (B) Coronal scan demonstrates bilateral hydronephrosis and dilated ureters; (C) Coronal scan of fetal pelvis shows dilated thick-walled urinary bladder (BL) between the umbilical arteries; (D) Fetal perineal scan showing the dilated posterior urethra (arrow). The anterior urethra is not dilated; (E) Fetal SMCUG with fetal micturition: The anterior urethra (arrowhead) is dilated up to mid shaft of penis

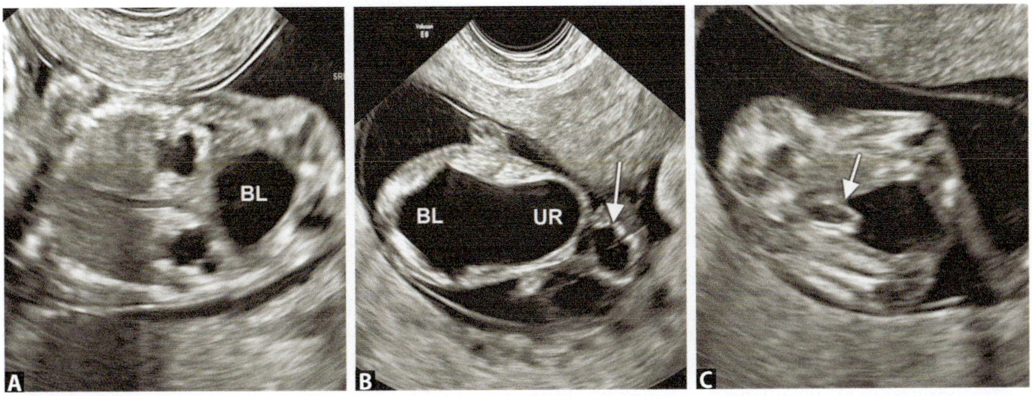

Figure 55: Anterior urethral atresia: (A) Coronal scan of fetal abdomen showing the bilateral hydronephrosis (arrows) and dilated urinary bladder (BL); (B) Oblique coronal scan of the fetal pelvis and cord insertion showing megacystis (BL), dilated urachus (UR) and allantoic cyst in the umbilical cord (arrow); (C) Scan of fetal perineum shows the penis with dilated anterior urethra (arrow) up to tip of penis

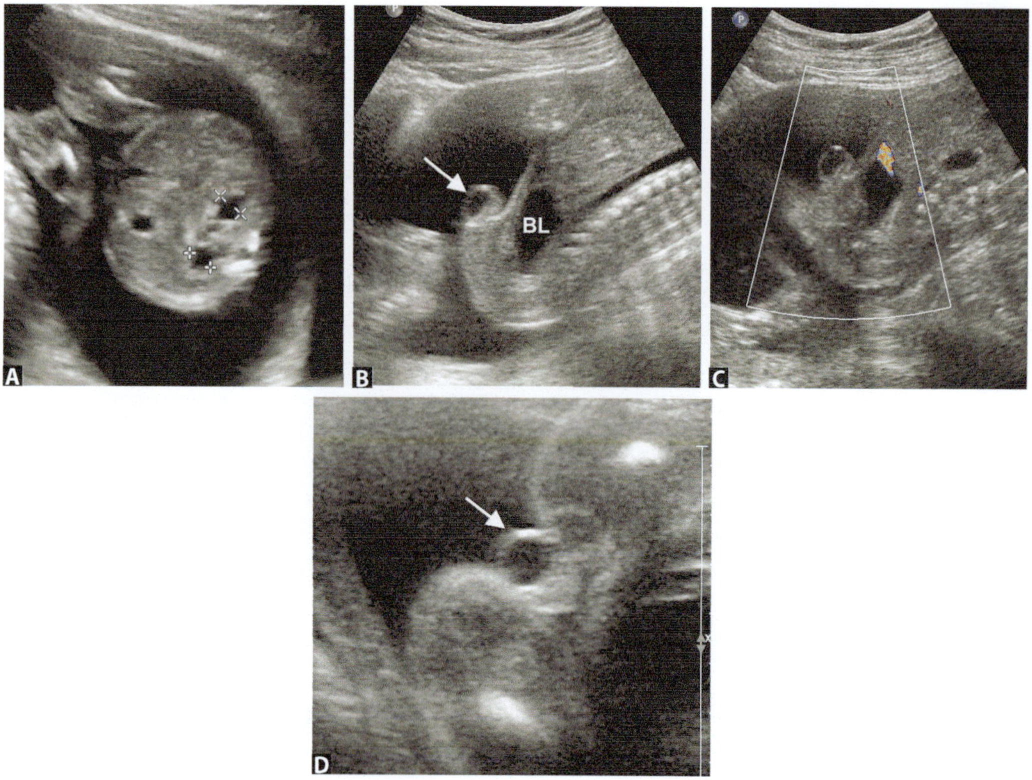

Figure 56: Megalourethra: (A) Axial scan of the fetal abdomen showing bilateral mild hydronephrosis; (B) Sagittal scan of the lower abdomen and perineum demonstrates the urinary bladder (BL) and scaphoid dilation of the penile urethra (arrow); (C) Color Doppler image shows absent flow in the urethra; (D) High frequency transverse scan of the penis demonstrates the dilated penile urethra (arrow) and absent corpus spongiosum

glandular urethra. Although severe narrowing of the meatus may cause complete anatomic urethral obstruction, no true anatomic obstructive defect has been indentified in cases of megalourethra.[38,39] Megalourethra is also associated with an exceedingly high rate of other congenital anomalies, frequently involving the gastrointestinal tract and spine. The long-term prognosis of cases of megalouretrhra is poor. Survivors are at risk of renal insufficiency, impotence and infertility, although most perinatal mortality associated with megalourethra is due to associated extraurinary malformation.[40] The confident prenatal diagnosis of megalourethra is established by the documentation of scaphoid dilatation of the penile urethra **(Figure 56)**. Color Doppler sonography is also used to rule out the presence of a loop or cyst of the umbilical cord, which can be mistaken as the dilated urethra. The differential diagnosis of the condition is anterior urethral atresia, where there is total obstruction with obstructive signs and severe oligohydramnios or anhydramnios. The dilated anterior urethra is tubular in anterior urethral atresia **(Figure 55)** in contrast to the scaphoid dilatation in megalourethra.

Megacystis Microcolon Intestinal Hypoperistalsis Syndrome (MMIHS)

Megacystis microcolon intestinal hypoperistalsis syndrome or Berdon syndrome, is a

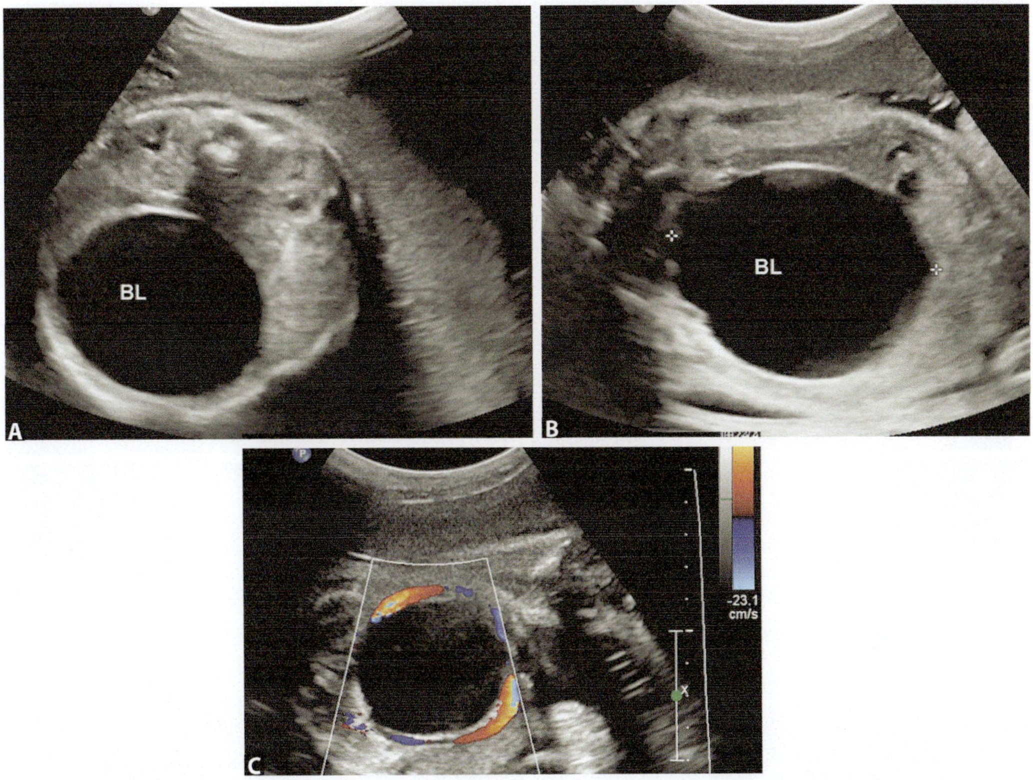

Figure 57: Megacystis microcolon intestinal hypoperistalsis: (A) Axial scan showing normal kidneys and overdistended urinary bladder (BL); (B) Coronal scan of overdistended urinary bladder; (C) Color Doppler study showing umbilical arteries skirting the urinary bladder. There was polyhydramnios. BL—urinary bladder

rare congenital autosomal recessive condition that is characterized by nonobstructive bladder distention, hydronephrosis, hydroureter, intestinal hypoperistalsis and microcolon.[41,42] The intestines are poorly developed, stenotic or atretic. In these cases, the amniotic fluid volume is normal or increased. MMIHS has a 4:1 female to male ratio.[42] On sonography, there is megacystis with mild hydronephrosis with normal or increased amniotic fluid volume **(Figure 57)**.

Megacystis Megaureter Complex

This is an association of large capacity thin walled urinary bladder and bilateral hydroureteronephrosis due to massive vesicoureteric reflux with normal amniotic fluid **(Figure 58)**. There may be hyperperistalsis of ureters. SFMCUG will reveal that the urethra and micturition are normal ruling out urinary bladder outflow obstruction **(Figure 58D)**. This condition is due to bilateral gross vesicoureteric reflux.

Prune Belly Syndrome

Prune Belly syndrome is a very rare congenital condition where there is aplasia of the detrusor muscles resulting in grossly dilated urinary bladder which stretches the anterior abdominal wall leading to secondary atrophy of the muscles of abdominal wall.[43,44] About 97% of cases occur in male fetuses. Postnatally when the urinary bladder collapses the abdominal wall reveals wrinkles resembling the prune fruit. On prenatal scan, there is grossly over distended urinary bladder with

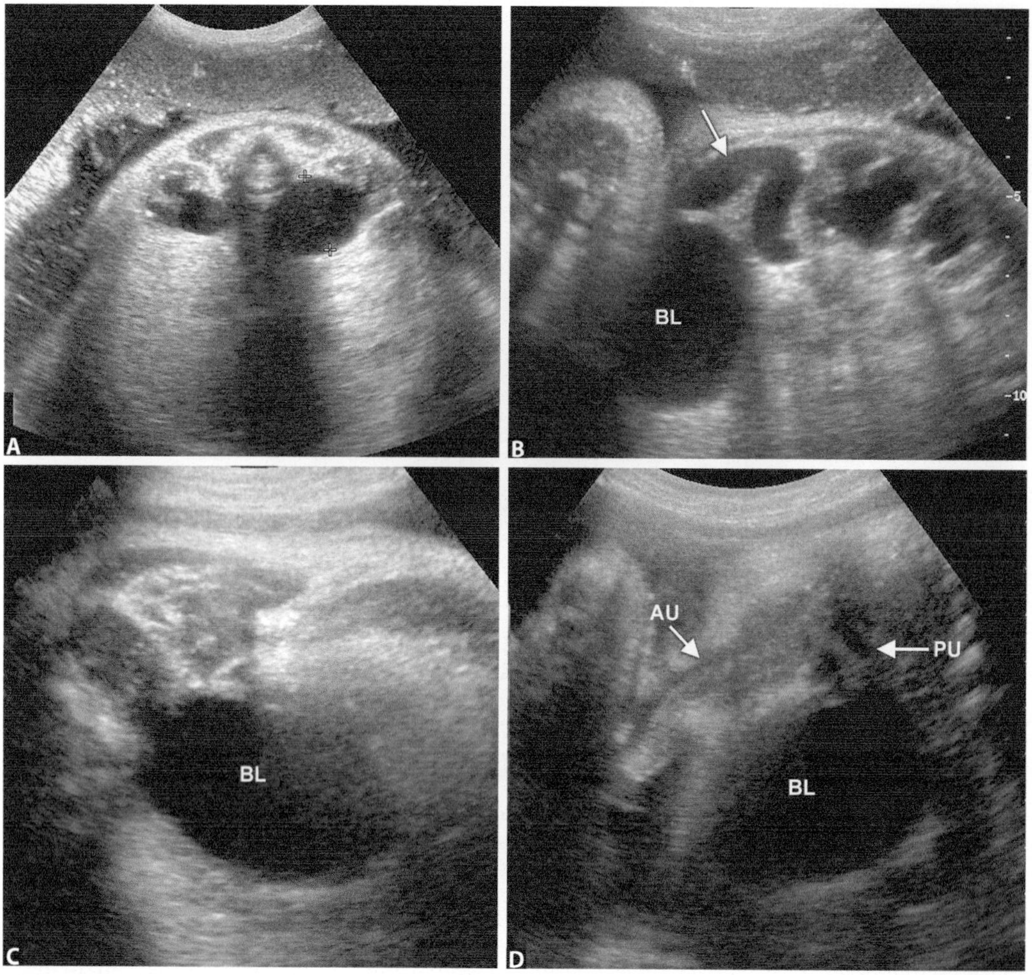

Figure 58: Megacystis megaureter complex: (A) Axial scan shows bilateral hydronephrosis; (B) Oblique scan shows dilated tortuous ureter (arrow); (C) Coronal scan of fetal pelvis showing the megacystis; (D) Fetal SMCUG shows slightly distended normal urethra. BL—urinary bladder AU—anterior urethra PU—posterior urethra. Postnatal MCU revealed bilateral gross vesicoureteric Reflux

bulging thin anterior abdominal. The thin anterior abdominal wall differentiates this condition from urethral atresia where the abdominal wall is thick **(Figures 59 and 55)**.

Rarely, there may be transient megacystis in third trimester without any other associated features and normal amniotic fluid volume. Postnatally, these newborns do well spontaneously or with an indwelling catheter of a few days.

Nonvisualized Urinary Bladder

When urinary bladder is not visualized, scan should be repeated a few times, since it may be physiological due to emptying cycles of fetal micturition. Nonvisualized urinary bladder is confirmed by the narrow space between the umbilical arteries on color Doppler study **(Figures 13B, 32B, 60D and 61C)**. If there is persistent nonvisualization,

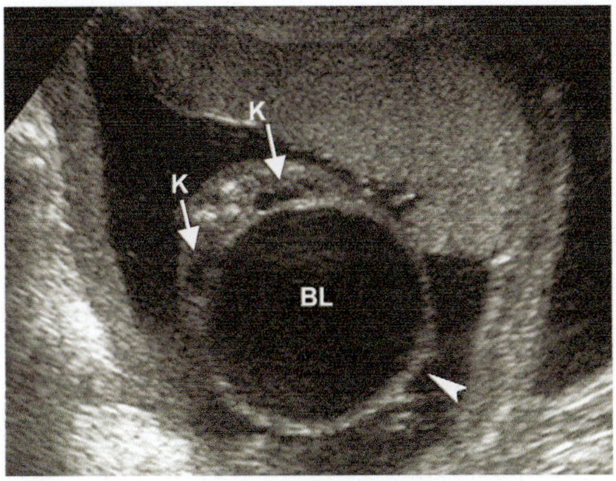

Figure 59: Prune Belly syndrome: Axial scan of fetal abdomen demonstrating bilateral hydronephrosis (arrows) and markedly overdistended urinary bladder (BL) completely filling the abdomen and bulging the anterior abdominal wall. The combined urinary bladder wall and anterior abdominal wall is extremely thin (arrowhead). There is Oligohydramnios

amniotic fluid volume has to be assessed. Nonvisualized urinary bladder with oligohydramnios/anhydramnios should lead to imaging of the fetal kidneys. The pathological conditions causing this may be bilateral renal agenesis, bilateral severe obstruction or bilateral cystic renal diseases which have been discussed already. The urinary bladder is persistently nonvisualized in rare conditions of renal tubular dysgenesis (RTD) and extrophy of urinary bladder.

Renal Tubular Dysgenesis

RTD is a rare autosomal recessive condition with severe disorder of renal tubular development characterized by early onset and persistent fetal anuria leading to severe

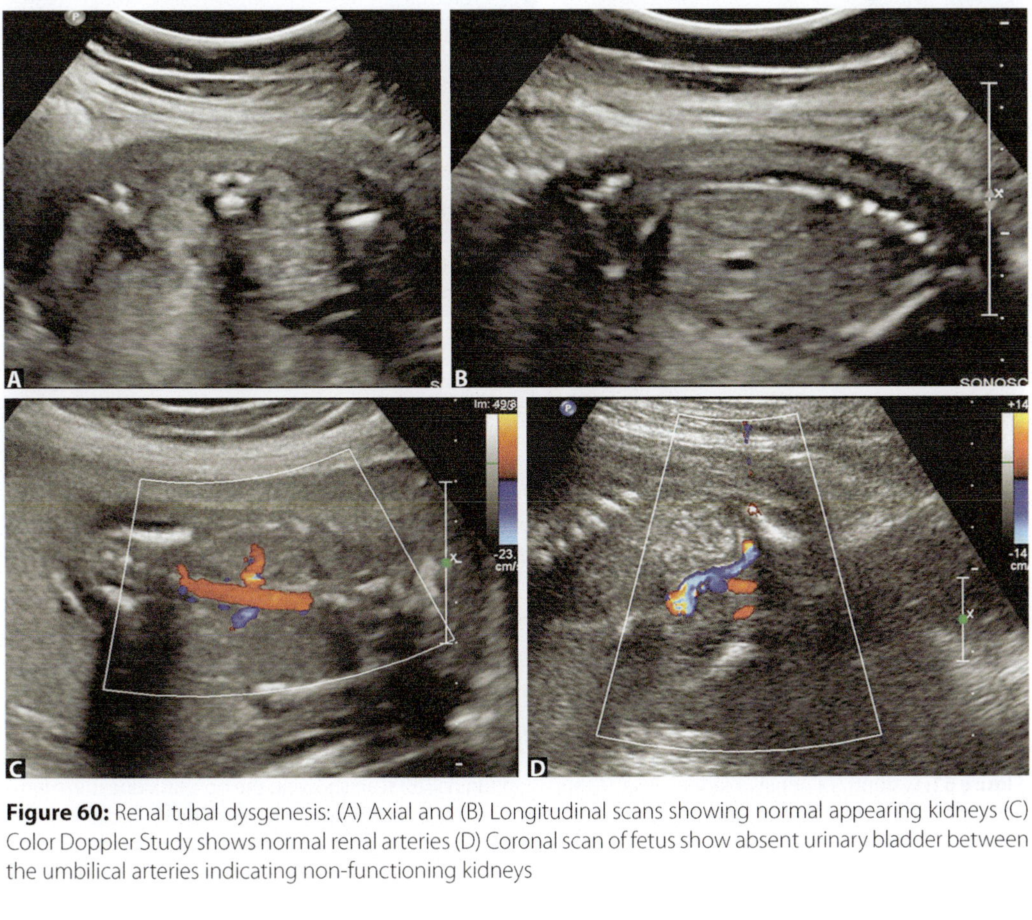

Figure 60: Renal tubal dysgenesis: (A) Axial and (B) Longitudinal scans showing normal appearing kidneys (C) Color Doppler Study shows normal renal arteries (D) Coronal scan of fetus show absent urinary bladder between the umbilical arteries indicating non-functioning kidneys

oligohydramnios. The disease is genetically heterogeneous and linked to mutation in the genes encoding any of the components of the renin angiotensin system (RAS).[45] It can manifest from as early as 20–22 weeks with oligohydramnios. Ultrasound shows normal kidneys or mild hyperechogenicity, poor corticomedullary differentiation (CMD) or moderate oligohydramnios with nonvisualized urinary bladder. Gross renal malformations are consistently absent **(Figure 60)**. Chronic oligohydramnios leads to Potter sequence. Fetuses may die in utero. The diagnosis is by histopathology of the kidneys.

Extrophy of Urinary Bladder

Bladder extrophy in a very rare congenital malformation in which the anterior wall of the bladder with anterior abdominal wall is absent and the posterior wall of the bladder is exposed to amniotic fluid.[1,46] It can occur as an isolated anomaly or be part of complex association of OEIS complex with extrophy, omphalocele, bowel anomalies, spina bifida and phallus bifidus. Incidence of bladder extrophy is 1/30,000 births with a 3:1 male to female ratio. The ultrasound signs are: nonvisualization of urinary bladder with an irregular soft tissue mass bulging from lower abdominal wall **(Figure 61)**. The amniotic

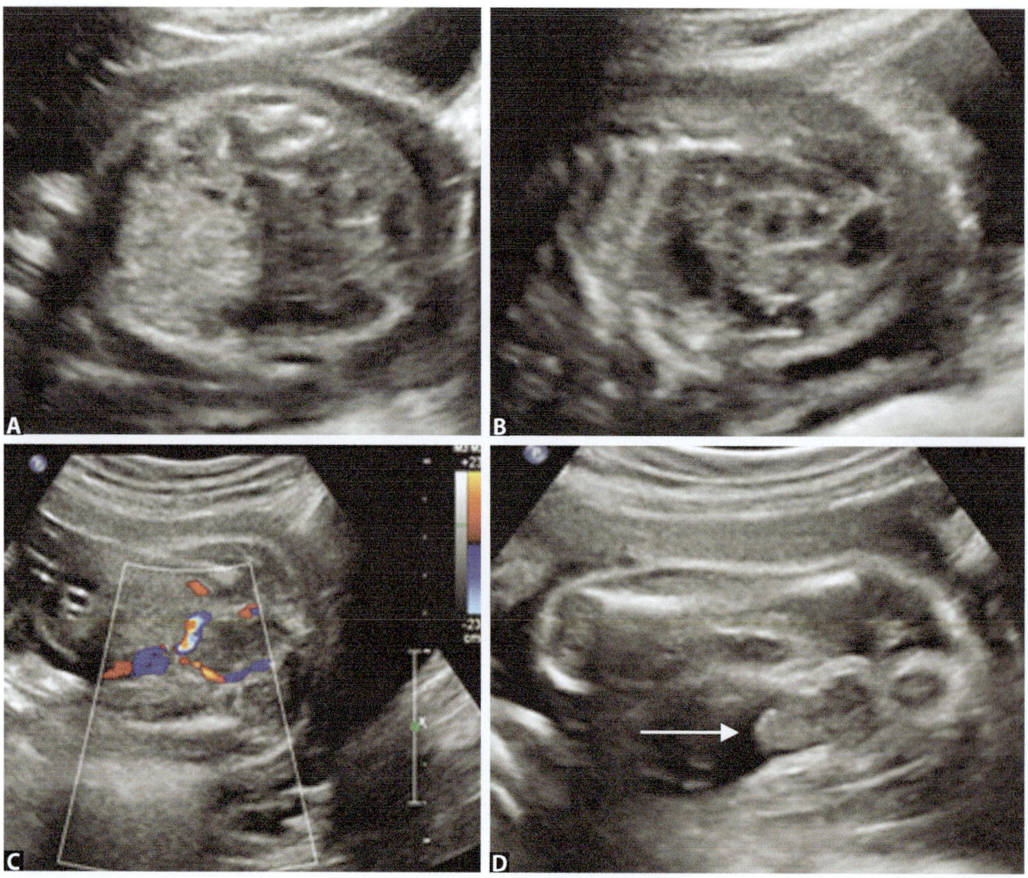

Figure 61: Extrophy of urinary bladder: Axial (A) and longitudinal; (B) scan showing the normal kidneys in a fetus with normal amniotic fluid volume; (C) Oblique coronal scan with color Doppler study of pelvis demonstrating absent urinary bladder between the umbilical arteries; (D) Oblique scan of fetal perineum and anterior abdominal wall demonstrating the irregular soft tissue mass (arrow) of lower abdominal wall below the cord insertion

fluid is normal. Minor findings include a low insertion of umbilical cord, widening of iliac crest and a small penis.

Duplication of Urinary Bladder

Duplication of urinary bladder can be partial or complete. Partial duplication is seen as a sagittal incomplete septum from fundus of urinary bladder. It is usually associated with ambiguous genitalia **(Figure 62)**. Complete duplication of the urinary bladder and urethra is extremely uncommon and is more frequent in males.[47] In complete bladder duplication, a septum divides the two bladders and orientation of the septum is variable. A sagittal septum is more common. Each bladder receives a ureter of its ipsilateral kidney and is drained by its own urethra lying side by side.[48] Associated anomalies are more common in children with the sagittal type of duplication.[49] In more than 50% of cases, there is also duplication of the hindgut. About 90% may demonstrate duplication of the genital tract.[50] In males, there may be duplication of the penis with bifid scrotum. In females duplication of the vagina and/or uterus is present. Various hypotheses have been proposed as an embryological explanation for duplication of urinary bladder.[48,51,52] Complete duplication of urinary bladder and urethra presents as two cysts in pelvis in between the two umbilical arteries. The two urinary bladders will show emptying independent of each other **(Figure 63)**. There will be varying degrees of duplication of external genitalia, internal genital organs and midgut.[53]

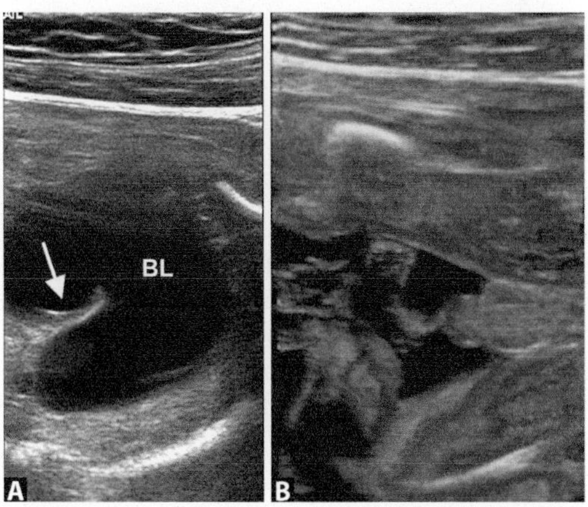

Figure 62: Partial duplication of urinary bladder: (A) Coronal scan of fetal pelvis showing the partially septated (arrow) urinary bladder (BL); (B) Scan of perineum demonstrating the ambiguous genitalia

URORECTAL MALFORMATION SEQUENCE (URSM) OR CLOACAL MALFORMATIONS

The lower portion of gastrointestinal and the genitourinary tracts develop from the caudal mesoderm—the primitive cloaca. Cloacal malformations are a spectrum of rare anomalies that results due to the failure of division of the primitive cloaca by the urorectal septum. Hence, these malformations are grouped under the term 'Urorectal Septum Malformation Sequence' (URSM). The incidence of URSM is reported to be 1 in 50,000 to 2,50,000 among liveborns with a female preponderance. Early in embryogenesis, during 5 to 7 weeks of gestation, the urorectal septum fuses with the cloacal membrane and then divides it into the anterior urogenital sinus and the posterior rectum. The urorectal septum then breaks down and leaves an open urogenital sinus and rectum. The urogenital sinus differentiates into the urinary and genital tracts. Arrest of this developmental process would lead to URSM, though a precise etiology has not been established. No familial inheritance has been reported. Recent evidence suggests the involvement of homeobox and sonic hedgehog signaling pathways in the pathogenesis of URSM.[54-59] Genetic cause has not yet been established.

Two types of URSM have been described. Complete URSM is characterized by the absence of anal and perineal openings, a smooth perineum and ambiguous genitalia.

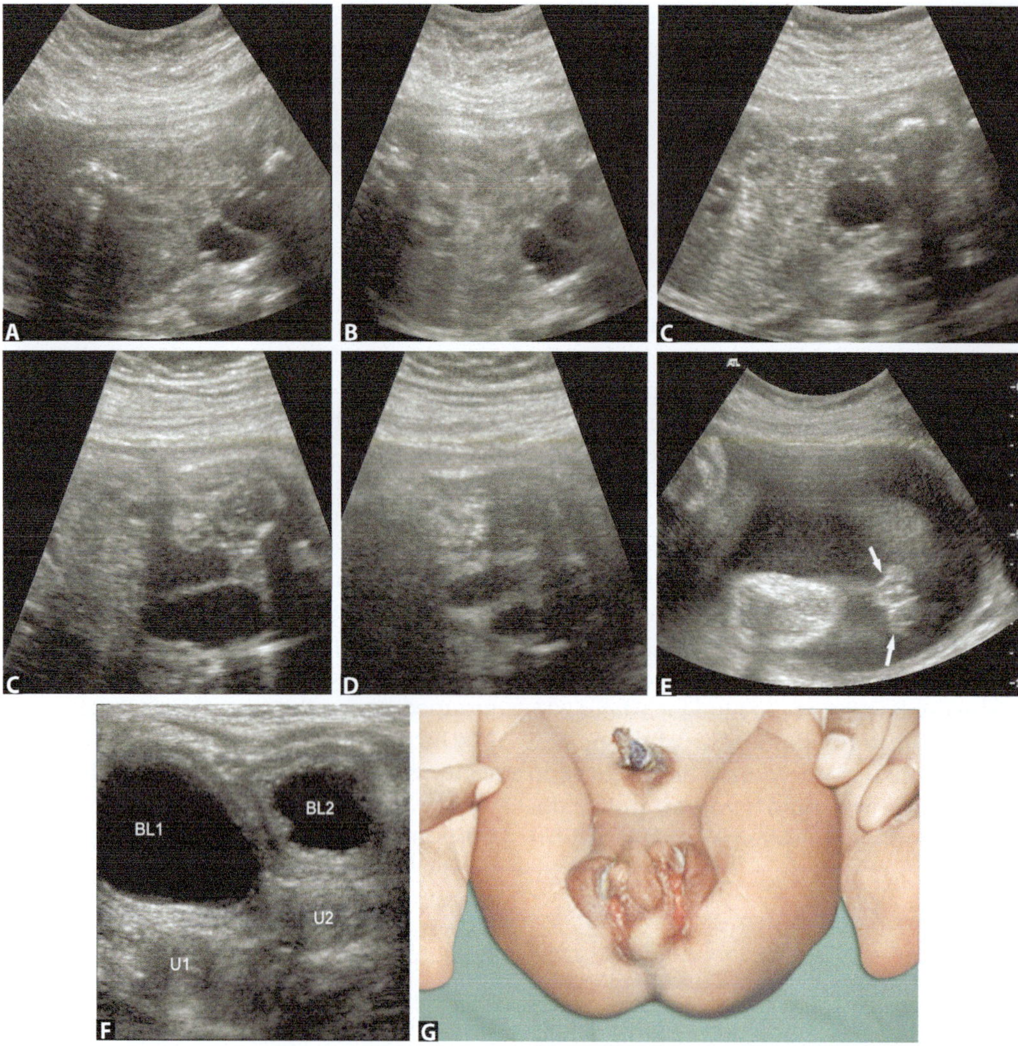

Figure 63: Complete duplication of urinary bladder: Serial coronal scans of fetal pelvis showing two urinary bladders emptying independent of each other. (A) Both bladders appear full; (B) Scan 5 minutes after first image shows partially contracted left bladder; (C) Scan 16 seconds after (B) showing left bladder completely emptied and right bladder alone is seen; (D) Scan 5 minutes after; (C) showing partially full left bladder and a full right bladder; (E) Scan 1 minute after; (D) showing partially emptied right bladder; (F) Scan of fetal perineum shows the two vulvae (arrows); (G) Postnatal transverse scan of pelvis of the newborn confirms the two bladders (BL1 & BL2) and also shows the two uteri (U1 & U2) posterior to them; and (H) Postnatal photograph confirms the two vulvae and two anal openings

It is a lethal anomaly and would result in stillbirths and perinatal mortality. Partial URSM is characterized by a single anal or perineal opening that serves a common conduit for gastrointestinal and genito-urinary tracts. It is a less severe variant. Differentiation of the types is not possible by prenatal ultrasonography. The association of URSM with other anomalies such as VACTERL and OEIS complex has been described. The following signs would suggest a URSM:

1. Nonvisualization of the anus on a tangential scan of the fetal perineum. Normally, the anus is visualized as a hypoechoic ring with an echogenic dot which represents the anal sphincter complex and lumen respectively **(Figure 64)**.[59]
2. Cystic mass with a fluid-debris level that funnels to the pelvis in a female fetus is one of the most consistent observations which represents the hydrocolpos **(Figure 65)**. The fluid-debris level is due to the urine admixed with meconium distending the vagina of the fetus. Mullerian duplication is noted in 60% of cases with URSM. The incidence

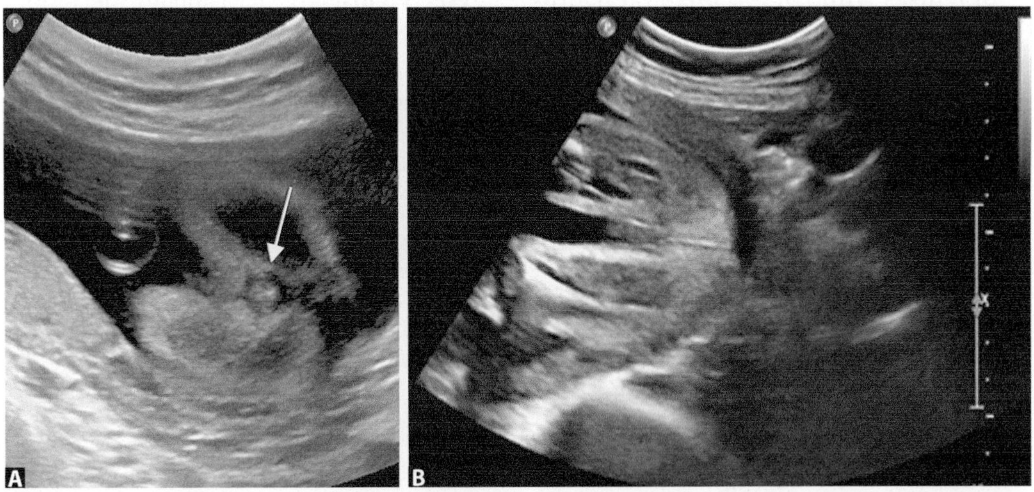

Figure 64: (A) Tangential axial section of fetal perineum showing the normal anus seen as an echopoor circle with an echogenic center (arrow); (B) Similar section in a fetus with nonvisualized anus as part of URSM sequence

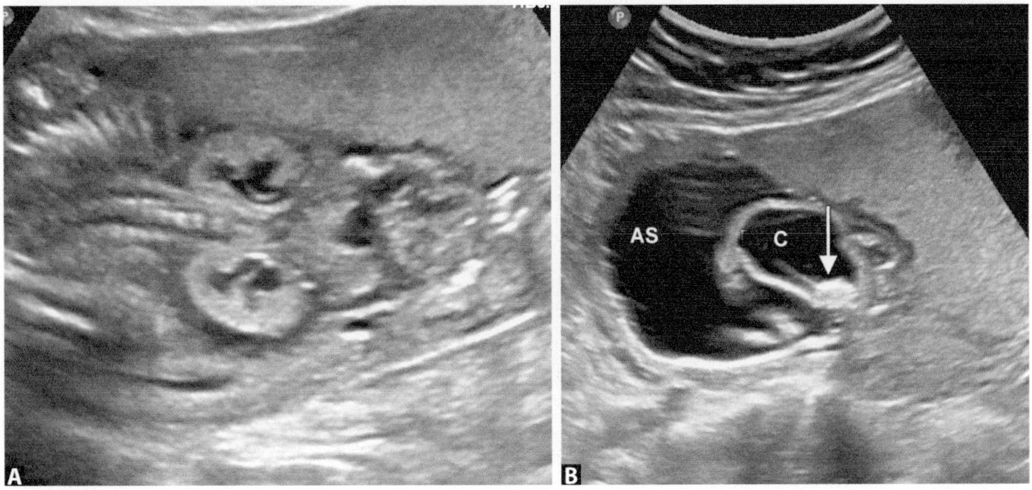

Figure 65: Urorectal malformation sequence (URSM):(A) Coronal scan of fetal abdomen reveals anhydramnios and bilateral hydronephrosis with echogenic parenchyma; (B) Demonstrates ascites and pyriform cystic mass (C) with debris (arrow)

increases to 80% in those cases where prenatal diagnosis of septated cystic mass is made, which represents hydrocolpos of duplicated vagina **(Figure 66)**. Hydrocolpos is highly diagnostic of URSM but its absence does not rule out URSM. Hydrocolpos may not be evident in upto 50% of fetuses with URSM.

3. Renal anomalies are reported in 90% of fetuses with URSM. Bilateral hydronephrosis is the most common, though other anomalies such as renal cystic dysplasia, pelvic kidney, horse-shoe kidney and crossed fused ectopia have also been noted. There may dilated colon with echogenic balls of meconium **(Figure 67).**
4. Presence of echogenic ascites due to the reflux of urine mixed with meconium through fallopian tubes into the peritoneum **(see Figure 66)**. Occasionally meconium

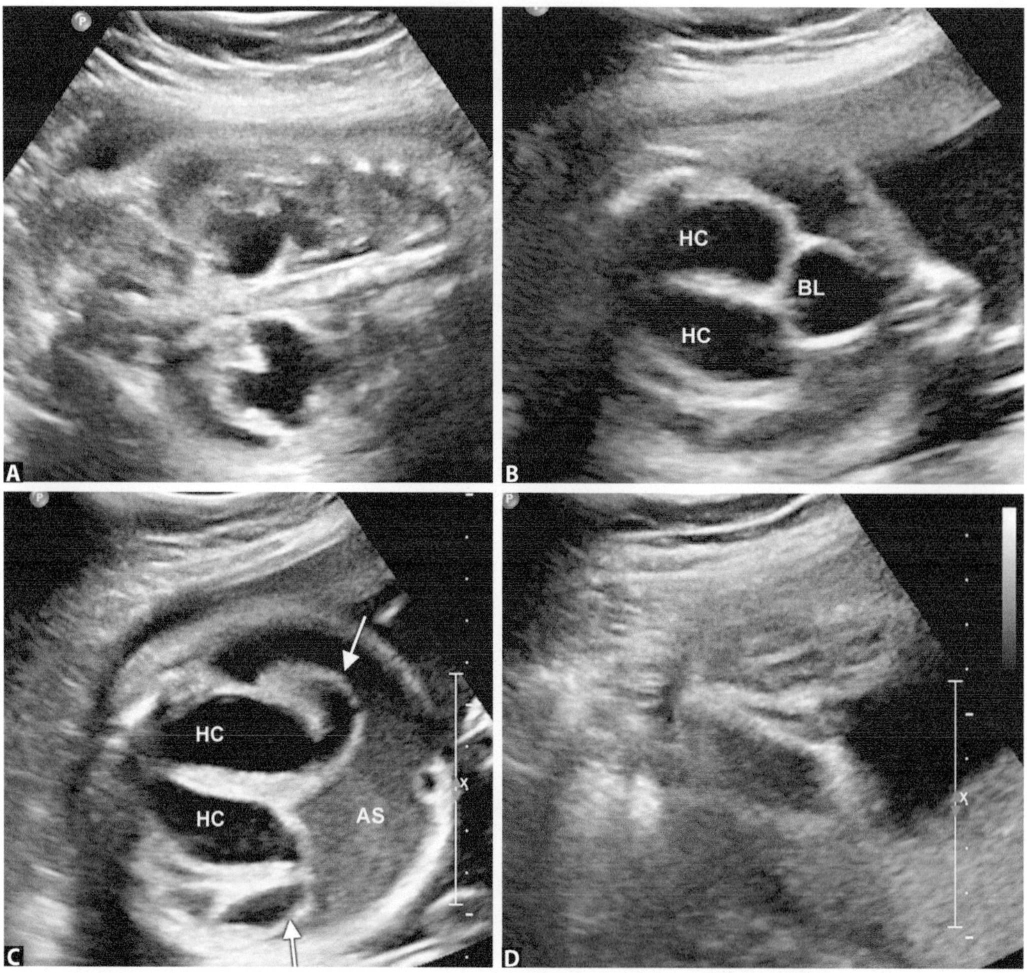

Figure 66: Urorectal malformation sequence (URSM): (A) Coronal scan shows bilateral hydronephrosis; (B) Axial scan of fetal pelvis shows a large septated cystic mass (HC) posterior to urinary bladder (BL); (C) Oblique Coronal scan of fetal abdomen demonstrates echogenic ascites (AS) and hydrocolpos (HC) of duplicated vagina with hydrometra of the duplicated uteri (arrows); (D) Tangential scan of fetal perineum demonstrates nonvisualized anus

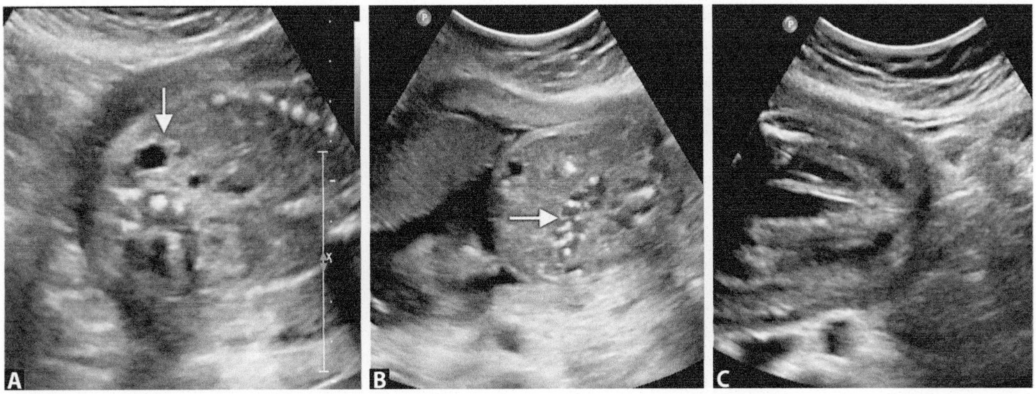

Figure 67: Urorectal malformation sequence (URSM): (A) Coronal scan reveals multicystic dysplastic of the kidney; (B) Axial scan of lower abdomen shows dilated colon with echogenic meconium balls; (C) Tangential scan of fetal perineum demonstrates nonvisualized anus

peritonitis may be visible as peritoneal calcification. Bowel may either be normal in caliber or dilated.

5. Spinal abnormalities such as hemivertebra or hypoplastic sacrum are frequently associated.
6. The degree of oligohydramnios depends on the severity and renal involvement. Complete URSM is associated with anhydramnios.

There could be other associated anomalies such as ambiguous genitalia and single umbilical artery. Antenatal recognition is important since it may provide the couple; the option of termination when diagnosis is established before the legal time limits of termination. URSM carries a guarded prognosis. Functional disturbances are often encountered in anorectal, urological and gynecological systems.

SIRENOMELIA

Sirenomelia sequence is a rare incidence of 1:60,000 births with a lethal pattern of congenital anomalies characterized by a number of hallmark skeletal anomalies including fusion of the lower extremities or a single lower limb with single or two femora, bilateral renal agenesis or dysgenesis with absent or hypoplastic renal arteries, oligohydramnios and the presence of aberrant vasculature.[60] Two separate systems of classification of sirenomelia have been proposed, one based on the number of feet and the other according to the fused bones. The pattern of sonographic anomalies that characterize sirenomelia, especially the single or fused lower limbs, often go undetected prenatally as ultrasonographic exploration of the fetus is hindered by the severe oligohydramnios or anhydramnios that occurs as a result of the bilateral renal agenesis.[61] When sirenomelia is suspected, it is confirmed by the features of a single stout femur **(Figure 68)**. When there are two femora, the diagnosis is facilitated by color Doppler to pick up vascular malformation and by high resolution scan. The most dominant vascular feature of sirenomelia is the presence of an aberrant umbilical artery derived from a persistent vitelline artery. The vascular steal theory describes this feature as the pathogenetic mechanism that causes

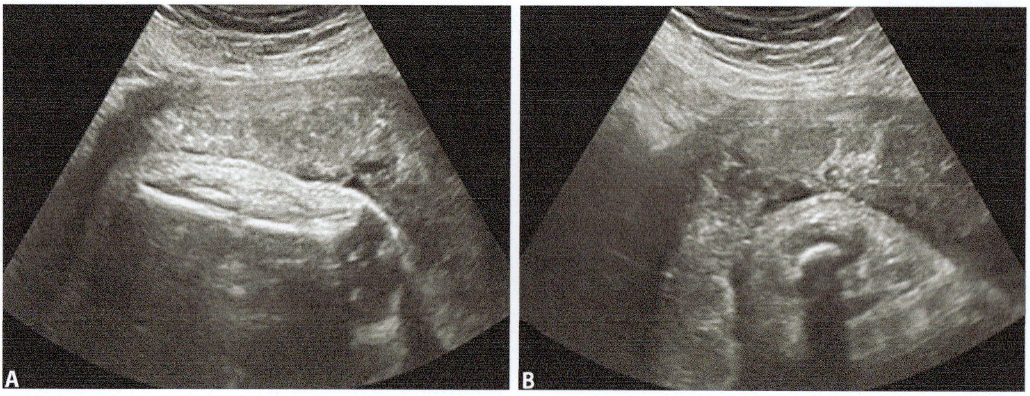

Figure 68: Sirenomelia:(A) Longitudinal and (B) axial scan of the single stout femur in a fetus with bilateral renal agenesis, single umbilical artery and anhydramnios, characteristic of sirenomelia

sirenomelia, attributing the lower limb abnormalities to hypoperfusion secondary to blood shunting into the dominant vitelline vessels and away from the absent or hypoplastic iliac arteries. Various vascular patterns associated with sirenomelia are described by Patel.[60] The prenatal use of color Doppler imaging in the presence of oligohydramnios is three-fold. First, it can be used to confirm the presence of bilateral renal agenesis when gray-scale images fail to detect the presence of renal tissue, especially when the adrenal glands take on a discoid configuration. Second, the caliber and patency of the aorta can be assessed in addition to the presence of normal umbilical arteries in fetuses with bilateral renal agenesis, not associated with sirenomelia. Third, it can detect both the origin of the aberrant vitelline artery in the fetal abdomen and the absence of the normal intimated relationship between the umbilical arteries and the side walls of the bladder **(Figure 69)**. In some types of sirenomelia, there are two femora with soft tissue fusion. High resolution sonography is useful to diagnose this type by revealing the continuous fused soft tissues around the two femora, when it is suspected in the fetus with features of bilateral renal agenesis and aberrant vitelline artery **(Figure 69)**.[32] The rarest form of sirenomelia is one where the soft tissue fusion is incomplete with a pterygium or web like band of fusion on posterior aspect of the lower limbs extending from the perineum to the foot with the knees in fixed flexion **(Figure 70)**. In contrast to diagnosis in second trimester, sirenomelia can be diagnosed with ease in first trimester. This is made possible because oligohydramnios is usually less severe in the first trimester on account of the smaller contribution of fetal urinary excretion to the amount of amniotic fluid, allowing clearer lower limb imaging by ultrasound **(Figure 71)**. Visualization of lower extremity anomalies consistent with sirenomelia sequence has been noted as early as 9 weeks of gestation.

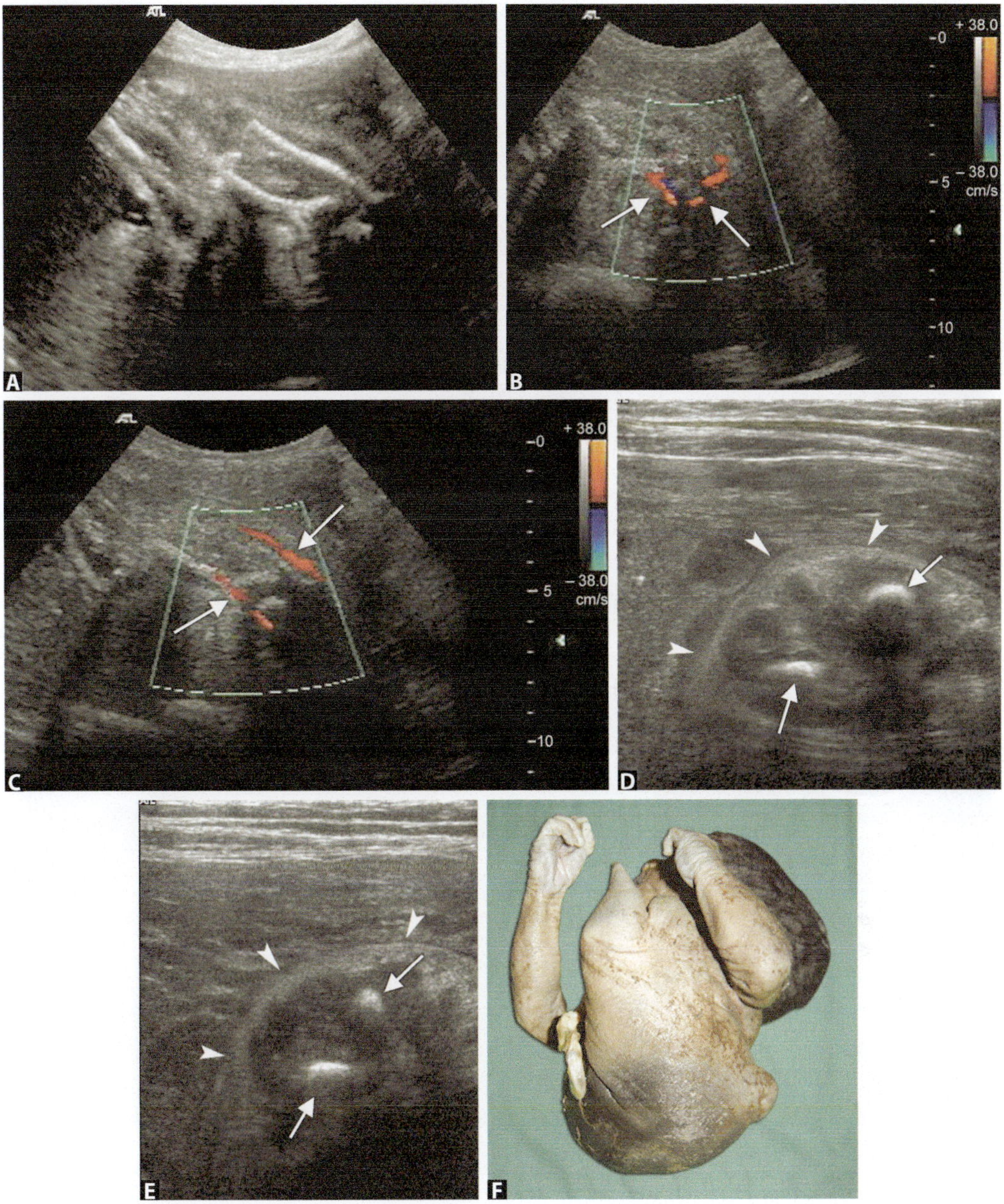

Figure 69: Sirenomelia: (A) Ultrasound image of the coronal plane of the thigh showing the two separate femora. Color Doppler images showing; (B) the two iliac arteries (arrows) in the pelvis; (C) Femoral arteries (arrows) in the thigh. High resolution transverse scans through the upper thigh; (D) Lower thigh; (E) Depicting the continuous skin line (arrowheads) over both the femora (arrows); (F) Picture of the abortus revealing sirenomelia

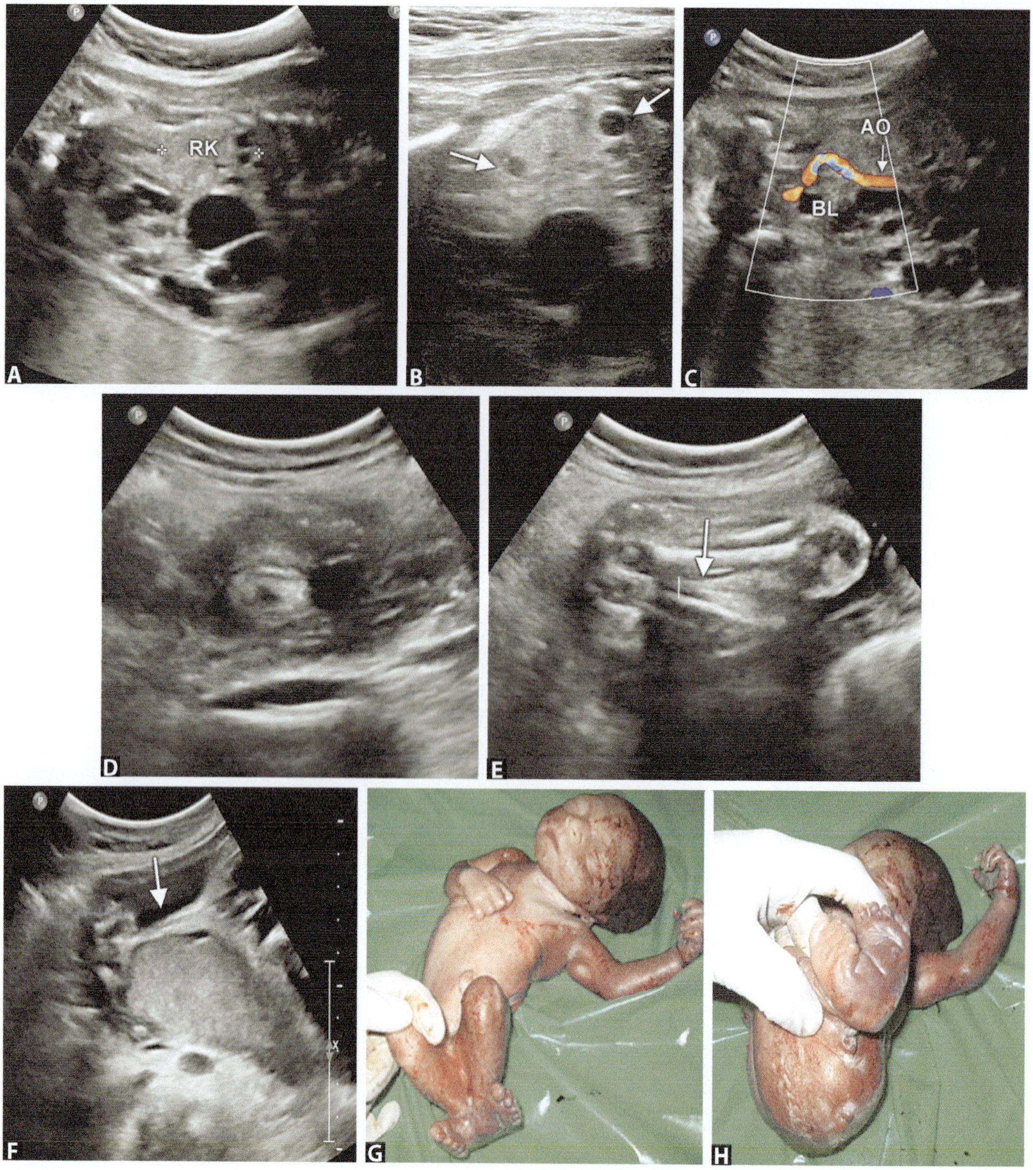

Figure 70: Sirenomelia: (A) Coronal scan demonstrating the multicystic dysplasia of both kidneys with anhydramnios; (B) High frequency scan of right kidney demonstrating the multicystic dysplasia; (C) Color Doppler study revealing the aberrant vitelline artery arising from the aorta (AO) BL—Urinary bladder; (D) Scan of perineum showing the nonvisualized anus; (E) Coronal scan of thigh shows the soft tissue fusion along the proximal aspect; (F) Web like fused soft tissue (arrow) along posterior aspect of thighs and legs extending from perineum to the feet; (G) and (H) Photographs of the abortus demonstrating the soft tissue fusion and flat fused gluteal region with absent anal opening

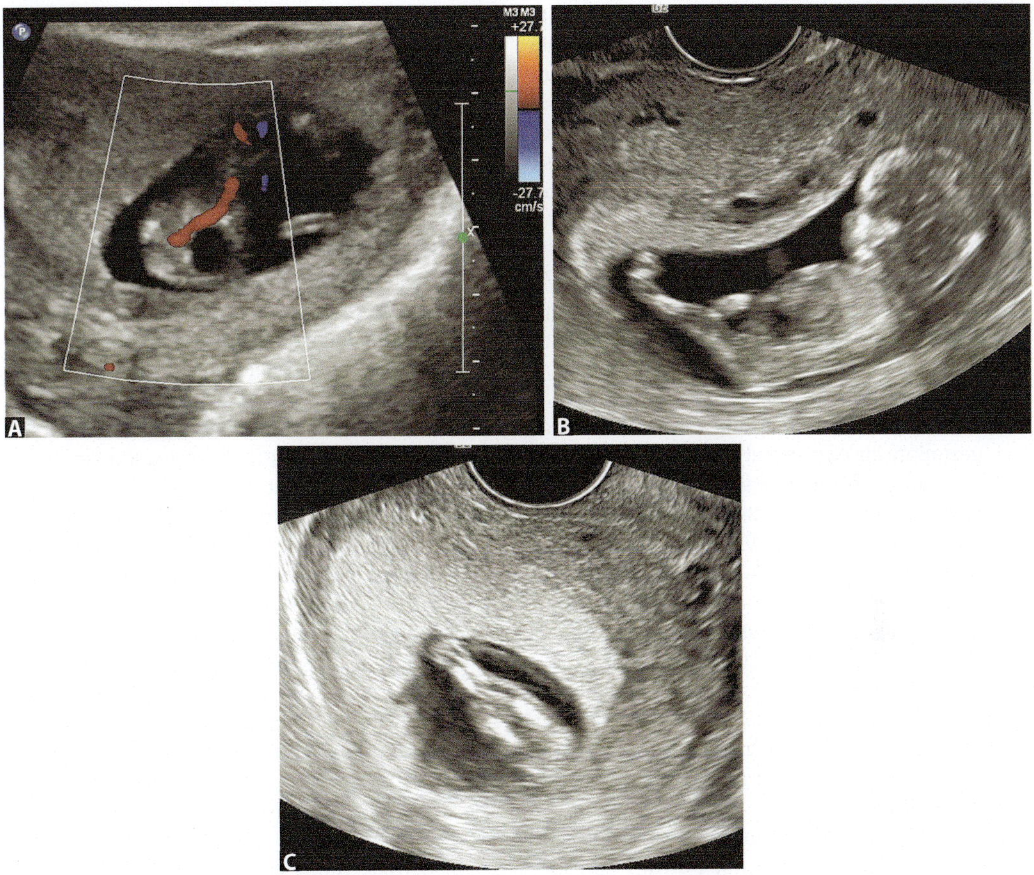

Figure 71: Sirenomelia in first trimester: (A) Color Doppler study showing the aberrant vitelline artery; (B) Longitudinal scan of the fetus shows the characteristic fixed posture of the fused lower limb; (C) Coronal scan of the fused lower limbs easily demonstrated because of adequate amniotic fluid in first trimester

ACKNOWLEDGMENTS

I wish to thank my wife Mrs Radhika Vijayaraghavan for her cooperation and Mr S Sreedharan, for his help in preparing this chapter.

REFERENCES

1. Van Allen MI. Urinary tract. In: Stevenson R, Hall J, Goodman R, (Eds). Human Malformation and Related Anomalies. Oxford: Oxford University Press; 1993.p.502-62.
2. Vijayaraghavan SB. Fetal perineal sonography in the diagnosis of ectopic ureteric opening. Ultrasound Obstet Gynecol. 2007;29(3): 347-51.
3. Boopathy VS. Sonography of fetal micturition. Ultrasound Obstet Gynecol. 2004;24(6): 659-63.
4. Nguyen HT, Benson CB, Bromley B, Campbell JB, Chow J, Coleman B, et al. Multidisciplinary consensus on the classification of prenatal and postnatal urinary tract dilation (UTD classification system). J Pediatr Urol. 10(6): 982-98.
5. Nguyen HT, Herndon CD, Cooper C, Gatti J, Kirsch A, Kokorowski P, et al. The Society for Fetal Urology consensus statement on the evaluation and management of antenatal hydronephrosis. J Pediatr Urol. 6(3):212-31.

6. Benacerraf BR, Mandell J, Estroff JA, Harlow BL, Frigoletto FD, Jr. Fetal pyelectasis: A possible association with Down syndrome. Obstet Gynecol. 1990;76(1):58-60.
7. Bromley B, Lieberman E, Shipp TD, Benacerraf BR. The genetic sonogram: A method of risk assessment for Down syndrome in the second trimester. J Ultrasound Med. 2002;21(10):1087-96; quiz 1097-8.
8. Carbone JF, Tuuli MG, Dicke JM, Macones GA, Odibo AO. Revisiting the risk for aneuploidy in fetuses with isolated pyelectasis. Prenat Diagn. 31(6):566-70.
9. Liao AW, Sebire NJ, Geerts L, Cicero S, Nicolaides KH. Megacystis at 10-14 weeks of gestation: chromosomal defects and outcome according to bladder length. Ultrasound Obstet Gynecol. 2003;21(4):338-41.
10. Nyberg DA, Souter VL, El-Bastawissi A, Young S, Luthhardt F, Luthy DA. Isolated sonographic markers for detection of fetal Down syndrome in the second trimester of pregnancy. J Ultrasound Med. 2001;20(10):1053-63.
11. Avni FE, Garel L, Cassart M, Massez A, Eurin D, Didier F, et al. Perinatal assessment of hereditary cystic renal diseases: the contribution of sonography. Pediatr Radiol. 2006;36(5):405-14.
12. Avni FE, Hall M. Renal cystic diseases in children: new concepts. Pediatr Radiol. 40(6):939-46.
13. Tsatsaris V, Gagnadoux MF, Aubry MC, Gubler MC, Dumez Y, Dommergues M. Prenatal diagnosis of bilateral isolated fetal hyperechogenic kidneys. Is it possible to predict long term outcome? Bjog. 2002;109(12):1388-93.
14. Chaumoitre K, Brun M, Cassart M, Maugey-Laulom B, Eurin D, Didier F, et al. Differential diagnosis of fetal hyperechogenic cystic kidneys unrelated to renal tract anomalies: A multicenter study. Ultrasound Obstet Gynecol. 2006;28(7):911-7.
15. Avni FE, Garel C, Cassart M, D'Haene N, Hall M, Riccabona M. Imaging and classification of congenital cystic renal diseases. AJR Am J Roentgenol. 198(5):1004-13.
16. Aslam M, Watson AR. Unilateral multicystic dysplastic kidney: long-term outcomes. Arch Dis Child. 2006;91(10):820-3.
17. Hains DS, Bates CM, Ingraham S, Schwaderer AL. Management and etiology of the unilateral multicystic dysplastic kidney: A review. Pediatr Nephrol. 2009;24(2):233-41.
18. Cassart M, Eurin D, Didier F, Guibaud L, Avni EF. Antenatal renal sonographic anomalies and postnatal follow-up of renal involvement in Bardet-Biedl syndrome. Ultrasound Obstet Gynecol. 2004;24(1):51-4.
19. Breysem L, Bosmans H, Dymarkowski S, Schoubroeck DV, Witters I, Deprest J, et al. The value of fast MR imaging as an adjunct to ultrasound in prenatal diagnosis. Eur Radiol. 2003;13(7):1538-48.
20. Bisceglia M, Galliani CA, Senger C, Stallone C, Sessa A. Renal cystic diseases: a review. Adv Anat Pathol. 2006;13(1):26-56.
21. Woolf AS, Feather SA, Bingham C. Recent insights into kidney diseases associated with glomerular cysts. Pediatr Nephrol. 2002;17(4):229-35.
22. Jain M, LeQuesne GW, Bourne AJ, Henning P. High-resolution ultrasonography in the differential diagnosis of cystic diseases of the kidney in infancy and childhood: preliminary experience. J Ultrasound Med. 1997;16(4):235-40.
23. Guay-Woodford LM, Galliani CA, Musulman-Mroczek E, Spear GS, Guillot AP, Bernstein J. Diffuse renal cystic disease in children: morphologic and genetic correlations. Pediatr Nephrol. 1998;12(3):173-82.
24. Ulinski T, Lescure S, Beaufils S, Guigonis V, Decramer S, Morin D, et al. Renal phenotypes related to hepatocyte nuclear factor-1beta (TCF2) mutations in a pediatric cohort. J Am Soc Nephrol. 2006;17(2):497-503.
25. Wilson PD. Polycystic kidney disease. N Engl J Med. 2004;350(2):151-64.
26. Brun M, Maugey-Laulom B, Eurin D, Didier F, Avni EF. Prenatal sonographic patterns in autosomal dominant polycystic kidney disease: a multicenter study. Ultrasound Obstet Gynecol. 2004;24(1):55-61.
27. Hildebrandt F, Zhou W. Nephronophthisis-associated ciliopathies. J Am Soc Nephrol. 2007;18(6):1855-71.
28. Salomon R, Saunier S, Niaudet P. Nephronophthisis. Pediatr Nephrol. 2009;24(12):2333-44.

29. Blowey DL, Querfeld U, Geary D, Warady BA, Alon U. Ultrasound findings in juvenile nephronophthisis. Pediatr Nephrol. 1996; 10(1):22-4.
30. Ickowicz V, Eurin D, Maugey-Laulom B, Didier F, Garel C, Gubler MC, et al. Meckel-Gruber syndrome: Sonography and pathology. Ultrasound Obstet Gynecol. 2006;27(3): 296-300.
31. Boopathy VS, Kamalam M, Raman ML. Prenatal sonographic appearance of congenital bile duct dilatation associated with renal-hepatic-pancreatic dysplasia. Ultrasound Obstet Gynecol. 2004;23(6):609-11.
32. Vijayaraghavan SB, Amudha AP. High-resolution sonographic diagnosis of sirenomelia. J Ultrasound Med. 2006;25(4): 555-7.
33. Fernandez MS, Estornell F, Reig C, Dominguez C, Martinez M, Garcia IF. [Ureteral ectopia in pediatric age: treatment and evolution in 55 cases]. Cir Pediatr. 1997;10(1):3-8.
34. Chowdhary SK, Lander A, Parashar K, Corkery JJ. Single-system ectopic ureter: a 15-year review. Pediatr Surg Int. 2001;17(8):638-41.
35. Cox CE, Hutch JA. Bilateral single ectopic ureter: a report of 2 cases and review of the literature. J Urol. 1966;95(4):493-7.
36. Jayanthi VR, Churchill BM, Khoury AE, McLorie GA. Bilateral single ureteral ectopia: difficulty attaining continence using standard bladder neck repair. J Urol. 1997;158(5):1933-6.
37. Mahony BS, Callen PW, Filly RA. Fetal urethral obstruction: US evaluation. Radiology. 1985;157(1):221-4.
38. Jones EA, Freedman AL, Ehrlich RM. Megalourethra and urethral diverticula. Urol Clin North Am. 2002;29(2):341-8, vi.
39. Stephens FD, Fortune DW. Pathogenesis of megalourethra. J Urol. 1993;149(6):1512-6.
40. Sepulveda W, Elorza C, Gutierrez J, Vasquez P, Castro V. Congenital megalourethra: outcome after prenatal diagnosis in a series of 4 cases. J Ultrasound Med. 2005;24(9):1303-8.
41. Berdon WE, Baker DH, Blanc WA, Gay B, Santulli TV, Donovan C. Megacystis-microcolon-intestinal hypoperistalsis syndrome: a new cause of intestinal obstruction in the newborn. Report of radiologic findings in five newborn girls. AJR Am J Roentgenol. 1976;126(5):957-64.
42. Osborne NG, Bonilla-Musoles F, Machado LE, Raga F, Bonilla F Jr, Ruiz F, et al. Fetal megacystis: differential diagnosis. J Ultrasound Med. 30(6):833-41.
43. Herman TE, Siegel MJ. Prune belly syndrome. J Perinatol. 2009;29(1):69-71.
44. Chen L, Cai A, Wang X, Wang B, Li J. Two- and three-dimensional prenatal sonographic diagnosis of prune-belly syndrome. J Clin Ultrasound. 38(5):279-82.
45. Gubler MC, Antignac C. Renin-angiotensin system in kidney development: renal tubular dysgenesis. Kidney Int. 77(5):400-6.
46. Lee EH, Shim JY. New sonographic finding for the prenatal diagnosis of bladder exstrophy: a case report. Ultrasound Obstet Gynecol. 2003;21(5):498-500.
47. Woodhouse CR, Williams DI. Duplications of the lower urinary tract in children. Br J Urol. 1979;51(6):481-7.
48. Abrahamson J. Double bladder and related anomalies: clinical and embryological aspects and a case report. Br J Urol. 1961;33:195-214.
49. O'Sullivan GJ, Hunter J, Dubbins PA. Case report: antenatal ultrasonic diagnosis of complete bladder duplication. Clin Radiol. 1996;51(11):818-9.
50. Kossow JH, Morales PA. Duplication of bladder and urethra and associated anomalies. Urology. 1973;1(1):71-3.
51. Uhlir K. Rare malformations of the bladder. J Urol. 1968;99(1):53-8.
52. Satter EJ, Mossman HW. A case report of a double bladder and double urethera in the female child. J Urol. 1958;79(2):274-8.
53. Vijayaraghavan SB, Nirmala AB. Complete duplication of urinary bladder and urethra: prenatal sonographic features. Ultrasound Obstet Gynecol. 2004;24(4):464-6.
54. Escobar LF, Weaver DD, Bixler D, Hodes ME, Mitchell M. Urorectal septum malformation sequence. Report of six cases and embryological analysis. Am J Dis Child. 1987;141(9):1021-4.
55. Gupta A, Bischoff A, Pena A, Runck LA, Guasch G. The great divide: septation and malformation of the cloaca, and its implications for surgeons. Pediatr Surg Int. 30(11):1089-95.
56. Liang X, Ioffe OB, Sun CC. Cloacal dysgenesis sequence: observations in four patients including three fetuses of second trimester gestation. Pediatr Dev Pathol. 1998;1(4):281-8.
57. Wheeler PG, Weaver DD. Partial urorectal septum malformation sequence: a report of

25 cases. Am J Med Genet. 2001;103(2): 99-105.
58. Winkler NS, Kennedy AM, Woodward PJ. Cloacal malformation: embryology, anatomy, and prenatal imaging features. J Ultrasound Med. 31(11):1843-55.
59. Vijayaraghavan SB, Prema AS, Suganyadevi P. Sonographic depiction of the fetal anus and its utility in the diagnosis of anorectal malformations. J Ultrasound Med. 30(1): 37-45.
60. Patel S, Suchet I. The role of color and power Doppler ultrasound in the prenatal diagnosis of sirenomelia. Ultrasound Obstet Gynecol. 2004;24(6):684-91.
61. Sirtori M, Ghidini A, Romero R, Hobbins JC. Prenatal diagnosis of sirenomelia. J Ultrasound Med. 1989;8(2):83-8.

10

CHAPTER

Skeletal Dysplasias and Abnormalities of Musculoskeletal System

Sonal Panchal, Sanjay Vasoya

Diagnosis of skeletal dysplasias and abnormalities of the musculoskeletal system of the fetus is a very difficult task, because it needs the evaluation of the entire fetus, the skull, spine, limbs and also the trunk for abnormalities of the ribs. Moreover, there is a huge variety of different skeletal dysplasias, as many as about 200, of which the common ones are very few, which we are going to discuss in this chapter. For the rest, it is best to refer to the online websites (where enteric the ultrasound findings can short list the diagnostic possibilities), as otherwise also it is impossible to remember even the names of all and naturally the diagnostic features also. Most skeletal dysplasias have a low risk of being associated with chromosomal disorders, except a small risk of trisomy 18, 13 and neuroarthrogryposis. But, in spite of that, most antenatally diagnosed skeletal dysplasias are lethal, and therefore, termination may be the choice of obstetric management. This means that to study the abnormalities of the fetal musculoskeletal system, it is essential to study the entire fetus—the four limbs, spine, thorax and skull.

For a systematic assessment, it is essential to follow a standard pattern of examination and documentation of each part to be assessed.

This is :

a. All four limbs, all three segments (proximal, middle, distal).
b. Long bone mineralization, shape, any fracture and measurement of the long bones. These are of special importance to categorize skeletal dysplasias.[1]
c. Fetal posture and fetal movements.
d. Assessment of small bones of had (carpals, metacarpals) and feet (tarsals, metatarsals).
e. Configuration and mineralization (echogenicity) of fetal head, spine, thorax and pelvic bones.
f. Joint contractures and dislocations.

Apart from the systematic examination, it is important to have a detailed history about the presence of any musculoskeletal abnormality in any other member of the family. This is essential because many musculoskeletal disorders have typical inheritance patterns and are familial.

NOMENCLATURE OF THE BONE DEFECTS

Abnormal Shapes of the Skull

1. *Clover-leaf skull:* It is due to very early closure of lambdoid, coronal and sagittal sutures, parietal bones are most severely affected. It is typical of thanatophoric dysplasia. It is best appreciated on coronal view.
2. *Acrocephaly or turricephaly:* It can be simply explained as pointed head or a tower head. It has increased craniocaudal diameter due to early closure of all sututres.
3. *Brachycephaly:* Early closure of the two coronal sutures leading to short antero-posterior diameter of the skull.
4. *Scaphocephaly:* Premature closure of sagittal suture leads to long occipitofrontal diameter of the skull.
5. *Plagiocephaly:* Unilateral premature closure of coronal and lambdoid suture leads to asymmetrical skull but is usually not seen antenatally.
6. *Trigonocephaly:* Triangular shape of the upper most part of the skull, due to closure of metopic suture.

Abnormal Spine

Platyspondyly: Flattened vertebral bodies and decreased distance between the end plates.

Abnormalities of the Limbs

- Shortening of the proximal portion of the limbs (femur and humerus) is *rhizomelia.*
- Shortening of middle portion of the limbs (forearm and leg bones) is *mesomelia.*
- Shortening of hand and feet bones is *acromelia.*
- Severe shortening of all portions of the limbs is called *micromelia.*
- Absent limb: *Amelia*
- Absence or deformity of distal part of limb/limbs: *peromelia*
- Absence of distal portion of one limb: *Hemimelia* (type of peromelia)
- Partial absence of a limb: *Meromelia*
- Poor development of proximal portions of limbs when hands and feet are directly attached to trunk: Phocomelia
- Hypoplasia of long bones of limb: *Ectromelia*
- Fused lower extremities: *Sirenomelia.*

Abnormalities of Extremities

- Pathological contracture of ankle: *Clubfoot*
- Pathological contracture of the hand: Ulnar deviation of the hand.
- Inwards bent of heel and foot: Varus
- Outwards bent of heel and foot: Valgus
- Abnormal hyperextension of the foot: Equinus.
- Polydactyly: An extradigit. It is called post-axial if the sixth digit is on the ulnar or fibular side (after fifth digit), and it is called preaxial, if it is on radial or tibial side (before thumb or toe), respectively in upper limb and lower limb.
- Absence of one or more digits: *Ectrodacyly*
- Fused fingers: *Syndactyly*
- Absence of one or both hands: *Acheiria*
- Absence of one or both feet: *Apodia*
- Absence of hands and feet: *Achieropodia*
- Absence of fingers or toes: *Adactyly*
- Subnormal number of fingers or toes: *Oligodactyly*
- Short fingers or toes: *Brachydactyly*
- Permanent medial or lateral deflection of one or more fingers: *Clinodactyly*
- Permanent flexion of fingers and toes: *Campodactyly*

Micrognathia

Arrested growth of mandible. If it is only anteroposterior restriction it is retrognathia and if the entire mandible is small it is micrognathia.

DIVIDED OF FETAL MUSCULOSKELETAL ABNORMALITIES

Fetal musculoskeletal abnormalities can be divided as follows:

A. Osteochondrodysplasias (skeletal dysplasias)
   1. Thanatophoric dysplasia
   2. Osteogenesis imperfect
   3. Achondroplasia
   4. Achondrogenesis
   5. Others
B. Redcutional defects
   1. Terminal defects
   2. Constriction band sequence
   3. Phocomelia
   4. Proximal femoral focal deficiency (PFFD)
   5. Splithand-split foot malformation (SHFM)
   6. Ectrodactyly

   Hand and foot deformities.
C. Polydactyly
D. Syndactyly
E. Hemivertebrae
F. Joint abnormalities
   - Fetal akinesia deformation syndrome. (FADS)
   - Diastrophic dysplasia
   - Club foot
   - Rockerbottom foot.
G. Other skeletal defects: patellar anterior luxation; teratogenic effects of drugs like Misoprost.

Osteochondrodysplasias

These are a group of about 350 different disorders, all distinctly identifiable. They all have hetrogeneous genetic basis.[1] Being a large group, for better understanding these are divided into subgroups depending on involvement of proximal, middle or distal portion of the limbs.[2]

Skeletal dysplasias can be very conveniently be studied by antenatal ultrasound.[3] The common ones are easier to identify on ultrasound than the less common ones.

These are[4]:

a. Thanatophoric dysplasia
b. Osteogenesis imperfecta
c. Achondroplasia
d. Achondrogennesis
e. Captomelic dysplasia
f. Spondylothoracic dysplasia
g. Atelosteogenesis
h. Others.

Incidence of skeletal dysplasias is about 3-4 in 10,000 and perinatal deaths in neonates with skeletal dysplasias is 9 in 1000. But, it is difficult to assess the incidence of individual skeletal dysplasia because there are some entities that mimic skeletal dysplasias, including dysmorphic syndromes and intrauterine growth restriction. Many of these dysplasias are lethal. When a skeletal dysplasia is suspected, the entire survey of the fetus, especially its skeleton is essential. X-ray was the modality used earlier but now the skeletal survey can be done with ultrasound, especially 3D ultrasound, fetal MRI or fetal CT.

The diagnosis is based on anatomo-morphological study assessing the characteristics of enchondral ossification line or by DNA assessment.[5]

Thanatophoric Dysplasia

This most common lethal skeletal dysplasia can be of two types, both caused by gene mutation with autosomal dominant inheritance.[6,7]

The gene affected is FGFR3. Its incidence is 0.69/10000 live births. It can be classified into two types: type I which is more common and is characterized by curved femur and type II which is characterized by straight femur but clover leaf skull.

It is severe rhyzomelic micromelia.

- All limbs are affected and all are short
- Bones are bowed especially in type I with metaphyseal cupping of femur **(Figure 1A)** and humerus (French telephone receiver deformity).
- Bone mineralization is normal

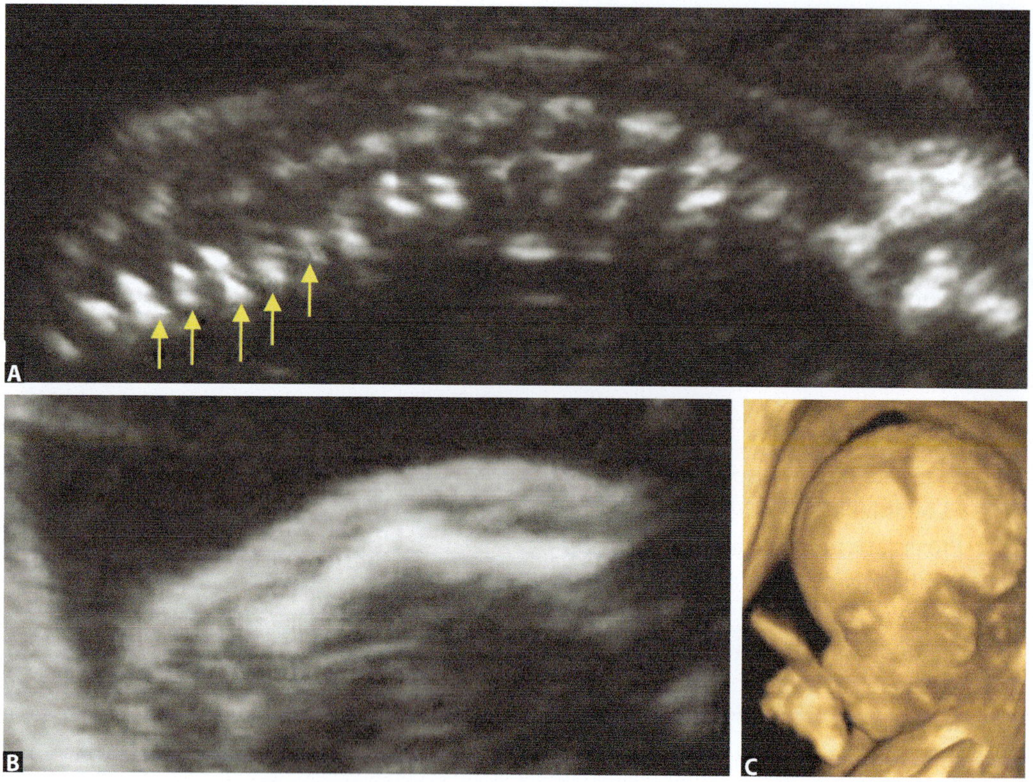

Figure 1: (A) Flattened vertebral bodies—platyspondyly (arrows); (B) Curved femur with normal ossification; (C) macrocrania with frontal bossing

- Ribs are short and platyspondyly **(Figure 1B)** lead to bell-shaped thorax. This also leads to pulmonary dysplasia and that makes this pathology lethal.
- Skull is large—macrocrania with frontal bossing and depressed nasal bridge **(Figure 1C).** But in type II, there is premature closure of cranial sutures giving it a cloverleaf configuration and appears trilobed on coronal section.

It is often associated with renal, cardiac and central nervous system anomalies. Polyhydramnios is seen in about 50% of cases.

Tips to differential diagnosis

- Achondrogenesis: Micrognathia and severe hypomineralization.
- Hypophosphatasia: generalized hypomineralization
- Osteogenesis imperfecta type II fractures
- Clover-leaf skull may be present in Pfeiffer syndrome, that has different skeletal anomalies and Cruzon's syndrome that has no limb shortening.

Osteogenesis Imperfecta

It is a genetic disorder that affects type I collagen. It is generally caused by a new gene mutation with an autosomal dominant inheritance. It is characterized by severe bone fragility, prenatal growth deficiency and blue sclera. Osteogenesis imperfecta can be classically divided into four types. Of these, type I and IV are not seen in fetus. Type III can sometimes be recognized in the third trimester. Type II (Vrolich type) is the most severe form and can be diagnosed by antenatal scans. This type II osteogenesis imperfecta is micromelic type. It is a uniformly lethal abnormality. This is believed to be due to pulmonary hypoplasia as a consequence of multiple rib fractures leading to thoracic hypoplasia.

On ultrasound: Severe bone fragility due to defective ossification leads to multiple fractures, leading to bone angulations (severe bone hypomineralization). Because of the bone fragility, there may also be skull damage and cerebral hemorrhage. But type III shows multiple fractures and kyphosis in third trimester or after birth. Though these patients survive till adult age, they have bad quality of life due to walking disability, fragile bones and otosclerosis. Oral bisphosphonates may help improve the bone quality. Stem cells have proved to be effective in experimental cases.[8] Incidence including all types of is 0.4/10,000 live births.

Tips to differential diagnosis

- Achondrogenesis: Micrognathia and no fractures
- Hypophosphatasia: Clavicle sparing hypomineralization.

Achondroplasia

This is a rhizomelic micromelia. Its incidence is about 1 in 10,000 live births. It may be homozygous or heterozygous type. The heterozygous type is usually due to new mutations and therefore carry a low recurrence risk, but with homozygous type (one/both parents affected) the recurrence risk is as high as 50-75%. If homozygous, it is lethal, but heterozygous cases have good global and intellectual prognosis. The gene that undergoes mutation is the fibroblast growth factor receptor (FGFR3) at 4p16.3. This mutation prevents binding of FGF to its receptors and in turn impairs bone growth.

Ultrasound features: This is typically late onset rhizomelia appearing at around 26-28 weeks of gestation.

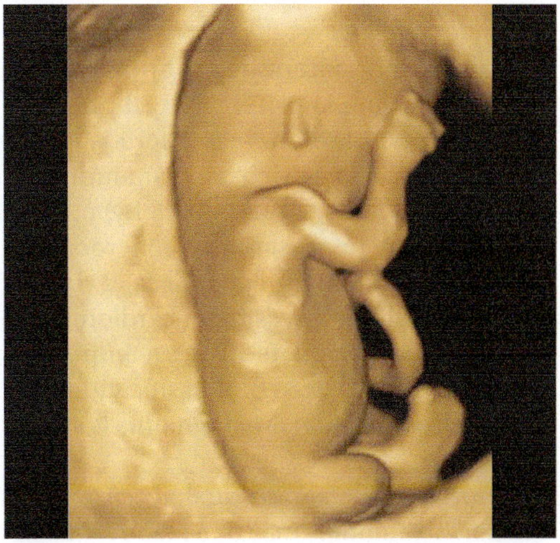

Figure 2: Typical image of achondroplastic fetus with macrocrania with frontal bossing (normal trunk and short limbs)

Normal bone mineralization and morphology with short femur and humerus (1-5th centile of the growth chart matching the ethnicity. Macrocrania and frontal bossing may be seen. This can be appreciated by abnormal HC/FL (head circumference/ femoral length) ratio or abnormal BPD/ FL (biparietal diameter/femoral length) ratio. The nasal bridge may be flat. Thorax is typically normal **(Figure 2).**

Trident hand (increased space between 3rd and 4th digit) may be present. Lack of widening of lumbar canal may be found in some cases. This during life may be a cause of peripheral neurological deficits.

Tips to differential diagnosis

- Trisomy 21: Nuchal fold thickness, and abnormal karyotype.
- Campomelic dysplasia: Bowed long bones and micrognathia.
- Chondroectodermal dysplasia (Ellis-Van-Crevald syndrome): Marked thoracic hypoplasia, polydactyly and congenital heart disease.
- Osteogenesis imperfecta (types I,I II, IV): late onset fractures and bowed long bones.

Achondrogenesis

It is a lethal osteochondroplasia with severe micromelia where long bones are very small and are curved. There is global bone hypoplasia which also includes rib hypoplasia leading to pulmonary hypoplasia. This gives an impression of macrocrania. Because of pulmonary hypoplasia at times it may give a false impression of cardiomegaly. Hypomineralization is also an important feature with poor vertebral ossification, and poor skull ossification. Micrognathia is almost always seen.

Associated gastrointestinal abnormalities and polyhydramnios may be a feature. Redundancy of subcutaneous tissues. (pseudohydrops) and generalized subcutaneous edema is more common in the patients in whom the disease is diagnosed early.

Achondrogenesis is of two typres:

- Type I: Parenti-Fraccaro type. Cranium looks disproportionately large due to soft tissue edema, lack of ossification of the skull and spine with short bones and thin ribs with rib fractures. It has autosomal recessive inheritance and is seen in about 25% of cases achondrogenesis.
- Type II: Langer-Saldino type. It is due to de novo mutations with autosomal dominant inheritance pattern. In some cases, it is mutation in COL2A1 gene coding for collagen type II. It is characterized by virtual absence of ossification in spine and pubic bones. But normal skull ossification and no rib fractures are seen. Outcome is fatal in neonatal life.

Tips to differential diagnosis:

- Thanatophoric dysplasia: Only mild hypomineralization
- Hypophosphatasia: No micrognathia
- Osteogenesis imperfecta type II: Constant occurrence of fractures.

Campomelic Dysplasia

This is an extremely rare always lethal disease, always a result of a de novo mutation (SOX9 allele that codes for SRY-box 9 protein, expressed in testis and skeleton). Sex reversal in affected male is characteristic with bifid scrotum and micropenis or ambiguous genitalia.

Ultrasound shows bones with abnormal curvature **(Figure 3A),** especially of the lower limbs, bell shaped narrow chest with eleven pairs of ribs and hypoplasia of mid-thoracic vertebrae and scapulae. Micrognathia may be present **(Figure 3B).**

It may be associated with hydronephrosis, hydrocephalus and cardiac anomalies. Sometimes, even fibular hypoplasia may be seen.

Though in most cases, it is fatal in neonatal life or infancy because of trachea-bronchomalacia and respiratory complications.

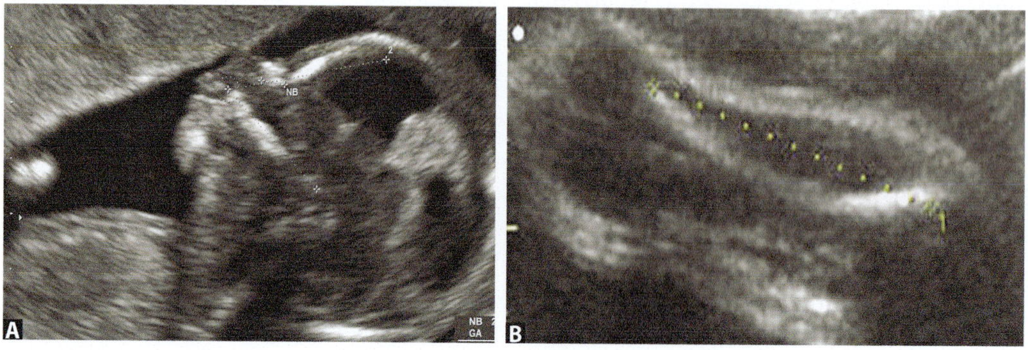

Figure 3: (A) Profile image of the fetal face showing micrognathia with hypodense culvarium; (B) curved hypodense femur

Tips to differential diagnosis:

Osteogenesis imperfecta types I,III,IV: Culvarial hypomineralization is the differentiating point.

Spondylothoracic Dysplasia Ijarcho-Levin Syndrome

It is characterized by delayed ossification of spine and ribs. Some cases though may be lethal, but the rest may reach adult life. It may be difficult to differentiate it from asphyxiating thoracic dysplasia (Jeune thoracic dysplasia), short rib-polydactyly syndrome, etc.

Atelosteogenesis (Spondylo-humero-femoral Dysplasia)

Ultrasound:

- Bent tibia/boomerang tibia **(Figure 4)**
- Absent fibula
- Short long bones.

Asphyxiating Thoracic dystrophy (Juene's syndrome)

It is a rare disorder with the locus on 15q13 genetically. It is diagnosed by thoracic hypoplasia with moderate rhizomelia and renal anomalies. If the anomaly is not severe it is nonlethal, and in that case, it may also be missed antenatally. Neonatal mortality is 60%.

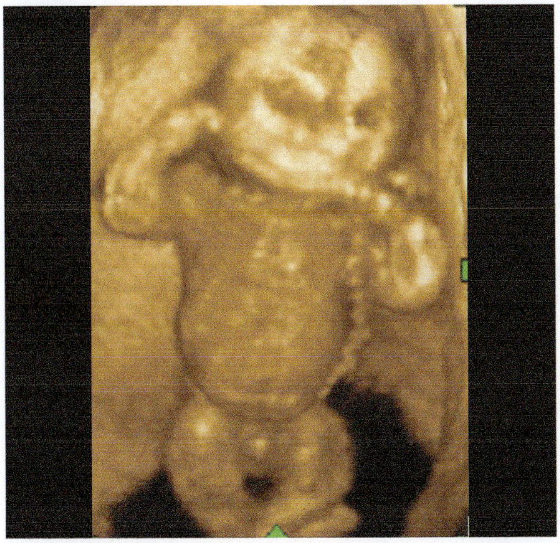

Figure 4: Bent legs and short long bones of atelosteogenesis

Tips for differential diagnosis:

- Chondroectodermal dysplasia: which may have cardiac defects and polydactyly
- All other disorders with thoracic hypoplasia like thanatophoric dysplasia, osteogenesis impercta type II, achondrogenesis and hypophosphatasia, also need consideration. These can be differentiated by associated limb bone dysplasias.

Chondroectodermal Dysplasia: (Ellis-van Crevald Syndrome)

It affects the cartilaginous layer between diaphysis and epiphysis and dysplasia of ectodermal tissues (nails and teeth). But these cannot be identified on antenatal ultrasound. It is rare abnormality (1 in 60,000 live births) due to mutation in chromosome 4p16. It has 50% infant mortality. It has an autosomal recessive inheritance and therefore 25% recurrence risk after an affected pregnancy.

Ultrasound shows acromesomelia, short ribs and moderate thoracic hypoplasia, postaxial polydactyly (always in hands and at times in feet). Congenital cardiac anomaly may be associated but the most common is atrial septal defect, which may be difficult to diagnose antenatally.

Tips to differential diagnosis:

- Asphyxiating thoracic dystrophy (Juene's syndrome) has significantly more thoracic hypoplasia, and there is no polydactyly or micromelia.
- Short-rib polydactyly syndrome also has more severe thoracic hypoplasia.

Hypophosphatasia

This also is a rare disorder and detected antenatally only if severe. It occurs because of defect in serum and tissue alkaline phosphatase. The genetic basis is defect of tissue nonspecific alkaline phosphatase gene mapping on 1p36.1-p34 chromosome.

Malfunction of the bone isoform correlates with the severity of phenotypic expression.

Severe micromelia, severe thoracic hypoplasia, diffuse mineralization (except clavicles), hydrops and subcutaneous edema are the diagnostic features on ultrasound.

Differential diagnosis from most other skeletal dysplasias are difficult.

Short Rib Polydactyly Syndrome

This is a skeletal dysplasia with autosomal recessive inheritance and 25% recurrence risk and is invariably lethal. This syndrome also has four subtypes: Saldino-Noonan type, Majewsky type, Verma-Naumoff, Beemer-Langer type. These are all characterized by micromelia, thoracic hypoplasia and postaxial polydactyly.

There may be associated cleft lip (in type II and IV), congenital heart disease (transposition of great arteries), **(Figure 5)** renal dysplasia (polycystic kidneys) and anophthalmia **(Figure 6)**. These are the diagnostic features on ultrasound also. It is always lethal.

Tips to differential diagnosis:

- Achondrogenesis
- Thanatophoric dysplasia
- Hypophosphatasia

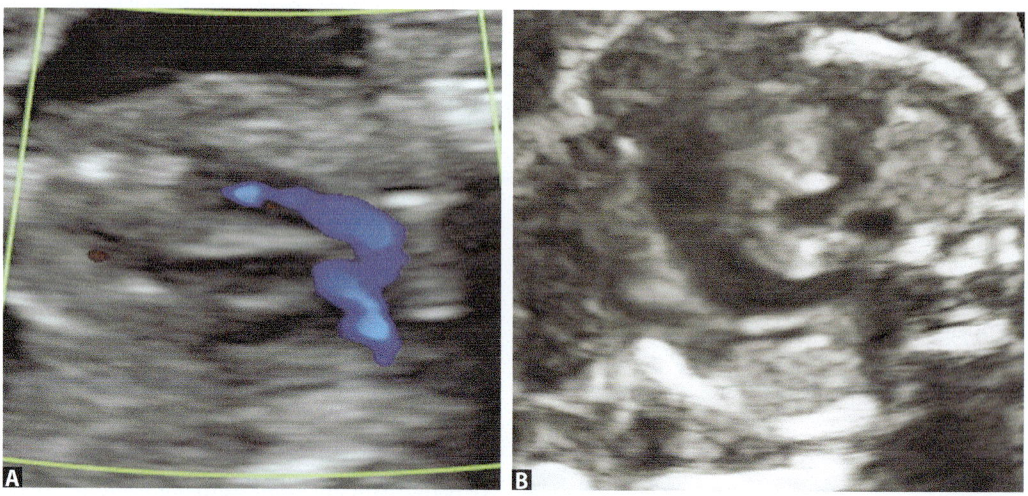

Figure 5: Transposition of great arteries, demonstrated by parallel outflow tracts, arising from two different chambers in the first image and curved outflow tract of right ventricular outflow tract

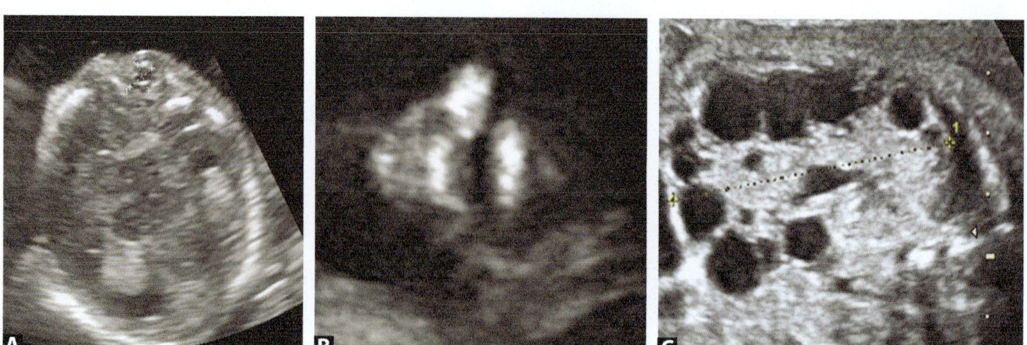

Figure 6: An/micro ophthalmia, cleft lip and polycystic kidneys

- Osteogenesis imperfecta type II
- Postaxial polydactyly present and hypomineralization is almost always absent in post rib polydactyly syndrome (SRPS).
- Chondroectodermal dysplasia has similar features but much less severe.

Other Osteochondrodysplasias

Nearly normal like bones except mild shortening is seen. Differential diagnosis is required from normal variant or IUGR. It is important to follow the growing pattern of the bones.

Reductional Defects

It is a hetrogeneous group of anomalies. There may be absence of any portion of the limb. According to EUROCAT definition, an intercalary reduction defect is represented by usually severe underdevelopment of one mesomelic bone segment only, whereas terminal transverse reduction defect is complete absence of terminal part of one limb (upper/lower). Transverse defects are congenital or acquired in utero.

These may be:

- Terminal defects
- Phocomelias
- Proximal focal femoral deficiency
- Split hand- split foot syndromes.

In, at least half the cases, there are isolated defects affecting only one limb and in another 25%, there may be more than one limb affected, but in the rest there are other structural defects also and may also show features of genetic syndrome. The outcome depends on the amount of compromise and the postnatal surgical outcome.

Terminal Defects

Usually affects the upper extremity. It is more common on the left side. It may be associated with other structural defects. These may also be associated with facial defects (microretrognathia) as a part of genetic syndrome.

Constriction band sequence: It is a sporadic entity. It may be due to amniotic band, constrictions, vascular compromise or interference of normal development of fetal extremities. Though it must be made clear here that placental septation is not the cause for constriction band sequence.

Asymmetric amputation of limbs is the only finding. No syndromic isolated defects of the limbs can involve all limbs at all levels. The reduction defects with syndromic risk are radial aplasia and focal femoral hypoplasia.

Terminal transverse reduction defects: The cause is interruption of the blood supply to the developing limb bud during organogenesis. But when it affects more than one limb, it may be associated with some syndrome. It may affect the mesomelic segment of the limb or the hand/ foot. Hand may be partially absent when hypoplastic digits are present on the terminal part of the wrist or metacarpus **(Figure 7).**

Femoral hypoplasia—unusual facies syndrome (FHUFS or femoral-facial syndrome: It may involve one or both femora with facial cleft and or micrognathia **(Figure 8).** It is a very rare abnormality, but a little more common in insulin-dependent diabetes mellitus mothers.

Hand malposition: Radial malposition of the hand may be associated with absent

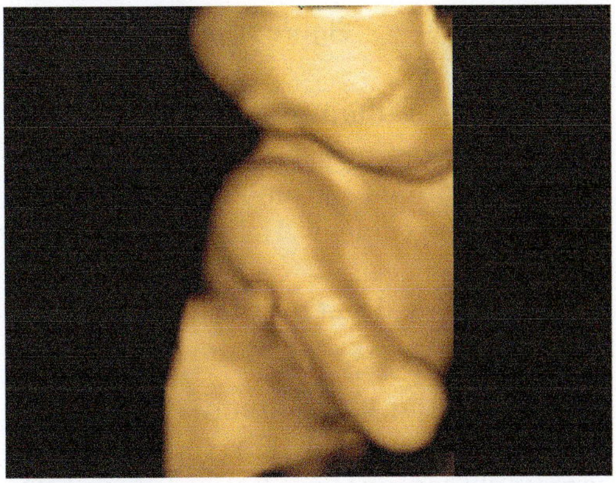

Figure 7: Absent forearm and partial absence of hand with small digits

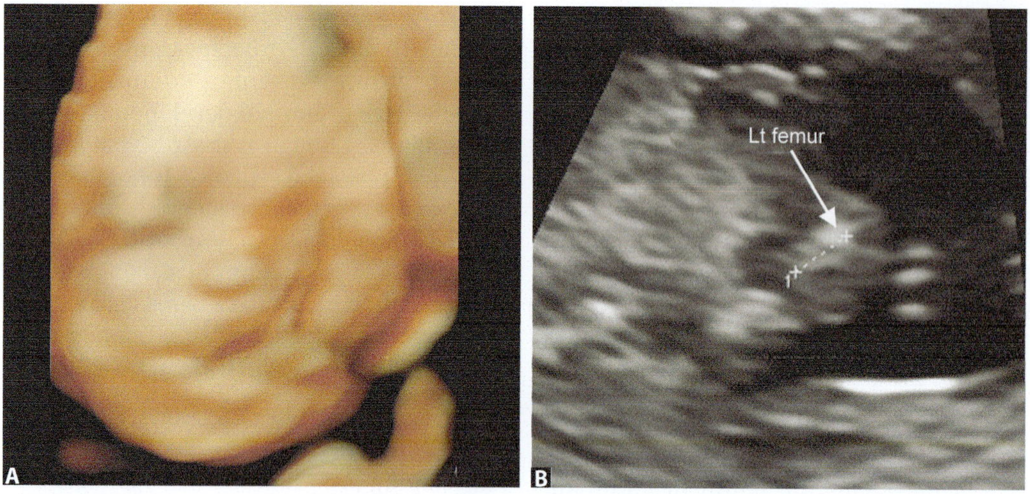

Figure 8: Facial cleft and hypoplastic femur

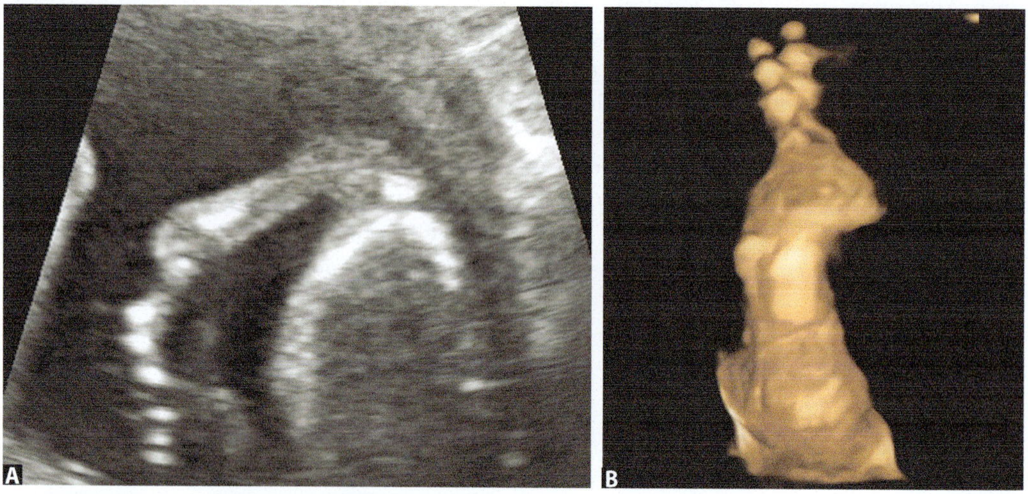

Figure 9: Abnormal forearm with absent radius and ectrodactyly

or hypoplastic thumb and also absent or hypoplastic radius. This may be a part of genetic syndrome, chromosomal anomalies, Fanconi's pancytopenia, Holt-Oram syndrome or scoliosis.

Malpositioned feet may also be associated with different types of syndromes.

Radial aplasia: It is commonly associated with ectrodactly (absent thumb, which represents terminal part of radial ray). On ultrasound the mesomelic component of the upper limb is abnormal **(Figure 9).**

Radius can be completely or severely hypoplastic.

Radial aplasia with or without ectrodatyly may also be seen in trisomy 18 (multiple anomalies + micrognathia), TAR (Thrombocytopenia with absent radius syndrome, also shows absent thumb), Holt-Oram syndrome (with syndactyly) and Robert's syndrome (phocomelia + cleft lip/palate). Unlike radial aplasia, all these also present with congenital heart disease. Nager syndrome and VACTERL association may also present with radial aplasia, wherein Nager syndrome has micrognathia and external ear anomalies, and VACTERL association also presents with vertebral and renal abnormalities and tracheo-esophageal fistula.

Phocomelia

This is a short limb syndrome with absent or hypoplastic terminal and middle part of the limbs. Phocomelia can occur sporadically or may be a part of genetic syndromes and even nongenetic syndromes like Holt-Oram syndrome, thrombocytopenia-absent radius (TAR) syndrome and Robert's syndrome (midface and limb anomalies presenting as microcefalia and growth restriction).

Proximal Femoral Focal deficiency (PFFD)

It may vary from marginally short femur to complete absence of femur. It may be unilateral or bilateral (in 10–15%) **(Figure 10).** PFFD is almost always isolated except its rare association with ipsilateral fibular hemimelia (sporadic) or ulnar hemimelia (genetic).

Split Hand and Split Foot Malformation (SHFM)(Ectrodacyly)[9]

It affects hand and feet in the form of syndactyly, median clefts of the hands and feet, aplasia and/or hypoplasia of phalanges, metacarpals and metatarsals **(Figure 11).** Typical isolated cases affect all four limbs

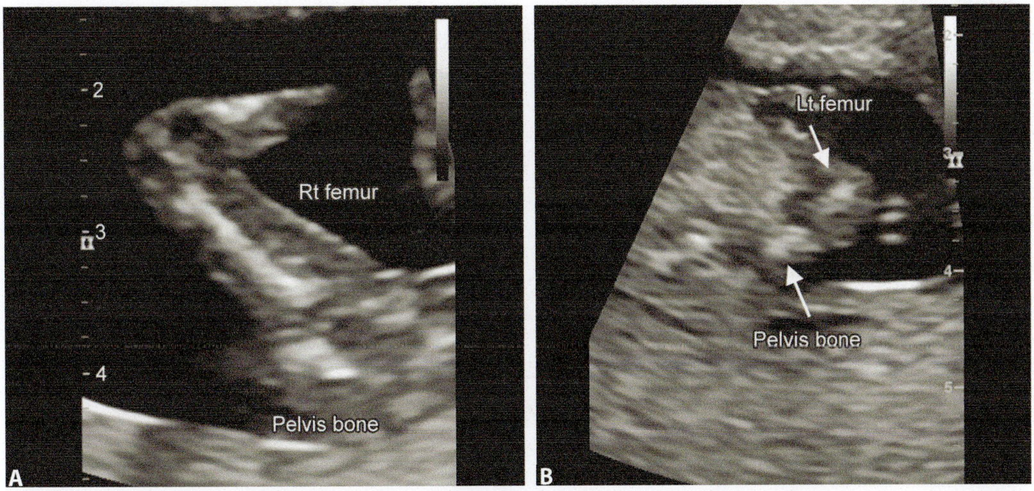

Figure 10: Severely hypoplastic left femur of the fetus

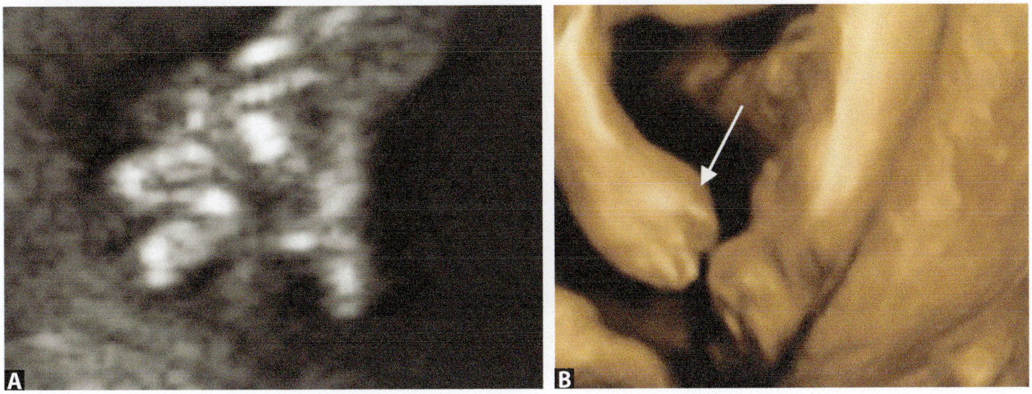

Figure 11: Ectrodactyly of fingers and toes

in "V" configuration and have a familial presentation. But atypical isolated cases may affect only one extremity in "U" configuration.

Polydactyly

It may be unilateral or bilateral. It may be seen in hand or feet. Extradigits may consist of only soft tissues or may contain even bony elements. It may be preaxial, post axial or central (when central three digits are affected). Preaxial polydactyly is more commonly associated with chromosomal disorders, while the post axial ones are usually isolated and have a good prognosis.

Syndactyly

The fusion of the digits may involve the soft tissues alone or both soft tissues and bones and may be complete (involving the complete finger) or incomplete. When syndactyly fuses more than two fingers, it gives either spoon hand or a mitten hand appearance. It may be associated with syndromes or constriction band sequence, but may also be sporadic with familial tendency.

Hemivertebrae

This is partial failure of formation of vertebral body. It may involve any part of the spine, though thoracolumbar segment involvement is the most common. This leads to abnormal curvature of the spine **(Figure 12).** It may be isolated and in that case the prognosis is good. But it may also be associated with other structural abnormalities or may also be a part of genetic syndromes like Klippel-Feil syndrome (fused cervical vertebrae with short neck).

Abnormalities of Joints

Fetal Akinesia Deformation Sequence (FADS)

Intrauterine fetal contractures of neurological, musculoskeletal or connective tissue origin leads to fetal akinesia. Typical features of the fetal akinesia deformation sequence (FADS) include fetal malposition, bilateral heel, knee and elbow deformities in flexion or extension **(Figure 13A).** The lesions may be symmetrical. It may be associated with polyhydramnios, thoracic hypoplasia, micrognathia **(Figure 13B)** and thick nuchal translucency. When generalized, it is lethal. Some features of FADS

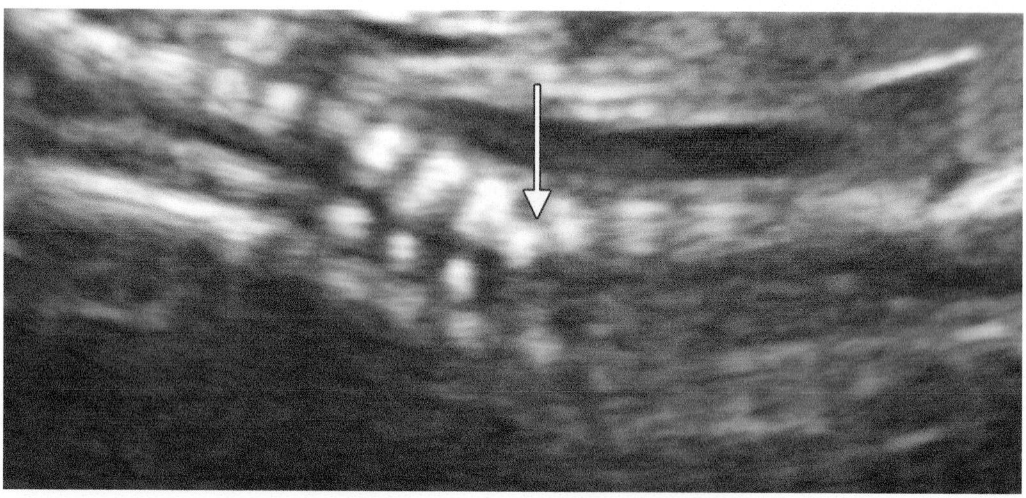

Figure 12: Abnormal spinal curvature due to absence of the ossification center of one of the two transverse processes of the vertebra marked by the arrow.

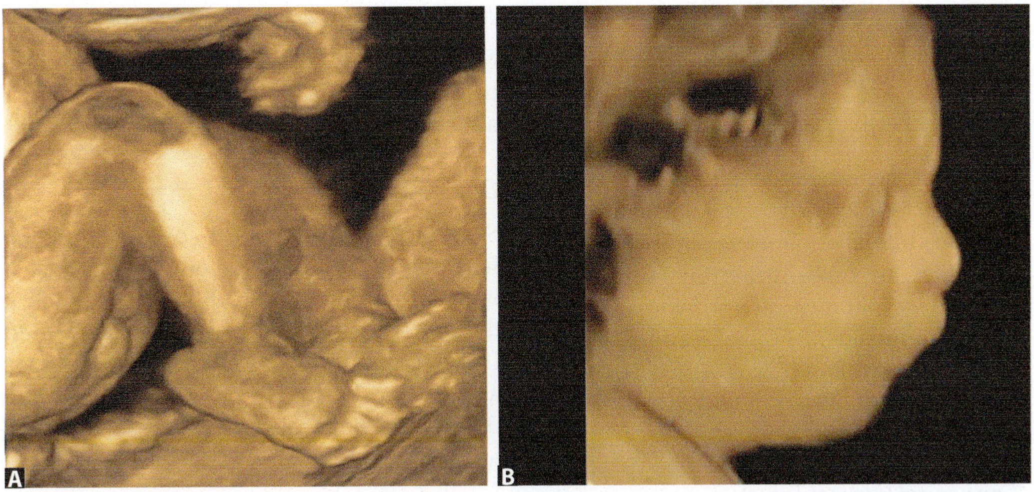

Figure 13: (A) Abnormal joint contractures of hand, ankle and feet; (B) Micrognathia

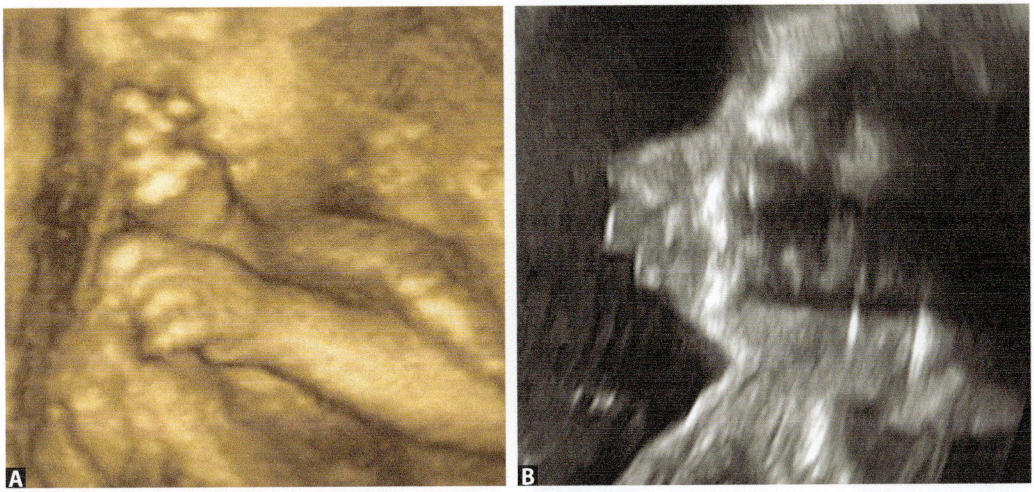

Figure 14: (A) Clenched fingers with ulnar deviation of hand; (B) Micrognathia

are present in other syndromes such as multiple lethal arthrogryposis, multiple pterygium syndrome and Pena-Shokeir syndrome. The differential diagnosis includes trisomy 18 and hypokinesia, secondary to severe oligohydramnios or to uterine malformation.[10]

Diastrophic Dysplasia

It is a rare skeletal dysplasia with postural abnormalities and joint contractures. It occurs due to DTDST gene mutation on 5q32-33.1 chromosome. It has autosomal recessive inheritance with 25% inheritance.

The diagnostic criteria on ultrasound are generalized joint contractures, 'hitch-hiker's thumb'(first digit fixed in extreme abduction) and other fingers clenched with ulnar deviation of hand **(Figure 14A).** Joint deformities also cause flexion contractures of elbows and talipes equinovarus. These fetuses also show severe rhizomelia and micrognathia **(Figure 14B).**

The only differential diagnosis required is from neuroarthrogryposis and the differentiating point is absence of rhizomelia.

Club Foot (Talipes Equino Varus) (Figure 15)

It can occur with isolated abnormality or may be seen in fetuses with neurological disorders like spina bifida, or neuromuscular disorders like FADS or environmental factors like ruptured membranes, uterine hypoplasia, etc. On ultrasound on the sagittal section of the leg and foot show different axis. And if isolated, it is a fully correctable surgery.

Rocker Bottom Foot (Congenital Vertical Talus)

It is characterized by calcaneus in equinus and valgus, hypoplasia and plantar flexion of the talus, abduction of the forefoot and all dorsal tendons tethered medial to the midline of the ankle. On ultrasound it is seen as convex plantar aspect of the foot **(Figure 16).** It may be commonly associated with trisomies 18 and 13.

Other Skeletal Defects

Patellar Anterior Luxation

Anterior flexion of the knee joint is secondary to patellar abnormality.

Teratogenic Effects

Misoprostol: Misoprostol used in the first trimester may be associated with distal limb abnormalities.

Differential Diagnosis

Skeletal dysplasias: Due to some overlapping features in different skeletal dysplasias, it is often confusing and difficult to reach a definitive diagnosis. This can be simplified if we consider certain distinct features as landmarks and then considering the differential diagnosis.

A. Severe micromelia:
   1. Thanatophoric dysplasia type II- thoracic hypoplasia ± cloverleaf skull
   2. Osteogenesis imperfecta type II- Ubiquitous fractures + hypomineralization
   3. Achondrogenesis - Thoracic hypoplasia ± hypomineralization
   4. Hypophospatasia - Severe ubiquitous hypomineralization except clavicle
   5. Short-rib polydactyly syndrome - Thoracic hypoplasia ± hypomineralization + congenital heart disease + polydactyly

B. Rhizomelia:
   1. Achondroplasia: Frontal bossing ± mild macrocrania

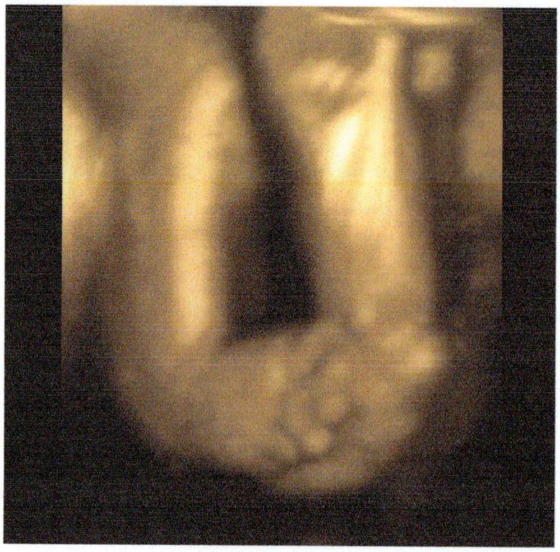

Figure 15: Clubfeet

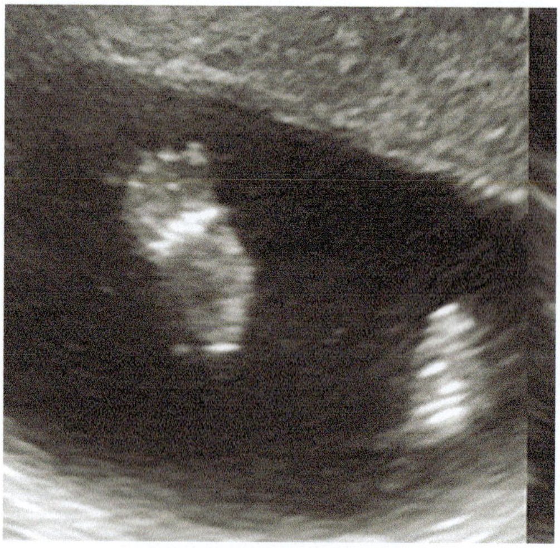

Figure 16: Rocker bottom foot

2. Asphyxiating thoracic dystrophy(juene's syndrome): thoracic hypoplasia ± Polydactyly ± renal anomalies
3. Diastrophic dysplasia: Postural deformities + 'Hitch-hicker's' thumb + micrognathia

C. Thoracic hypoplasia:
1. Thanatophoric dysplasia type II
2. Asphyxiating thoracic dystrophy (Juene's syndrome)
3. Achondrogenesis
4. Hypophosphatasia
5. Short-rib polydactyly syndrome

D. Hypomineralization:
1. Osteogenesis imperfecta type II
2. Hypophosphatasia
3. Achondrogenesis
4. Short-rib polydactyly syndrome

E. Micrognathia
1. Achondrogenesis
2. Campomelic dysplasia : Bowed tibia and femur + club foot + hypoplastic scapula
3. Diastrophic dysplasia
4. Fetal akinesia deformation sequence (FADS): Arthrogryposis + clubfoot ± hydrops
5. Cerebro-oculofacio-skeletal syndrome: Arthrogryposis (lower limbs)+ micro-opthalmia
6. Femoral hypoplasia-abnormal facies syndrome: Focal femoral hypoplasia + club foot

Differential Diagnosis: Abnormalities of Extremities

A. Polydactyly:
1. Short-rib polydactyly syndrome
2. Trisomy 13
3. Asphyxiating thoracic dysplasia
4. Meckel-Gruber syndrome: Polycystic kidney + cephalocele
5. Chondroectodermal dysplasia (Ellis van Creveld syndrome): Congenital heart disease + acromesomelia.

B. Ectrodacyly:
1. Robert's syndrome: Phocomelia + cleft lip/palate
2. Trisomy 18: Radial aplasia + micrognathia + multiple anomalies
3. Ectrodactyly-Ectodermal dysplasia (EEC): Cleft lip/palate or malar hypoplasia
4. Nager syndrome: Micrognathia + external ear abnormality
5. Split hand- split foot syndrome.

Differential Diagnosis of Joint Abnormalities

A. Arthrogryposis:
1. Cerebro-occulofacial skeletal syndrome:
2. Trisomy 18: Arthrogryposis (lower limbs) + congenital heart disease + exomphalos + cleft lip/palate + holoprosencephaly, etc.
3. Neu-Laxova syndrome: Upper and lower limbs both involved + microcephaly + agenesis of corpus callosum + cerebellar hypoplasia + cataract + syndactyly.
4. FADS: upper and lower limbs both involved + micrognathia + hydrops.
5. Multiple pterygium syndrome: Upper and lower limbs both involved + club foot + micrognathia + hydrops + pterygia

B. Clubfoot :
1. Lower spine neural tube defects: Neural tube defects
2. Campomelic dysplasia
3. Femoral hypoplasia-abnormal facies syndrome: Focal femoral hypoplasia + micrognathia
4. Multiple pterygium syndrome
5. FADS.

These anomalies present with involvement of different parts of fetal body and therefore for the simultaneous demonstration of all 3D ultrasound may be a more effective imaging tool. 3D ultrasound is also a preferred imaging modality for the assessment of the cranial sutures and also for the assessment of the joint contractures and anomalies. Even for assessment of shortened limbs or limb parts is more evidently demonstrated by 3D ultrasound in relation to other body parts.

ACKNOWLEDGMENT

I convey my special thanks to Dr. Paresh Lathiya and Dr. Kuldip Jasoliya for providing almost all images of this chapter.

REFERENCES

1. Ruano R, Molho M, Roume J, et al. Prenatal diagnosis of fetal skeletal dysplasias by combining two-dimensional and three-dimensional ultrasound and intrauterine three dimensional helical computer tomography. Ultrasound Obstet Gynecol. 2004;24(2):134-40.
2. Kos M, Hafner T, Funduk-Kurjak B, et al. Limb deformitiesand three dimensional ultrasound. J Perinat Med. 2002; 3-(1):40-7.
3. Garjian KV, Pretorius DH, Budorick NE, et al. Fetal skeletal dysplasia: three-dimensional US initial experience. Radiology 2000;214(3):717-23.
4. Kenelly MM, Moran P. A clinical algorithm of prenatal diagnosis of radial ray defects with two and three dimensional ultrasound. Prenat Diagn. 2007;27(8):730-7.
5. Cassart M, Massez A, Cos T, et al. Contribution of three dimensional computed tomography in the assessment of fetal dysplasia. Ultrasound Obstet Gynecol. 2007;29(5):537-43.
6. Dighe M, Fligner C, Cheng E, et al. Fetal skeletal dysplasia: an approach to diagnosis with illustrative cases. Radiographics. 2008;28: 1061-77.
7. Krakow D, Lachman RS, Rimoin DL. Guidelines for the prenatal diagnosis of fetal skeletal dysplasias. Genet Med. 2009;11(2):127-33.
8. Millington Ward S, Mc Mahon HP, Farrar GJ. Emerging therapeutic approaches for osteogenesis imperfect. Trends Mol Med. 2005;11:299-305.
9. Cassart M. Suspected fetal skeletal malformations or bone diseases: how to explore. Pediatr Radiol. 2010;40:1046-51.
10. Carreras E, Toran N, Ediciones Mayo. Atlas de malformaciones fetales congenitas.

11
CHAPTER

Abnormalities of Placenta and Umbilical Cord

Sonal Panchal

Placenta is the chief circulatory unit that supports the growing fetus through its low resistance blood flow.

FORMATION AND DEVELOPMENT OF THE PLACENTA

With implantation of the embryo in one of the endometrial lips there are several changes occurring in the endometrium that chiefly include proteolytic and immunosuppresion mechanisms for acceptance of the foreign body—the embryo. Progesterone secretion from the corpus luteum and hCG produced by the implanting embryo, together lead to the formation and development of the chorionic tissue, which is the first step towards placentation. In the earlier stages the chorionic tissue is all around the gestational sac but as the embryo grows there is a self selection of the most vascular area expected. It is in this area of the endometrium that the chorionic tissue tries to invade deeper and therefore appears more thick. The chorionic tissue in the rest of the area surrounding the gestational sac starts regressing. The regressing part of the chorionic tissue then is known as chorion leave, whereas the part which becomes thicker and penetrates deeper and is functionally active in allowing the uterine blood flow to reach the embryo is known as chorion frundosum **(Figure 1)**. It is the chorion frundosum that will develop ultimately into placenta.

After 3-4 weeks of implantation, intermediate trophoblast invades maternal spiral arteries. This leads to disruption of extracellular matrix and replacement of

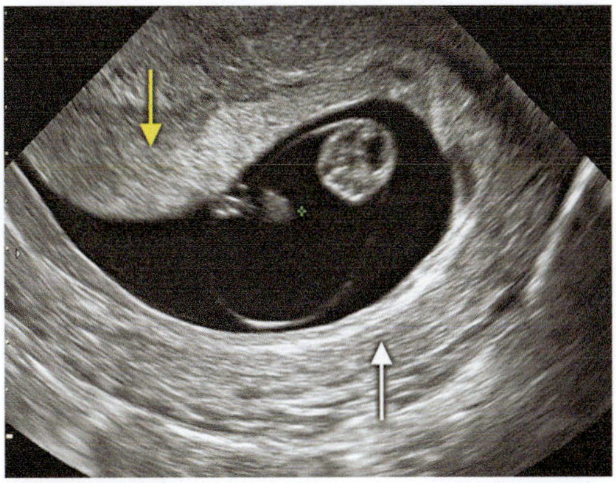

Figure 1: B-mode image of the gestational sac showing thickened chorion frundosum (yellow arrow) and thin chorion leave (white arrow)

maternal endothelium by cells of trophoblastic origin. This leads to development of low resistance vascular bed with large capacitance.[1] There is conversion of highly muscular spiral vessels into nonmuscular placental vessels **(Figure 2)**. Conversion of the vasculature occurs in two phases. First phase starts at around 8 weeks and the second one at around 18 weeks. The fall in resistance is fast till 12 weeks, with the initial phase of conversion in the type of vasculature and then slows down till 22 weeks. Beyond 22 weeks till term further changes in the placental vasculature in terms of lowering resistance is minimal.

Failure of this conversion of high resistance to low resistance vascular system leads to secretion of vasoactive substances from placenta and induces maternal hypertension **(Figure 3)**. Though a complete failure of this conversion will lead to first trimester abortions most commonly due to inability to support the vascular and nutritional needs of the growing fetus, partial failure of conversion will lead to pregnancy-induced hypertension (PIH) and

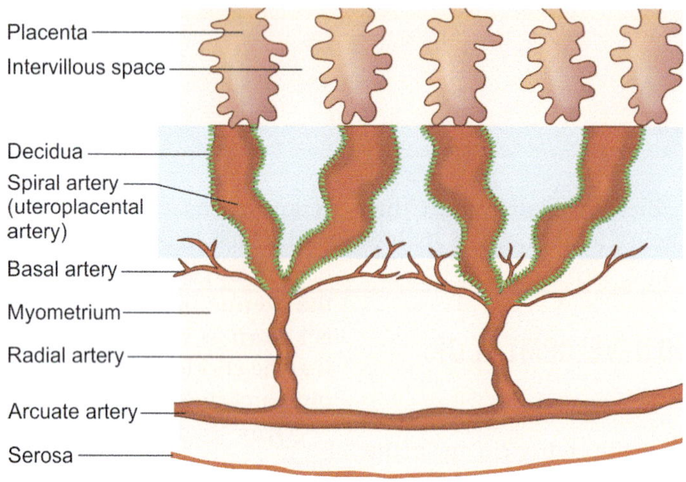

Figure 2: Diagrammatic representation of vascular changes of normal placentation

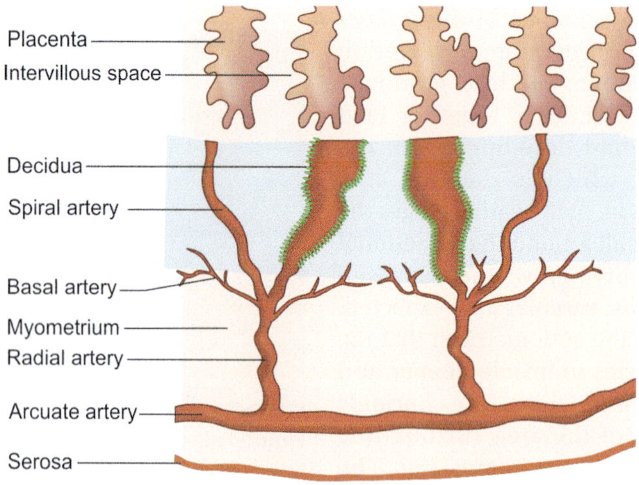

Figure 3: Diagrammatic representation of vascular changes of abnormal placentation

intrauterine grwoth retardation (IUGR) in late second and third trimester, depending on the severity.

It is a consequence of multiple factors:
- Primary defect in invasive trophoblasts
- Endocrine, immunological and inflammatory phenomena which regulate the interplay between maternal and fetal factors.

The pathophysiology that works in development of IUGR is as follows:

Inadequate trophoblastic invasion, which leads to nondilatation of the uterine vessels as a result the placental perfusion is reduced, leading to inadequate villous circulation in turn leading to low oxygen levels in umbilical cord blood and therefore vascular changes in the fetus as a result of stimulation of chemoreceptors. This means the cause is diagnosed by high resistance in the uterine arteries and the results are shown as vascular changes in umbilical cord and fetal vessels.

Though this chapter is dedicated to abnormalities of placenta and the umbilical cord and not on PIH and IUGR, no mention about the vascular abnormalities may leave the discussion incomplete.

During pregnancy there is a persistent fall in the resistance of uterine and umbilical arteries, whereas there is a slow but steady rise in the resistance of middle cerebral artery (MCA) which is considered a representative of fetal circulation. A reverse trend in any of these vessels is indicative of placental insufficiency and may lead to PIH or IUGR **(Figures 4 and 5)**.

Placenta has about 50% reserve and so these changes will become evident only when there is compromise of more than 50% of placental circulation. In the initial phases, it is only dilatation of the middle cerebral arteries and reduced resistance that compensates for increased resistance of the umbilical arteries. When umbilical artery resistance increases significantly and the diastolic flow is significantly reduced the resistance index ratio of MCA to umbilical artery (CPR) becomes one or less than one. This can be taken as a cut off for prediction of bad pregnancy prognosis. An absent or reverse diastolic flow in the umbilical artery is taken as a strongly suggestive sign of fetal morbidity and a high risk of fetal mortality **(Figures 6 to 9)**. MCA resistance persistently falls to compensate for this reduced oxygenated blood supply through the umbilical cord, but fails at a certain point. When this happens, there is lactic acidosis, cerebral edema and paradoxical reversal of MCA resistance to normal. This phase is considered to be an irreversible stage of fetal cerebral damage. There is also a circulatory

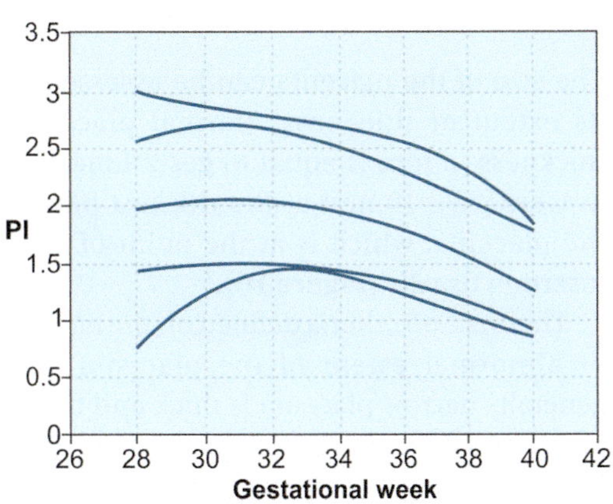

Figure 4: Nomogram of values of middle cerebral artery pulsatility index (PI) with changing gestational age

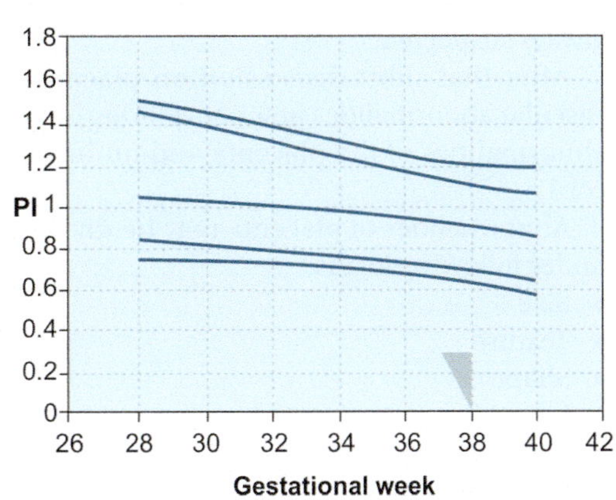

Figure 5: Nomogram of values of umbilical artery pulsatility index (PI) with changing gestational age

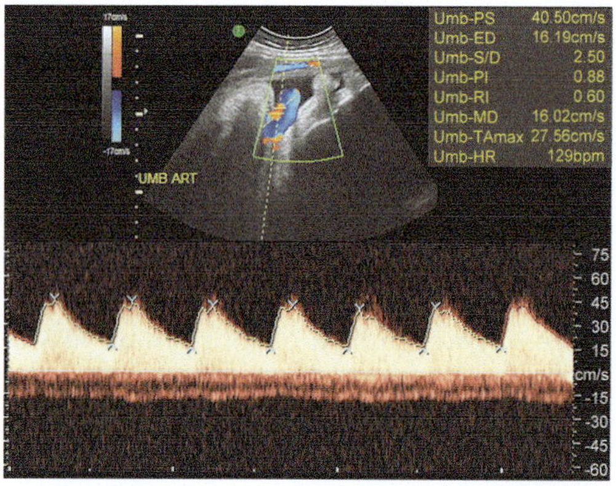

Figure 6: Normal umbilical artery flow pattern

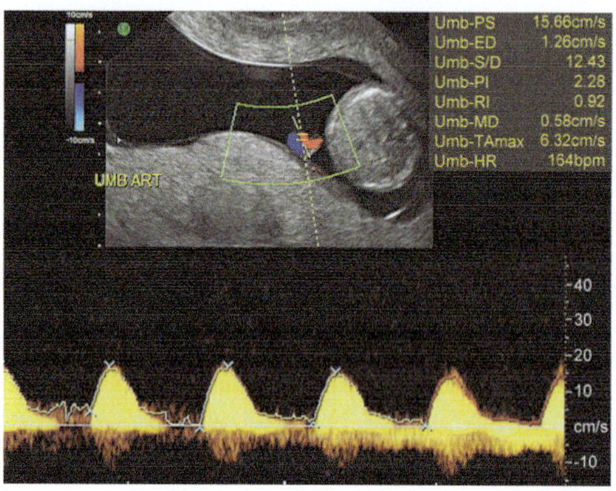

Figure 7: Absent diastolic flow in umbilical artery

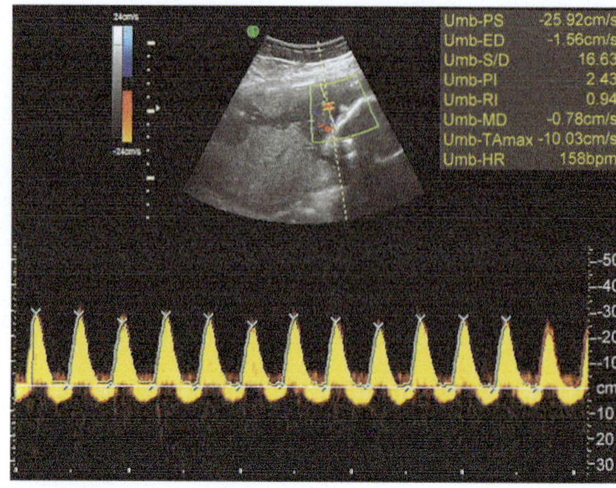

Figure 8: Reversed diastolic flow in umbilical artery

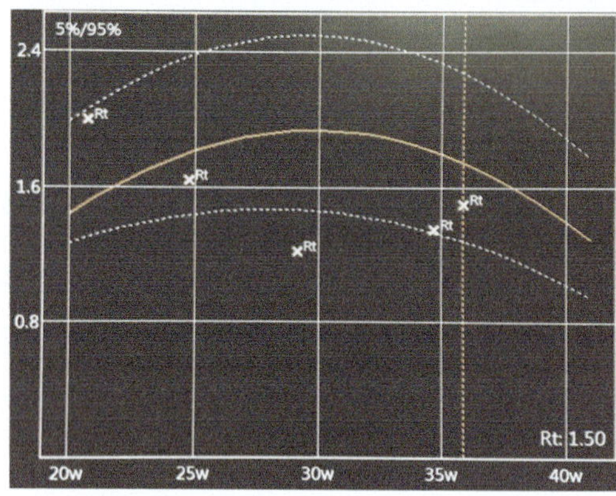

Figure 9: Plotting of MCA PI on the nomogram shows paradoxical reversal (rise) of the MCA resistance

paralysis and fetal or neonatal death is almost always suspected.

After that short discussion on placental vascular abnormalities now considering other abnormalities of the placenta and umbilical cord.

Abnormalities of placenta may be divided under following heads:

- Size
- Texture
- Shape
- Location
- Penetration
- Cord attachment.

ABNORMALITIES OF PLACENTAL SIZE

The size of the placenta can be assessed as its extent or thickness. Normal placental thickness in mm is equal to gestational age in weeks +/- 10 mm at the thickest part of the placenta, which is at the point of cord insertion usually **(Figure 10)**.[2]

There are no criteria defined on the normal or abnormal extent of the placenta, but generally narrow placenta is thick and broad placenta is thin. Ideally both parameters must be combined.

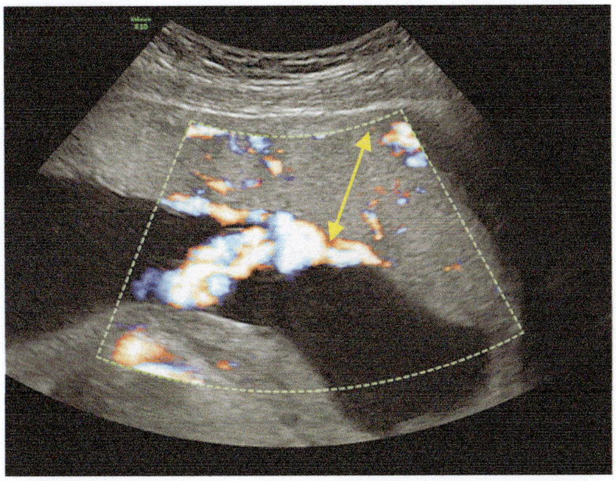

Figure 10: Normal placenta with cord insertion. Measurement of placental thickness is shown by double sided arrow

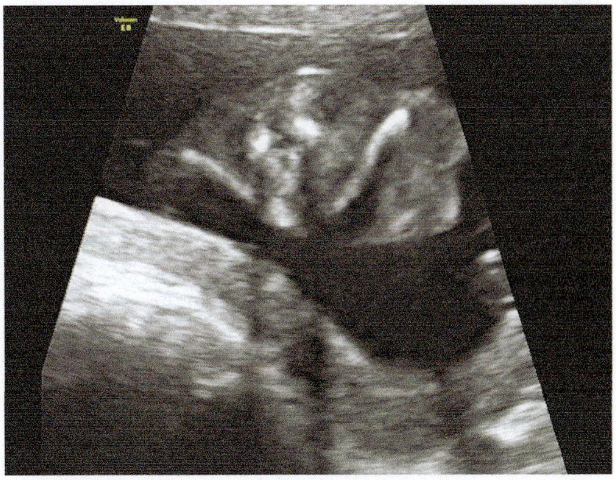

Figure 11: B-mode ultrasound image shows thin placenta

Three-dimensional (3D) ultrasound can be used to calculate placental volume.

Small Placenta

Small placenta is seen in:

- Intrauterine infections—chronic
- First trimester or preconceptional diabetes mellitus or glucose intolerance
- Chromosomal abnormalities
- IUGR of any cause
- Severe polyhydramnios—in these patients pacenta is not actually thin but because of abundant fluid, it gives an erroneous feel of thin placenta **(Figure 11)**.

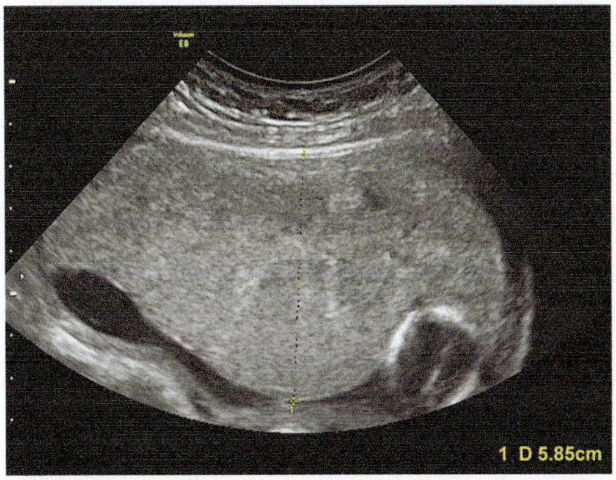

Figure 12: B-mode ultrasound image of thick—large placenta

Large Placenta

Large placenta is seen with (Figure 12):

- Fetal hydrops
- Acute gestational infections
- Maternal anemia
- Placental mesenchymal dysplasia: These patients have a high incidence of growth restriction and fetal demise. The placenta shows anechoic areas due to cystic changes in stem villi.
- Aneuploidies
- Triploidy
- Placental hemorrhage
- Molar pregnancy
- Beckwith-Wiedemann syndrome—macrosomia, macroglossia, visceromegaly increased susceptibility to childhood tumors.

TEXTURE ABNORMALITIES OF THE PLACENTA

Normal placenta has a homogenous texture. Abnormal texture may be in the form of:

- Calcifications
- Lakes

Placental Calcification and Grading

Calcifications in the placenta was thought to be related with the circulatory status of the placenta. It is known that towards the end of the third trimester as a preparatory process for delivery of the fetus and the placenta, the placental vasculature starts regressing by calcification of the vascular walls. This means more calcification in the placenta means more mature placenta and this can be graded as **(Figure 13)**

- Grade 0: Homogenous placenta
- Grade 1: Indentations in chorionic plate
- Grade 2: Basal stippling of placenta
- Grade 3: Calcification (is more commonly seen in smokers and in patients on aspirin or heparin prophylaxis).

Stating placental grading is not required in current scenario as calcification is no longer regarded as consistently associated with growth restriction, fetal distress in labor, PIH, diabetes or lung maturity.[3]

Placental Lakes (Figure 14)

Placental lakes are anechoic areas in the placenta. These are almost universally seen after 25 weeks and are of no clinical significance. Lakes are formed by fibrin deposits that are a result of pooling of blood in perivillous spaces. These are more common in peripheral parts of placenta.

But anechoic areas in the placenta may be also due to:

- Subchorionic hematoma
- Intervillous thrombosis
- Septal cysts
- Infarcts from retroplacental hematoma

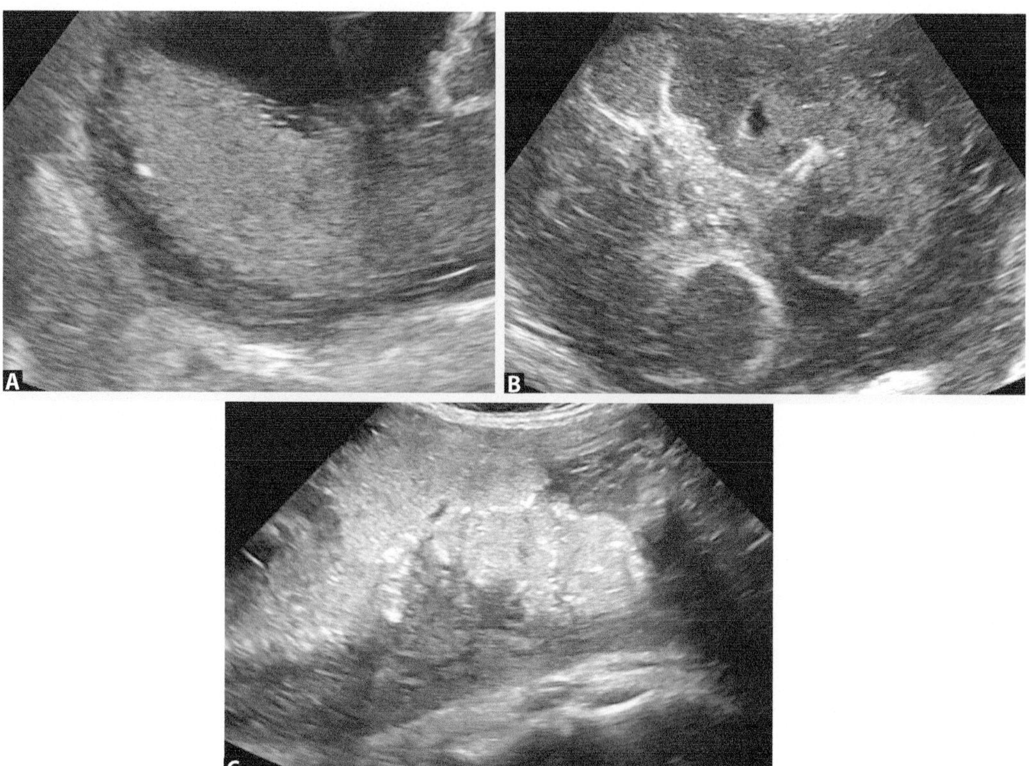

Figure 13: Placenta grade 0, 1, 2 (A through C)

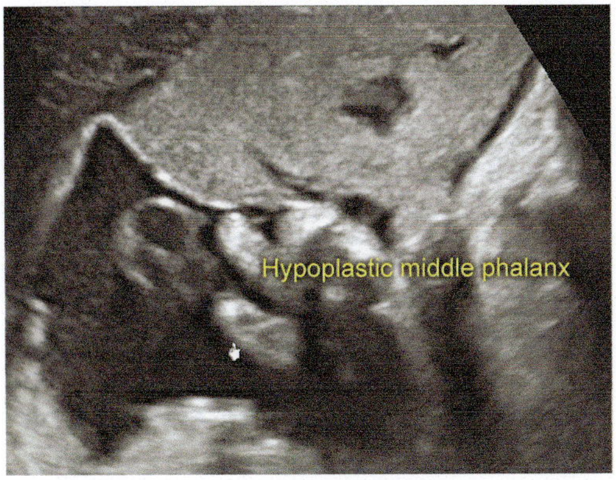

Figure 14: Anechoic areas in the placenta—known as placental lakes

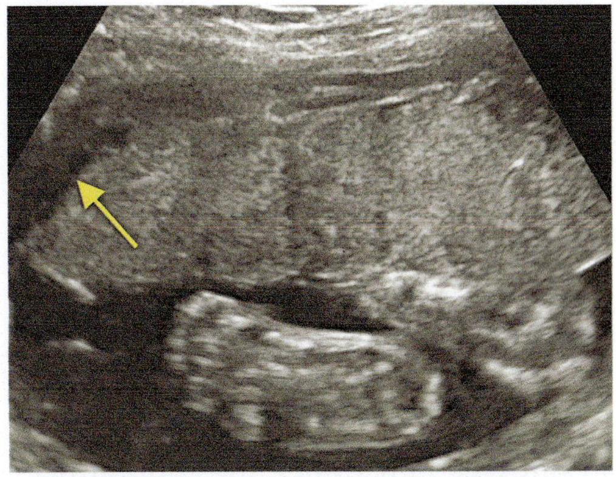

Figure 15: Anechoic area seen between the placenta and the myometrium—retroplacental hematoma

Subchorionic Fibrin Deposits

These are triangular or rectangular hypoechoic spaces with convex borders. These are of no clinical significance.[4]

Intervillous Thrombosis

This is due to fetal hemorrhage in intervillous spaces. These are of significance in fetuses with Rh incompatibility.[5]

Septal Cysts

Septal cysts are cystic areas in between cotyledons and again are of no clinical significance. Though if larger than 45 mm across, these may be associated with growth restriction.

Placental Infarcts

Infarcts in the placenta may result from retroplacental hematomas or thrombotic occlusion of fetal arteries.

Small ones are of no clinical significance but the larger ones may cause severe growth restriction and sometimes also fetal demise **(Figure 15)**.[6] These are echogenic when fresh but become anechoic later. During the transition process these may be at times difficult to identify on scan. Some of these may also calcify and become densely hyperechoic.[6]

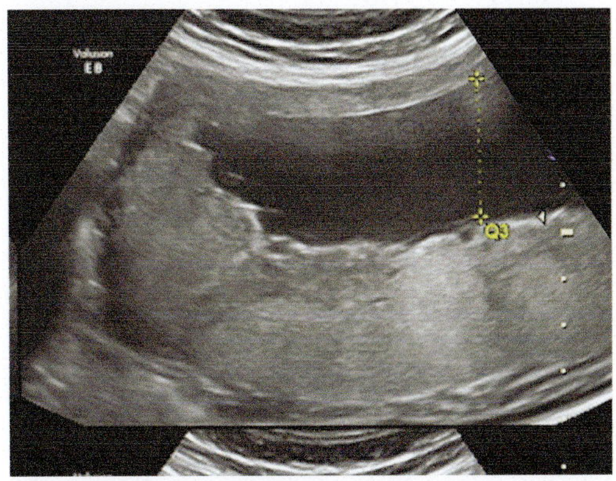

Figure 16: Normal placenta

PLACENTAL SHAPE

Normal shape of the placenta is biconvex, with one surface attached to the uterine wall and another convex surface is its free surface **(Figure 16).** It is thickest in the center, which is where the umbilical cord is normally attached and thins out towards periphery.

Abnormalities of the Placental Shape

Abnormalities of the placental shape may be:
- Placenta membranacea
- Circumvallate placenta
- Horseshoe placenta
- Annular or ring-shaped placenta.

Placenta Membranacea

This is a rare entity. The entire chorion is covered by villi and large part of this placenta is dysfunctional.[7] About 1/3rd of these placentas are abnormally adherent. It often covers the internal os. Because of these two reasons, these placentas are commonly associated with recurrent antepartum heamorrhage, growth restriction and postpartum hemorrhage.[8]

Circumvallate Placenta

In this type of placenta, the chorion plate is smaller than basal plate and therefore membranes insert close to the center instead of at periphery **(Figure 17)**. It may be complete or partial.

Partial variety is clinically insignificant. The complete variety may lead to placental abruption, growth restriction, perinatal mortality and fetal growth restriction.[9]

It has thickened rolled ridge of membranes with uplifted placental shelf.[10] It often shows lucent areas in the extrachorial part of placenta due to infarcts and hematomas.

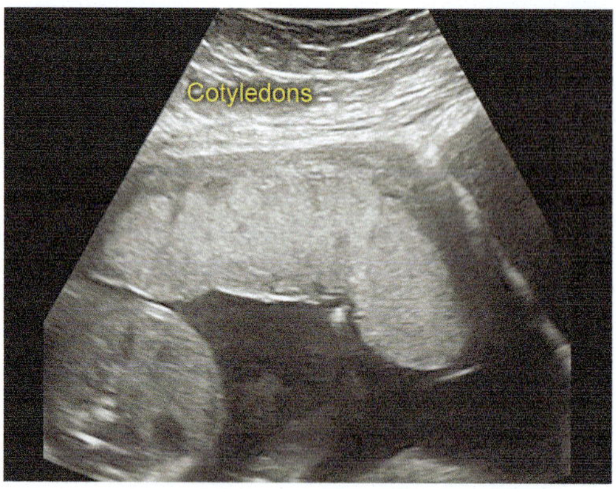

Figure 17: Circumvallate placenta

PLACENTAL LOCATION

Normally the placenta is located in the fundus or upper part of the body of the uterus. In this region of the uterus it may be located anteriorly, posteriorly or on the sides. Positions other than this are considered abnormal. When located in the lower segment of the uterus, these placenta have higher risk of hemorrhagic complications. These placentas are known as placenta previa.

Depending on how low the lower edge of the placenta extends, these placentas may be graded as **(Figures 18 and 19):**

- Grade 0: Lower segmental—distance from internal os <10 mm.
- Grade 1: Marginal, when the lower margin of the placenta is at the margin of the internal os.
- Grade 2: Incomplete, when the lower margin of the placenta, partially covers the internal os.
- Grade 3: Complete, when the internal os is fully covered by the placenta.

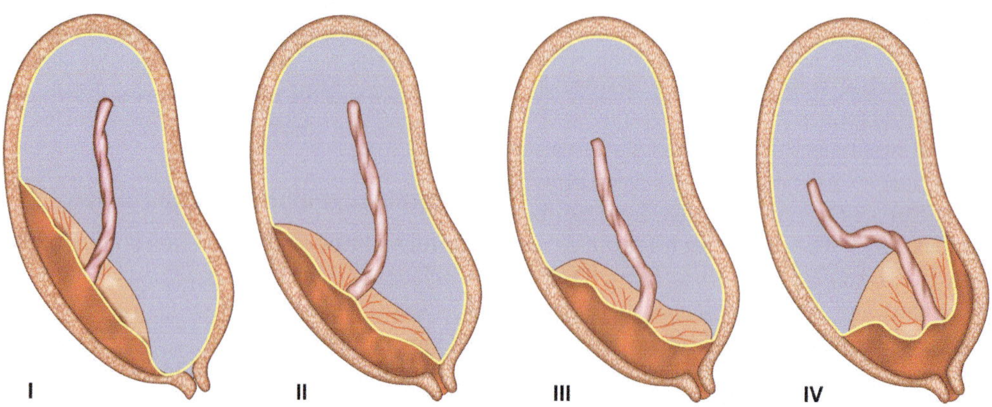

Figure 18: Diagrammatic representation of grades of placenta previa

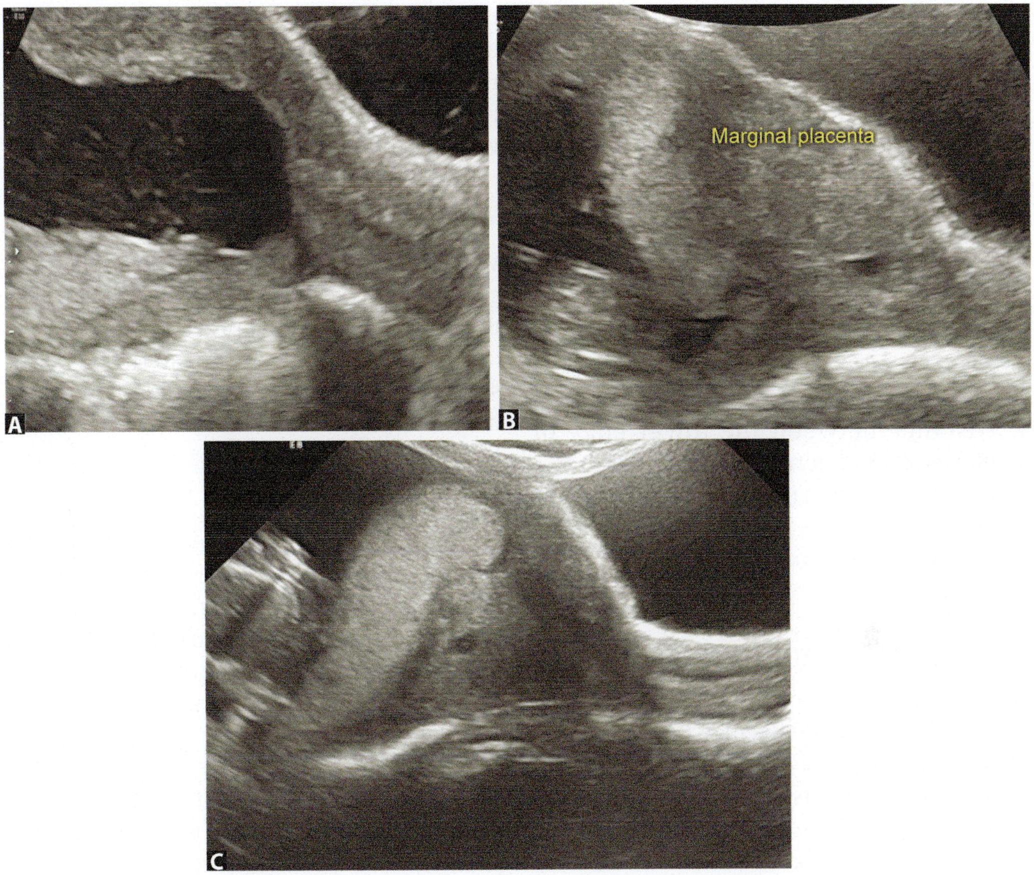

Figures 19: (A) Low lying placenta;(B) Marginal placenta preavia; (C) Complete placenta previa

Risk of postpartum hemorrhage (PPH) is higher when the distance between the internal os and lower edge of placenta is <4 cms.[11]

Risk of placenta preavia is more with:

- Previous CS
- Previous surgeries on uterus
- Previous vigorous curettage
- Multiparity
- Advanced maternal age.

But approximately 90% of low lying placentas at 20 weeks have a tendency to migrate up to normal position at term. Therefore, diagnosis of placenta previa and its grade must not be made before the end of 2nd trimester.[12] Placentas with thin lower edge are less likely to migrate as compared to those with thick edge.[13]

Placental Migration

Placental migration is a consequence of:

- Formation of lower uterine segment
- Placental trophotorphism.

Placental Trophotorphism

This term is used to describe preferential proliferation of trophoblastic villi in regions of better endometrial supply and atrophy of the villi in the region of poor blood supply.[14]

This theory can explain regression of placenta previa, succenturiate placental lobes and abnormal cord insertions in placenta.

When placenta migrates, the raw/ just opened up surface of the uterus may bleed leading to antepartum hemorrhage.

But bleeding with placental migration is not life-threatening and will not lead to the need of premature delivery usually. Antepartum bleeding can be more correlated with the cervical length and presence of echo-free space in lower edge of placenta, overlying the internal os.[15]

MANAGEMENT STRATEGY FOR PREGNANCIES WITH LOW LYING PLACENTA

- Distance between the lower edge of placenta and internal os if it is >20 mm—vaginal delivery is possible
- But if the distance is between 10 mm and 20 mm—most times vaginal delivery is possible.

Succenturiate Placental Lobe (Figure 20)

This means a lobe of the placenta distant from main placenta. This may be a lobe with vessels not commencing out of this lobe. But at times fetal vessels may commence from these lobes to merge with main placenta to form the cord.[16] These vessels are more likely to rupture at labor or at the time of rupture of membranes and can lead to fetal demise. This is especially likely because these vessels may be close to or pass over the internal os and get damaged and also because these may not be protected by Wharton's jelly. Retained placenta and PPH are common complications with succenturiate lobe of placenta.[16]

Vasa Previa (Figure 21)

When the cord vessels are the presenting structures it is known as vasa previa. It is different from placenta previa.

This is commonly associated with succentuariate lobe, velamentous or marginal cord insertion.

Placental Invasion

Normally the placenta is attached to the myometrium of the uterus, but a clear interface is always seen between the placenta and the myometrium and this is known as retroplacental space **(Figure 22).** Retroplacental space is a hypoechoic space of 10–20 mm in thickness.

Retroplacental space is irregular or interrupted in conditions like retroplacental hematoma, placental abruption and placental adherence. The retroplacental space becomes irregular in placental hematomas and abruption but is obliterated in abnormal placental invasion and abrasion.

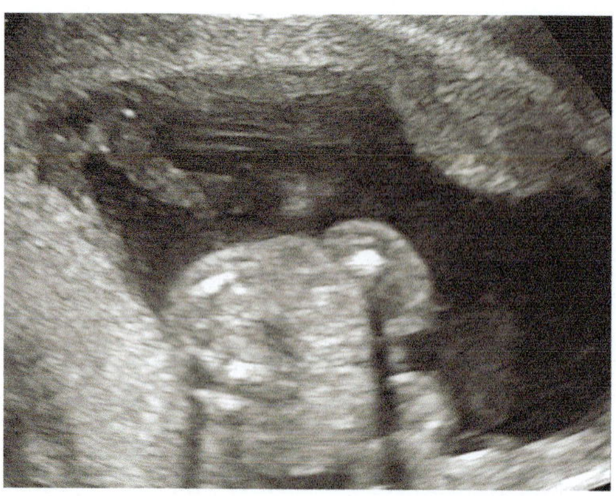

Figure 20: Succenturiate lobe of placenta seen on the anterior wall with the main placenta on posterior wall

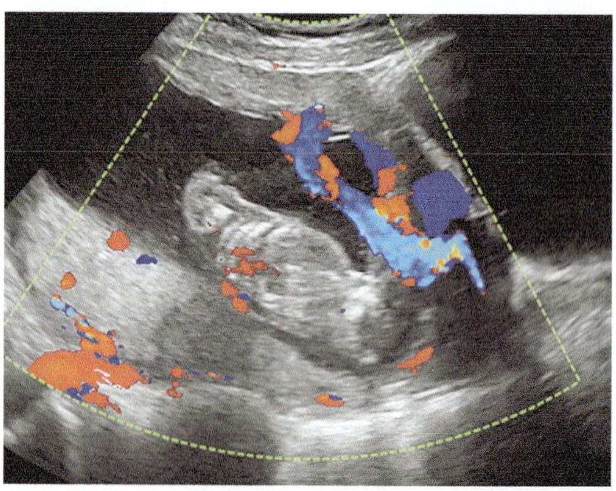

Figure 21: Vasa previa

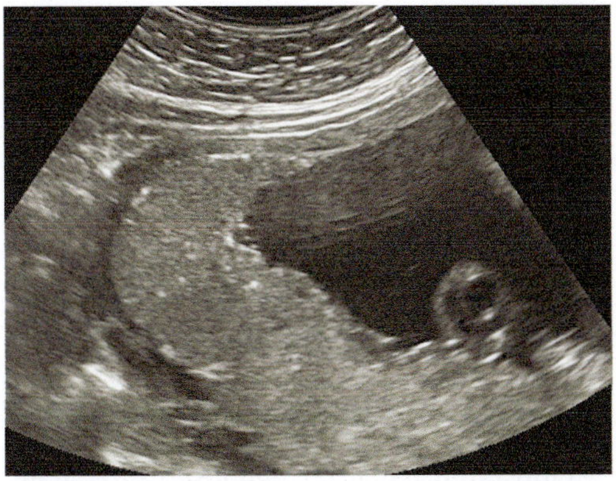

Figure 22: Normal placenta with intact retroplacental space (hypoechoic area between placenta and myometrium)

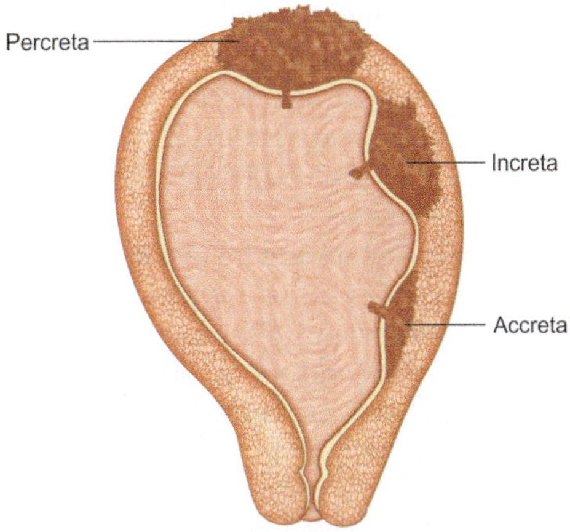

Figure 23: Diagrammatic representation of types of placental invasion

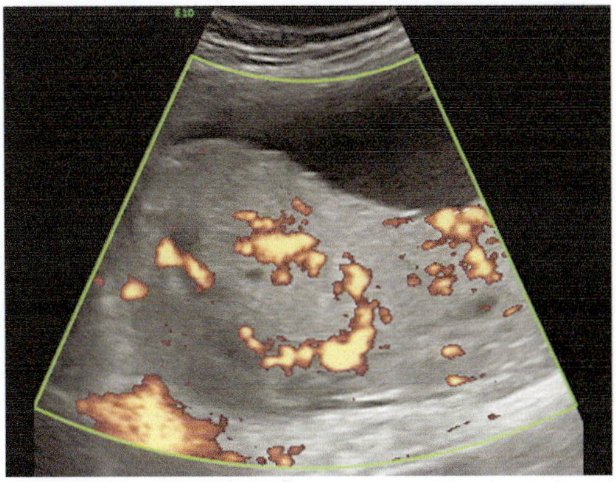

Figure 24: Placenta increta

Whenever this space is not consistent, assessment of the underlying myometrium is mandatory to exclude myomas, adenomyosis or calcifications. Myomas need to be differentiated from uterine contractions, which disappear in 20–60 minutes.

Placental Invasion Abnormalities (Figure 23)

- Placenta accreta
- Placenta percreta
- Placenta increta **(Figure 24).**

Placenta Accreta

Abnormal adherence of the placenta to myometrium. The placenta is adherent to but not invading the myometrium.

It is consequential to a defect in the fibrinoid (Nitabuch's) layer of decidua underlying the placenta.[17] Placenta previa is more commonly seen in patients with placenta accreta.

Diagnosis of placenta accreta on ultrasound

- Normal retroplacental hypoechoic space is 10–20 mm thick, this reduces to <2 mm
- Interface between placenta and myometrium is lost
- Multiple anechoic lacunae are seen in the placenta
- Blood vessels running perpendicular to the myometrial vessels in a normal placenta are also seen running across into the myometrium.[18]

Placenta Percreta

When the placental tissue invades into the myometrium, it is called placenta percreta. On ultrasound the retroplacental space is obliterated and on Doppler, placental vessels that are perpendicular to myometrial fibers and myometrial surace are seen penetrating into half or more thickness of the myometrium.

Placenta Increta

When the placental tissue invades the entire thickness of the myometrium through to serosa and beyond, it is called placenta increta. Ultrasound diagnosis is by obliteration of the retroplacental space and extention of placental vessels across the myometrium, through to the serosa and may be even to the surrounding tissues.

Placenta percreta and increta are the more worse forms of an adherent placenta. These placental abnormalities may often cause uterine inversion and severe bleeding. These may almost always demand a hysterectomy at delivery of the baby.

Accuracy of ultrasound for antenatal detection of invasive placenta is fairly high and diagnosed antenatally can plan deliveries better and also save the mother from fatal complications.

The diagnostic accuracy of adherent placenta on B-mode and color Doppler studies are as follows:

B mode

- Sensitivity 90.72%
- Specificity 96.94%
- Positive LR 11.01
- Negative LR 0.16.

Color Doppler

- Sensitivity 90.74%
- Specificity 87.68%
- Positive LR 7.77%
- Negative LR 0.17%.

HEMATOMAS AROUND PLACENTA

- Retroplacental hematoma
- Subamniotic hematoma
- Subchorionic hematoma
- Concealed hematoma

Retroplacental Hematomas

Hematoma seen between basal plate of placenta and uterine wall is called a retroplacental hematoma. The fresh ones are isoechoic to placenta and difficult to identify. But the old ones are hypoechoic and cause evident widening of the retroplacental space on ultrasound. These may lead to villous infarction.

Subamniotic Hematoma (Figure 25)

Hematoma between amnion and chorion is called a subamniotic Hematoma. The commonest location is at the placental cord insertion. It often occurs as a result of pulling of cord during delivery and therefore not an antenatal ultrasound diagnosis.

Only rarely it may be diagnosed antenatally and when large it is termed as Breus mole. This is commonly associated with growth restriction and fetal demise. On US it appears as an avascular hypoechoic lesion between chorion and amnion[19].

Subchorionic Hematoma

Hematoma between fetal aspect of placenta and overlying chorionic membrane is termed as a subchorionic hematoma. It is more often seen in patients with cocaine abuse, smoking habits, hypertension, preeclampsia, anticardiolipin antibodies and may also occur due to blunt trauma. Its clinical presentation and significance is related to size of hematoma and gestational age. It is associated with uterine irritation due to blood and may lead to preterm labor.[20]

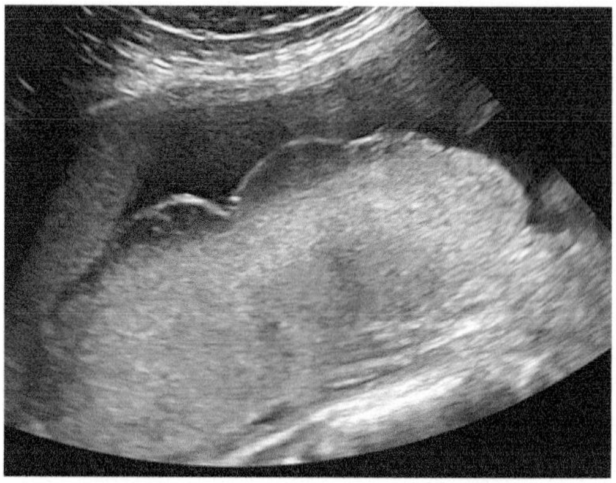

Figure 25: Subamniotic hematoma

Patients with subchorionic hematoma have a higher risk of abortion, IUGR, preterm labor, placental abruption or fetal distress, when associated with vaginal bleeding or uterine contractions.[20]

It can be treated with tocolytics and progesterone.

PLACENTAL TUMORS

These can be divided into:

- Nontrophoblastic tumors
- Gestational trophoblastic disease
  - Complete or partial moles
  - Invasive mole
  - Choriocarcinoma.

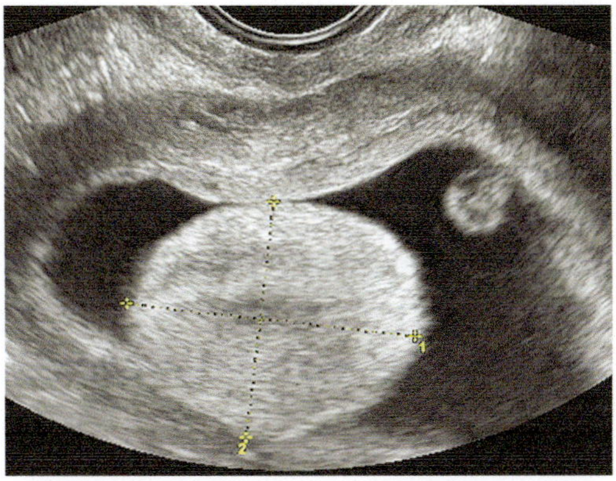

Figure 26: Chorioangioma

Nontrophoblastic Placental Tumors

- Chorioangiomas
- Placental teratomas : are cystic and solid lesions, variably vascular and on surface of placenta. These may represent an unsuccesful twin pregnancy.[21]
- Metastasis from melanoma, lymphoma, leukemia and breast lesions, though very rare may be seen in the placenta.[22]

Chorioangiomas (Figure 26)

These are the most common of nontrophoblastic placental tumors. These are benign tumours. The usually arise fron close to the cord attachment on the placenta. These are well-defined tumors but variably vascular. The smaller ones are nonsignificant, but the larger ones, especially those larger than >50 mm across may lead to nonimmune hydrops, fetal cardiomegaly, polyamnios or growth restriction.[23]

UMBILICAL CORD

Umbilical cord is the vascular and nutritional link between the mother's uterus and the fetus. It chiefly constitutes of two umbilical arteries and an umbilical vein and Wharton's jelly and all these covered in a single layer of amniotic epithelium. It has a helical structure with arteries and vein arranged as a spiral **(Figure 27)**. At term it is about 50-60 cm long and has a helical course with 10-11 coils in all.

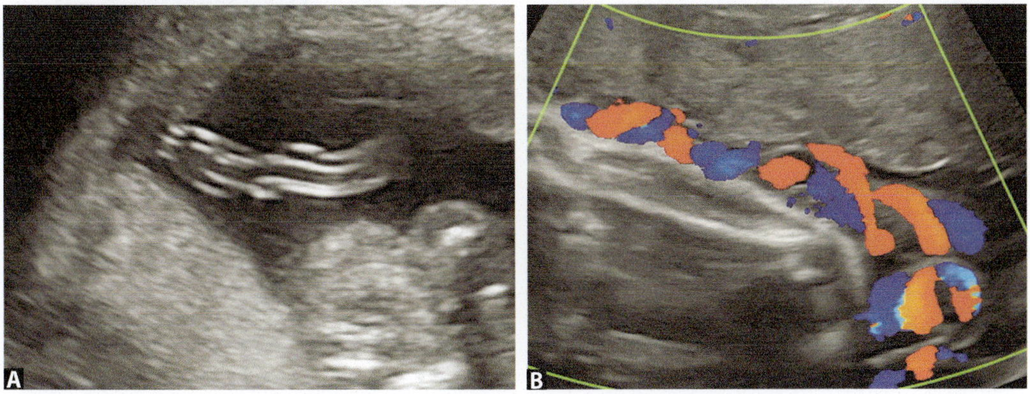

Figure 27: Normal umbilical cord on B mode and color Doppler

Structure of the umbilical cord can be influenced by:

- Gestational age
- Amniotic fluid amount
- Composition of amniotic fluid
- Fetoplacental hemodynamics
- Maternal complications.

Like all other fetal parts, umbilical cord also follows a sort of a growth pattern and has a definitive consistent pattern that it follows. Its diameter progressively increases till 32 weeks and then plateaus. Its thickness is because of the caliber of arteries and the vein and also because of the amount of Wharton's jelly. The umbilical cord vessels also have an increasing caliber with the growing pregnancy **(Figure 28)(Table 1)**.

Wharton's Jelly

Wharton's jelly consists of a collagen fibrillar network formed by canalicular structures and cavernous and perivascular spaces.[24] It is also supposed to have contractility comparable to smooth muscle cells and so participates in regulation of blood flow in the cord vessels.

It may have a role in bidirectional transfer of fluid and metabolites between amniotic fluid and cord vessels and also has metabolic functions. It protects the umbilical vessels from external pressure changes and minor injuries.

Abnormalities of the Umbilical

Abnormalities of the umbilical cord may be:

- Abnormal cord thickness
- Abnormal number of umbilical arteries
- Discordant umbilical arteries
- Abnormal length of the cord
- Abnormal coiling pattern of the cord

Abnormal Cord Thickness

Cord may be thin because of thin vessels and less amount of Wharton's jelly **(Figure 29).** It is known that thin umbilical cord vessels means less blood flow to the fetus.

Table 1: Diameter of umbilical vessels parameters in IUGR

	16 weeks	*At term*
Umbilical artery	1.2 +/–0.4 mm	4.2 +/– 0.4 mm
Umbilical vein	2.0 +/– 0.6 mm	8.2 +/– 0.8 mm

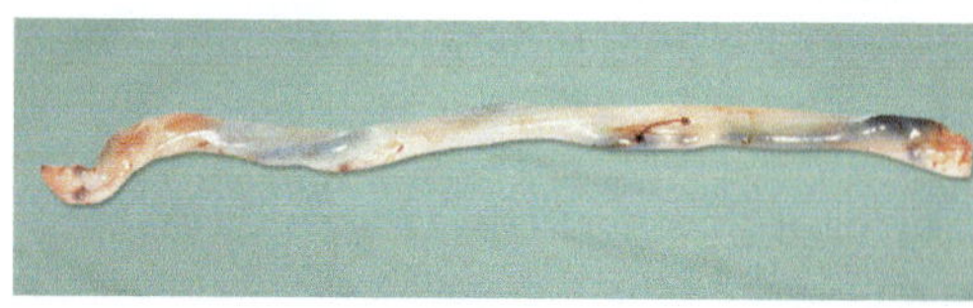

Figure 29: Thin umbilical cord

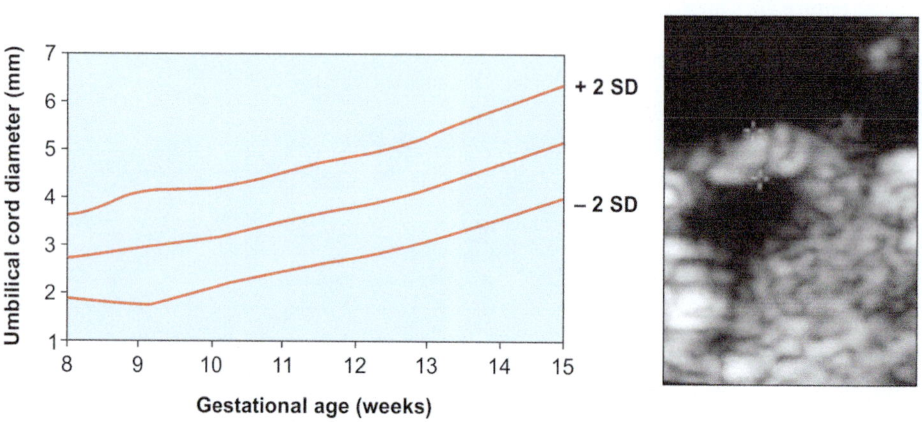

Figure 28: Graph showing increasing umbilical cord diameter with increasing gestational age

Cord mophology in normal and thin cord:[25] Refer Table 2.

Table 2: Cord morphology in normal and thin cord[25]

Characteristics	Normal cord	Lean cord	p
Cord length (cm)	57.6 ± 10.3	57.2 ± 11.5	NS
Coiling index	0.29 ± 0.09	0.18 ± 0.08	<0.001
Cord area (mm^2)	200.6 ± 34.6	87.6 ± 5.1	<0.001
Art area (mm^2)	14.3 ± 5.4	13.3 ± 5.3	NS
Vein area (mm^2)	50.5 ± 20.2	35.2 ± 11.5	<0.01
Jelly area (mm^2)	122.1 ± 33.4	25.7 ± 10.3	<0.001

Flow parameters in normal and thin cord:[25]

Table 3: Flow parameters in normal and thin cord

Characteristics	Normal cord	Lean cord	p
Artery PI	0.83 ± 0.14	0.85 ± 0.09	NS
Absolute vein blood flow	423.5 ± 93.2	293.6 ± 81.8	<0.001
Vein flow for fetal weight	126 ± 23.4	93.7 ± 17.8	<0.001
Vein flow velocity	9.0 ± 3.6	6.6 ± 2.7	<0.05

Table 4: Cord parameters in IUGR

Cord parameters	Normal	IUGR normal doppler	IUGR abnormal doppler
Wharton's jelly	49.4 ± 2.2	40.4 ± 3.7	33.4 ± 2.6
Vessel areas	7.8 ± 0.3	6.6 ± 0.3	4.8 ± 0.3
Art wall thickness	654 ± 20	645 ± 23	525 ± 24
Vein wall thickness	465 ± 18	465 ± 18	390 ± 14

Lean umbilical cord after 20 weeks of gestation had **4.4 fold higher risk of having a SGA infant** than the one with normal cord (95% confidence interval, 2.16–8.85).[26] Cord thickness of **<10th centile for gestational age is an early marker of SGA infant and occurrence of intrapartum complications.**[27]

It is shown in this study by Bruch et al. that fetuses with thin cord and IUGR have significantly less amount of wharton's jelly and also smaller vessels as compared to normal fetuses.[28]

Amount of Wharton's jelly may be reduced due to reduction in extracellular fluid or matrix in patients with hypertensive disorders and gestational diabetes.

Thick cord may be due to:

- Cord tumor
- Urachal cysts
- Mucoid degeneration of cord
- Omphalomesenteric cyst
- It has also been used as one of the parameters to predict fetal macrosomia.[29]
- Increased amount of Wharton's jelly is seen in patients with gestational diabetes mellitus (due to increased accumulation of fluid and plasma proteins and is seen after 24 weeks of gestation).[30]

Abnormal Number of Umbilical Arteries

This is almost always a single umbilical artery. More than two umbilical arteries are not known. Single umbilical artery can be picked up on long section of the umbilical cord also, but is always better demonstrated on the transverse section of the cord. The normal cord that has two umbilical arteries and one umbilical vein shows a typical mickey mouse face appearance on transverse section **(Figure 30).** This is not seen in case of a single umbilical artery **(Figure 31).**

Incidence of single umbilical artery is:

- 0.5–2.9% in euploid fetuses
- 1.5–7% in aborted fetuses
- 9–11% in aneuploid fetuses

There have been several studies on consequences of single umbilical artery and various studies have shown higher risk of chromosomal abnormalities and higher risk of IUGR. As for the risk of chromosomal abnormality the current concept is that as an isolated finding, this is of not much importance but when associated with other soft markers may increase the risk of chromosomal abnormalities.

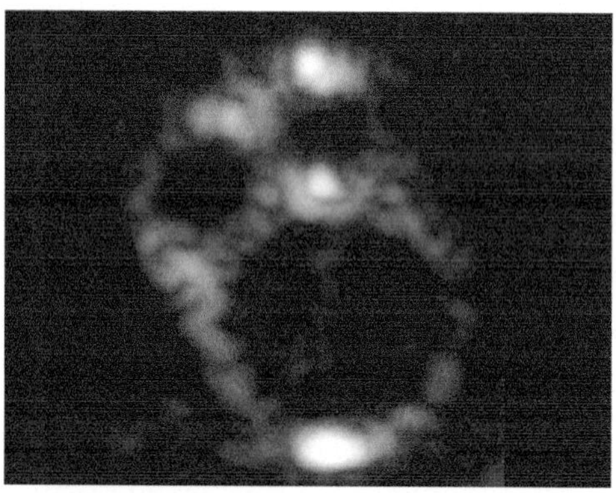

Figure 30: Normal cord in transverse section

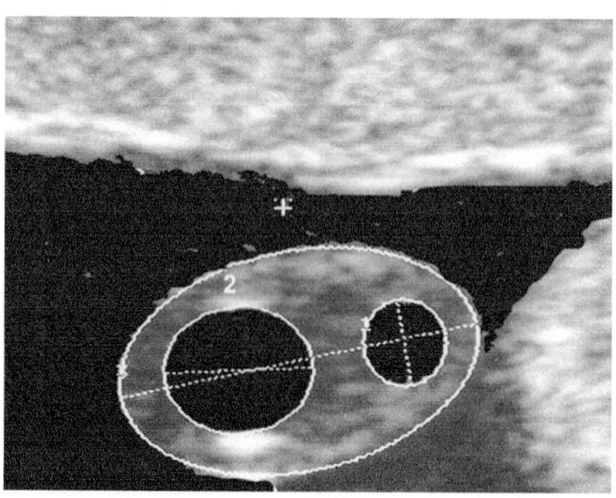

Figure 31: Cord with single umbilical artery in transverse section

Fetuses with single umbilical artery have a higher risk of:

- IUGR (controversial): As for the risk of IUGR, the current concept does not agree that single umbilical artery increases the risk of IUGR. Though fetuses with single umbilical artery have been shown to have a higher risk of intrapartum accidents and still births.
- Risk of congenital anomalies is calculated to be approximately 7 times higher. But unfortunately only 37% of these anomalies can be identified on prenatal scans.[31]
- Intrauterine death, the risk is more in third trimester.
- There is also an increased risk of intrapartum death.

Intrauterine death and intrapartum death may be attributed to two reasons. First is the absence of Hyrtl anastomosis, therefore no safety valve mechanism to fight sudden severe pressure changes. Second is that these cords have less Wharton's jelly, which further decreases in third trimester.

Single umbilical artery actually is thought to be an extreme form of discordant umbilical arteries.[31]

Discordant Umbilical Arteries (Figure 32)

Difference in diameter of umbilical arteries of at least 1 mm in three different parts of cord. These arteries also show difference in impedence to blood flow.[32] But discordant

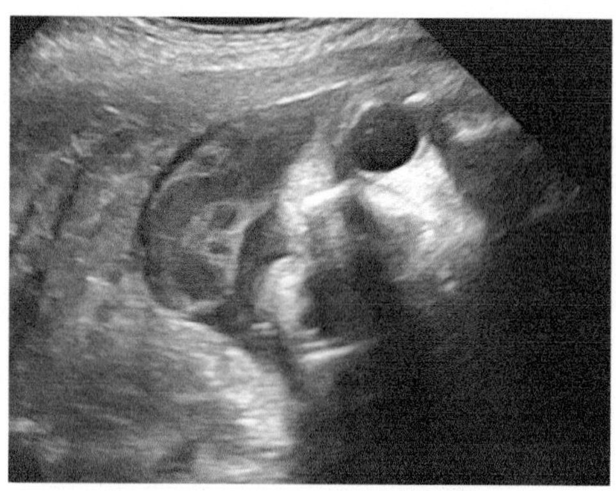

Figure 32: Discordant umbilical arteries

umbilical arteries have not shown effect on the development of the fetus.

Discordant umbilical arteries are common with:

- Placenta bipartite (placenta divided into two parts)
- Placenta succenturiata (succenturiate lobe of placenta)
- Absent Hyrtl anatomosis
- Marginal cord insertion in placenta
- Velamentous cord insertion.

Hytrl anastomosis: Hyrtl anastomosis is the only vessel that connects the two umbilical arteries or their branches on placental surface, close to the site of cord insertion and equalizes the blood pressure between the territories of two arteries **(Figure 33).** As it equalizes the pressure in the two umbilical arteries it actually works as a pressure release valve and protects the fetus and the cord from damages due to pressure changes. It is present in 95% of normal placentas. Absent Hyrtl anastomosisis is more frequently seen apart from fetuses with single umbilical artery, in patients with discordant umbilical arteries and in fetuses with velamentous cord insertion.

Hypothesis on the function of Hyrtl anastomosis:

1. It equalizes the pressure between the two umbilical arteries.
2. It allows uniform distribution of blood in the different regions of the placenta.
3. It acts as a safety valve for the placenta in case of compression or occlusion of one of the umbilical arteries or during uterine contractions.

Hyrtl anastomosis can be of three different types and are shown in the **Figure 34.**

Velamentous cord insertion: Velamentous insertion of the cord is insertion of the cord in the membranes distant from placenta with vessels running in the membranes without being protected by Wharton's jelly **(Figure 35).**

Helical pattern of the umbilical cord: Umbilical cord starts coiling at 8 weeks. Number of coils at the end of 1st trimester are the same as at term. More cords are left twisted, though the significance of side is not yet understood.

Single coil is distance between the right outer surface of consecutive arterial coils.

Umbilical coil index (UCI) is reciprocal of this value and represents the number of

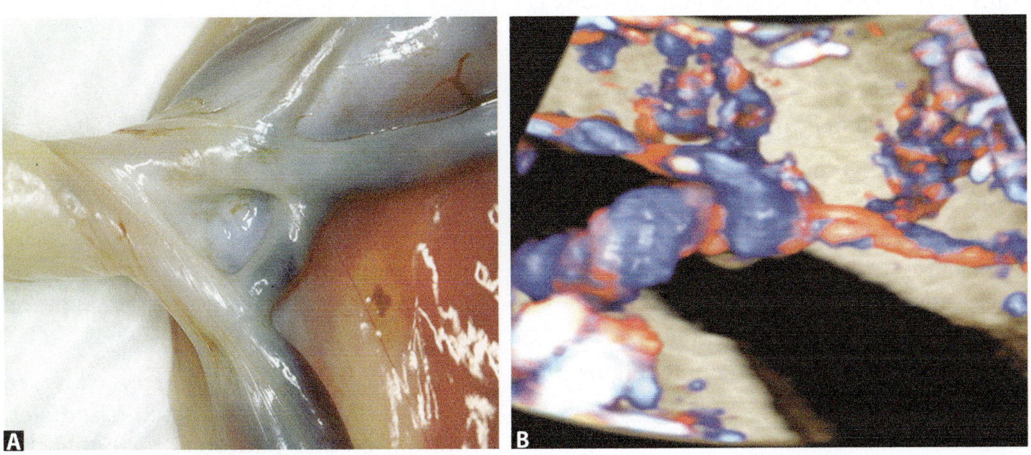

Figure 33: Normal Hyrtl anastomosis on dissection and on ultrasound

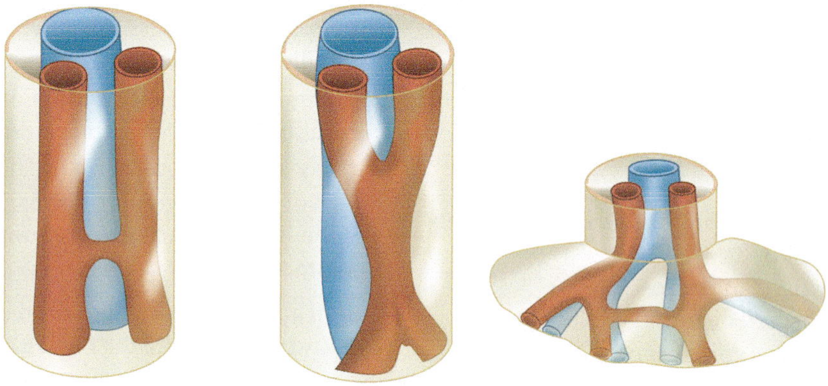

Figure 34: Diagrammatic demonstration of three types of Hyrtl anastomosis

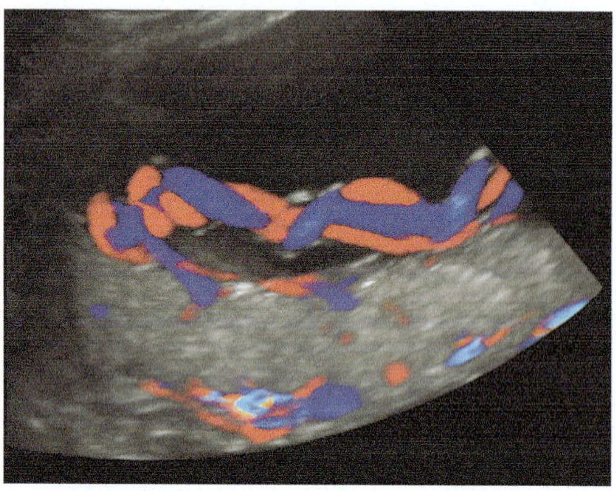

Figure 35: Velamentous insertion of cord.

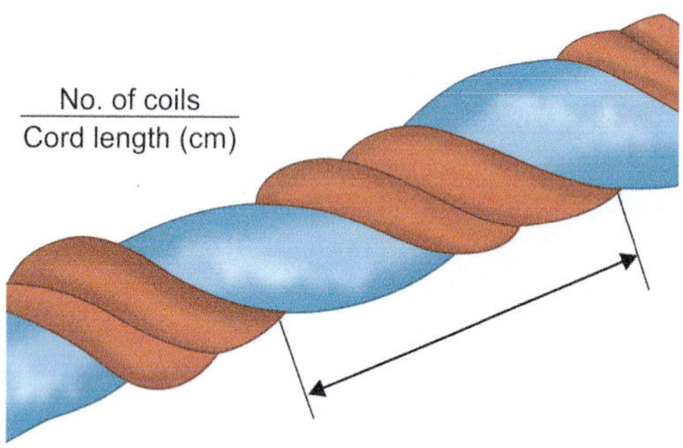

Figure 36: Calculating umbilical cord coiling index

coils in the cord. Umbilical coiling index is calculated as: Number of coils/cord length in cms **(Figure 36)**.

Abnormal Coiling Pattern (Figure 37)

- Uncoiled: No coils—straight umbilical arteries

  Uncoiled or hypocoiled cords are more seen in fetuses with IUGR, maternal hypertensive disorders and aneuploidies
- Hypocoiled: UCI <10th centile
- Hypercoiled: UCI >90th centile **(Figure 38)**
- Atypical coiling:
  - Uncoordinated or aperiodic coiling
  - Supercoiling or spring like cord.

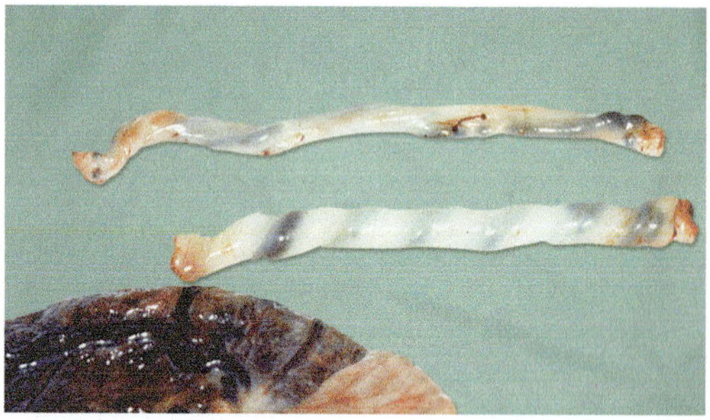

Figure 37: Less coiled and highly coiled cord at birth

Though no definite correlations to pathologies have been established yet, abnormal coiling patterns are thought to influence perinatal outcome.

Supercoiled cords can be associated with pathologic intra-abdominal process leading to increase in resistance at umbilical ring and venous congestion in extra-abdominal umbilical vein.

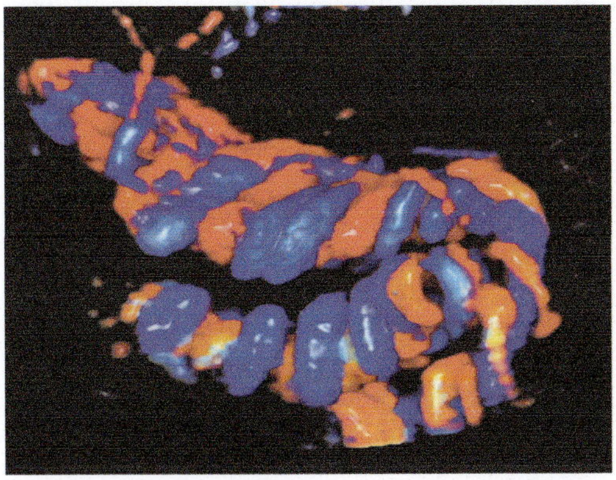

Figure 38: Hypercoiled cord

Cord Cyst (Figure 39)

Cysts may be seen in the cord. These are of not much clinical significance, though was once thought to be a soft marker for T21.

Cord Round the Neck

This is commonly seen. Single loop is not of much importance as usually is not a complete circle. When there are two or more loops **(Figure 40)**, it can strangulate the fetus. But at times even a single loop can cause strangulation when there is a knot **(Figure 41)**.

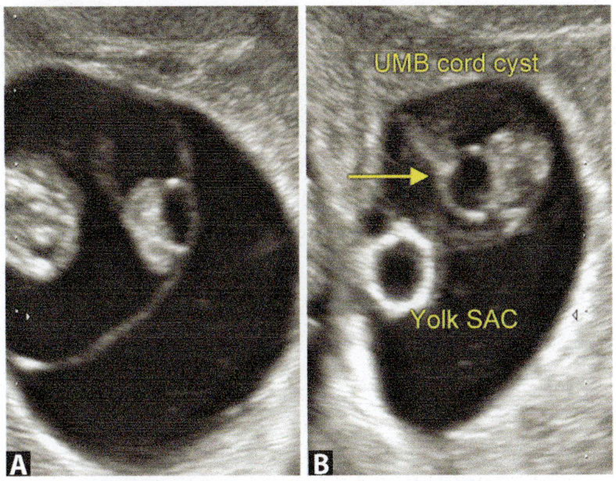

Figure 39: Umbilical cord cyst (arrow)

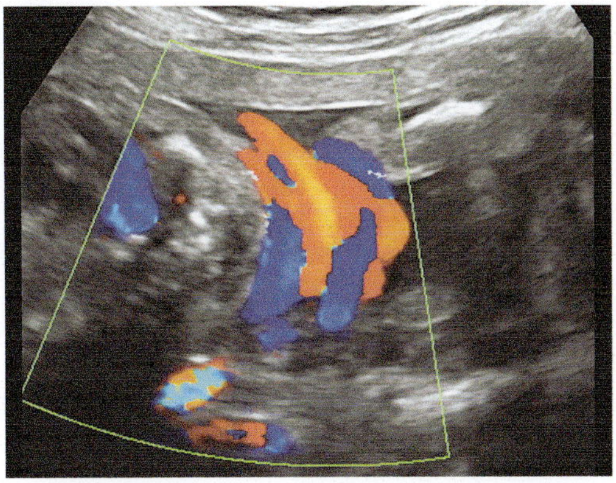

Figure 40: two loops of cord round the neck

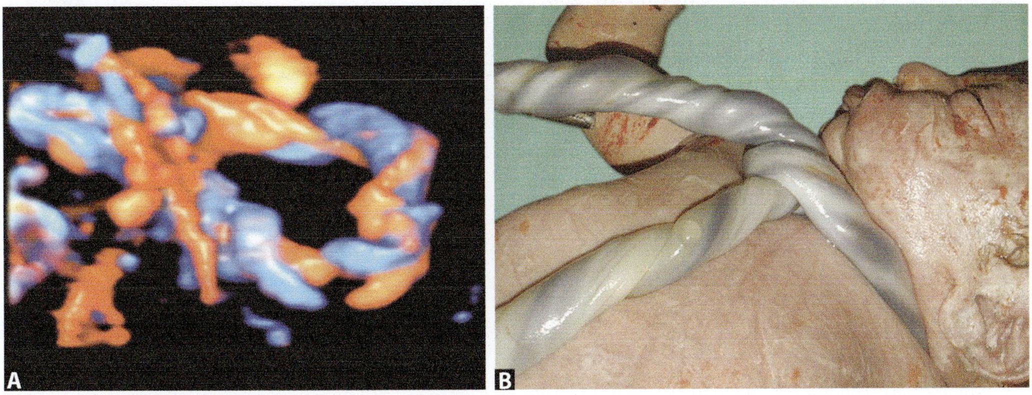

Figure 41: Single loop of cord round the neck with knot on color Doppler and in the neonate

Knot in the cord may lead to severe fetal hypoxia and intrapartum death. This is usually difficult to identify on B-mode image. Though 3D power Doppler can be diagnostic. But it is important to remember that it must be suspected to identify. Very important sign that would suggest a possibility is intermittent fetal bradycardia.

To conclude, placenta and the cord, though most times neglected on the scan can be important indicators of fetal status and must become a part of routine anomaly scans.

REFERENCES

1. Kliman HJ. Am J Pathol. 1993;143(2):332-6.
2. Harris RD, et al. In: Ultrasound in Obstetrics and Gynecology, 4th edition. WB Saunders Co; 2000.pp.597-625.
3. McKenna D, et al. Acta Obstet Gynecol Scand. 2005;8491:7-10.
4. Spirt BA, et al. In: Diagnostic Ultrasound: a logical approach, 1st edition. Lippincott-Raven Publishers; 198. pp. 181-200.
5. Salaa Cm, et al. Am J Obstet Gynecol. 1995;17394:1049-57.
6. Jauniaux E, et al. J Clin Ultrasound. 1991;19: 58-61.
7. Greenberg JA, et al. Obstet Gynecol. 1991;78(3 pt 2):512-4.
8. Wilkins BS, et al. Br J Obstet Gynecol. 1991; 98(7):675-9.
9. McCarthy J, et al. J Ultrasound Med. 1995; 14(1):21-6.
10. Oppenheimer L. J Obstet Gynecol Can. 2007; 29(3):261-73.
11. Oyelese Y. Ultrasound Obstet Gynecol. 2009; 34(2):123-6.
12. Ghourab S. Ultrasound Obstet Gynecol 2001; 18(2):103-8.
13. Predanic M, et al. J Ultrasound Med. 2005; 24(6):773-80.
14. Ghi T, et al. Ultrasound Obstet Gynecol 2009; 33(2):209-12.
15. Saitoh M, et al. Gynecol Obstet Invest. 2002; 54(1):37-42.
16. Hata K, et al. Gynecol Obstet Invest. 1988; 25(4): 273-6.
17. Mazouni C, et al. Placenta. 2006;28(7):599-603.
18. Shih JC, et al. Ultrasound Obstet Gynecol. 2009; 33(2);193-203.
19. Bromley B, et al. J Ultrasound Med. 1994;13(11): 883-6.
20. Nagy S, et al. Obstet Gynecol. 2003;102:94-100.
21. Ahmed N, et al. J Clin Ultrasound. 2004;32(2): 98-101.
22. Altman JF, et al. J Am Acad Dermatol. 2003; 49(6):1150-4.
23. Prapas N, et al. Ultrasound Onstet Gynecol. 2000;16(6):559-63.
24. Vizza E, et al. Reprod Fertil Dev. 1996;8(5):885-94.
25. Di Naro, et al. Umbilical vein flow in fetuses with normal and lean umbilical cord. Ultrasound Obstet Gynecol. 2001;17:224-8.
26. Raio L, et al. Ultrasound Obstet Gynecol. 1999;13(3):176-80.
27. Ghezzi F, et al. J Clin Ultrasound. 2005;33(1): 18-23.
28. Bruch, et al. Human pathlogy. 1997;28(10): 1139-45.
29. Cromi A, et al. Ultrasound Obstet Gynecol. 2007;30(6):861-6.
30. Weissman A, et al. J Ultrasound Med. 1997;16(10):691-4
31. Persutte WH, et al. Ultrasound Obstet Gynecol. 1995;6(3):216-29.
32. Raio L, et al. Obstet Gynecol. 1998;91(1):86-91.

12
CHAPTER

Fetal Hydrops

KV Sridevi, Sonal Panchal

Fetal hydrops is defined as an excess of total body fluid. The term hydrops should be used when excessive fluid is present in two of the body cavities (i.e. pleural, pericardial, peritoneal) or in one of the body cavities, in the presence of skin and subcutaneous thickening, due to edema (fluid collection).[1] When excessive fluid is limited to one of the body compartments, the condition may be named as an isolated finding,[2] e.g. isolated ascites.

Hydrops fetalis is thus not a disease a descriptive term used for abnormal fluid collection in different body cavities and compartments. Hydrops can be due to severe causes but these are chiefly divided as hydrops due to immune causes and hydrops due to nonimmune causes.

IMMUNE HYDROPS

Maternal Rh alloimmunization occurs when a pregnant woman develops an immunological response to a paternally derived red blood cell antigen (D) that is foreign to the mother and is inherited by the fetus from the father.

PATHOPHYSIOLOGY

The incidence of RhD negative blood group varies worldwide. About 15% of Caucasians are RhD negative. The incidence drops to <1% in Chinese and Japanese. Approximately, 5% of Indian population are RhD negative.[3] The RhD polypeptide is an integral membrane protein expressed exclusively on erythrocytes.[4] Individuals with Rh factor are 'RH positive'; others who lack it are 'Rh negative'. Rh factor is inherited and the Rh gene is located on the short arm of chromosome 1. Only two genes are identified, an RhD gene and an Rh CE gene with 5 major antigenic loci, D, C, c, E, e, each of which has many minor variants.[4] The D antigen is the most potent among the Rh antigens and is clinically the most important. Individuals who are homozygous dominant (DD) or heterozygous (Dd) are "Rh positive". Those who are homozygous recessive (dd) are "Rh negative"(i.e they do not have the D Rh antigen).

A heterozygous father has 50% chance of passing one Rh negative gene to the offspring; in such a case, the child of an Rh negative mother has 50% chance of being Rh negative

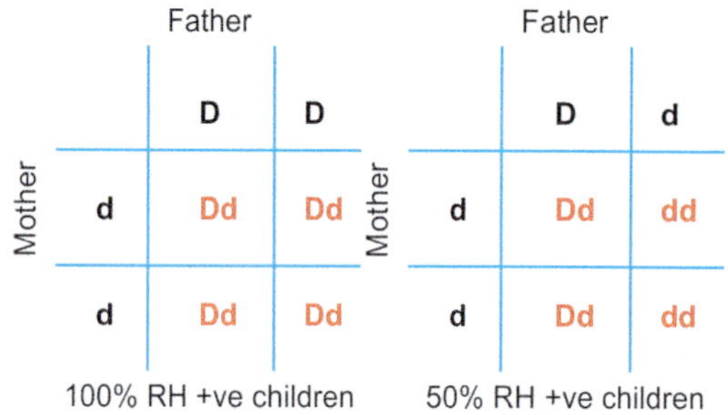

Figure 1: Chances of children of being Rh-negative or Rh-positive according to their parental category

and therefore being unaffected by any immune response **(Figure 1).**

Paternal and fetal genotyping is performed when anti-D antibodies are detected in the maternal circulation. Fetal genotype can be determined by using (i) cell-free fetal DNA from maternal blood,[5] (ii) amniocentesis, or (iii) fetal blood sampling.

ISOIMMUNIZATION

Isoimmunization has been defined as the process in which antibodies are produced in an individual in response to the injection of antigen (that is foreign to the recipient) from another individual of the same species.[6] Because this antigen belongs to the same spices it is called 'isoimmunization. There are two possible methods by which isoimmunization can occur: the first one is by transfusion of blood that has non-matching antigens. The second is when an Rh negative mother is carrying Rh positive fetus.

When the blood of an Rh negative mother comes in contact with blood from an Rh positive fetus, the Rh negative mother produces antibodies against the Rh factor. A person with RhD negative blood group who makes anti -RhD antibodies is called "**Rh sensitized**."

During pregnancy, small volumes of fetal red cells continually get into the maternal circulation. This trafficking of fetal red cells increases as gestation progresses. Bowman et al. showed at least 0.01 mL of fetal cells in 3%,12%.and 14% of women in each trimester.[7] This load of RhD antigen on fetal erythrocytes does not stimulate the mothers immune system because fetal red cells are rapidly cleared by reticuloendothelial system. However, in certain sensitising events like bleeding during pregnancy or interventions, when a large volume of fetal blood enters the maternal circulation, her immune system is stimulated and anti-D antibodies are produced leading to Rh-isoimmunization.[8]

The initial IgM Anti-D immunoglobulin response is short lived with a rapid switch over to IgG production. Unlike IgM, IgG antibodies cross the placenta and destroy fetal erythrocytes. This represents the basic pathogenetic mechanism responsible for Rh hemolytic disease of fetus and newborn. In the fetus in response to immunological fetal red cell destruction, extramedullary erythropoiesis takes place in the liver leading to hepatic dysfunction, portal and umbilical venous hypertension resulting in ascites and placental edema. Amino acid synthesis and transfer are impaired due to liver dysfunction and placental edema that leads to generalized edema and anasarca.

Many different antibodies (AntiD, anti-Kell, anti-C, anti-E, etc.) can cause hemolytic disease of the fetus/neonate; this chapter covers the management of pregnancies affected with RhD alloimmunization. The principles of management are similar regardless of the type of antibody involved, although care needs to be taken with pregnancies complicated by Kell alloimmunization, where antibody concentration does not always correlate with the severity of the disease.[9,10]

MANAGEMENT OF THE FIRST ALLOIMMUNIZED PREGNANCY

A women's first pregnancy complicated by RhD alloimmunization shows low anti-D titers at the beginning of the pregnancy. Severe fetal anemia may not develop or develop in the late second trimester or the third trimester.

In subsequent affected pregnancies fetal anemia usually is more severe and develops earlier in gestation.

Finding out which fetus is at risk is the initial step. An RhD negative fetus is not risk for complications from RhD alloimmunization. Therefore, when a pregnant woman is found to be RhD-negative, it is important to know the Rh status of the partner. If he is RhD negative, no further investigations are required. If the partner is RhD positive, then his genotype needs to be assessed, the maternal serum should be tested for presence of anti-RhD antibodies and the level (titer) should be determined. The presence of red cell antibodies in the mother signifies that alloimmunization has occurred as a result of a previous pregnancy or a previous blood transfusion. Maternal cell free fetal DNA testing-noninvasive assessment of fetal RhD using cell free DNA can used to know the fetal status.

ESTIMATION OF MATERNAL ANTI- D ANTIBODY TITERS IS DONE BY INDIRECT COOMBS TEST (ICT)

A "critical titer" is one at which there is significant risk of fetal hydrops, typically between 1:8 and 1:32 dilutions which varies in different laboratories (as it is a semi-quantitative visual test). Maternal antibody titers are screening tests and do not accurately predict the severity of fetal anemia. These have value only till a critical titer is reached. Beyond that serial middle cerebral artery peak systolic velocity is assessed to estimate the severity of fetal anemia **(Flowchart 1)**.

Anti-D levels if not detected at the initial visit a repeat assessment should be done at 28weeks.[11,12] Once detected, Anti-D levels should be measured every 4 weeks up to 28 weeks of gestation and then every 2 weeks then until delivery.[9,11]

Flowchart 1: Algorithm for the management of red-cell alloimmunization

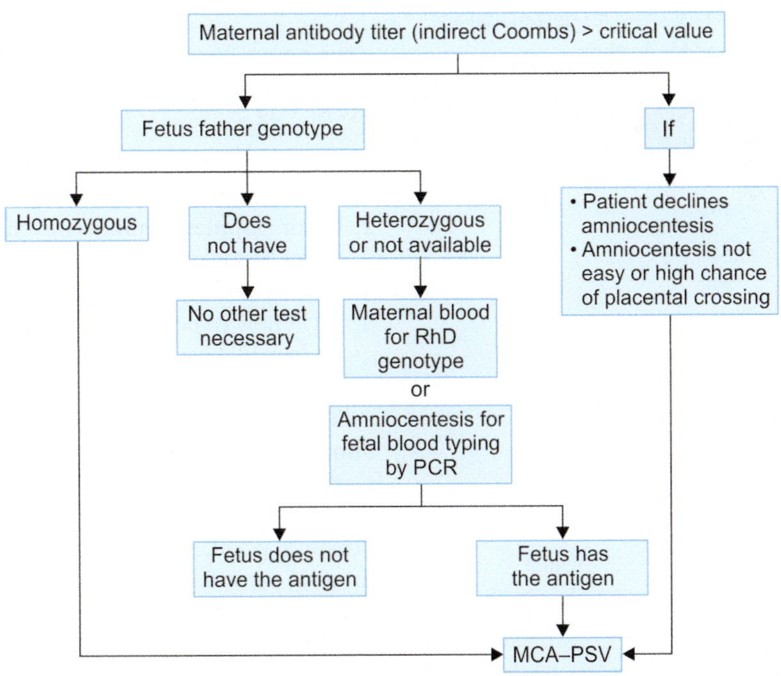

Abbreviation: MCA-PSV, middle cerebral artery peak systolic velocity; PCR, polymerase chain reaction; RhD, rhesus D16

Once there are rising antibody titers, or if the titers are above a specific threshold, or if ultrasound features are suggestive of critical fetal anemia, the fetuses are opted for definitive treatment and specialized care. Traditional technique of serial amniocentesis for delta OD 450 has now been superseded by Doppler velocimetry of middle cerebral artery peak systolic velocity (MCA - PSV). A fall in the fetal hemoglobin leads to increased cardiac output and decreased blood viscosity. As a consequence MCA-PSV increases as the fetal hemoglobin falls. In the year 2009, systematic reviews and many studies showed that Doppler of MCA-PSV performs well as a screening tool for severe fetal anemia of any etiology and sensitivity and specificity reached 75.5 and 90.8%. Sensitivity of increased MCA–PSV (>1.5 MoMs) for the prediction of moderate to severe anemia was 100%, either in presence or absence of hydrops, with a false positive rate of 12%, positive-predictive value of 53% and negative-predictive value of 98%.[9,13-15]

Table 1: Put the table here for gestational age and MCA values

	MCA–PSV (cm/s)	
GA (weeks)	***Median***	***1.5 MoM***
14	19.3	28.9
15	20.2	30.3
16	21.1	31.7
17	22.1	33.2
18	23.2	34.8
19	24.3	36.5
20	25.5	38.2
21	26.7	40.0
22	27.9	41.9
23	29.3	43.9
24	30.7	46.0
25	32.1	48.2
26	33.6	50.4
27	35.2	52.8
28	36.9	55.4
29	38.7	58.0
30	40.5	60.7
31	42.4	63.6
32	44.4	66.6
33	46.5	69.8
34	48.7	73.1
35	51.1	76.6
36	53.5	80.2
37	56.0	84.0
38	58.7	88.0
39	61.5	92.2
40	64.4	96.6

Reference range of fetal middle cerebral artery peak systolic velocity (MCA-PSV) median and 1.5 multiples of the median (MoM) values during pregnancy, GA, gestational age[19]

STEPS FOR CORRECT MEASUREMENT OF MCA–PSV[15]

1. Axial section of the head is obtained at the sphenoid bones.
2. Color Doppler identifies the circle of Willis
3. Color box is placed around the MCA.
4. The MCA is zoomed.
5. MCA flow velocity waveforms are displayed and the highest point of the waveform (PSV) is measured.

The waveforms should be all similar. The above sequence is repeated at least three times in each fetus.

MCA-PSV should be sampled at its proximal point, soon after its origin from the internal carotid artery, avoiding the need for angle correction, because measurement at this point is associated with lowest intra- or inter-observer variability. Sample volume should be placed at the center of the vessel.

Why MCA and not any other vessel?

MCA supplies more than half of the cerebrum and so is most representative of the cerebral circulation. Moreover, studying the MCA-PSV is that it is easy to obtain an angle of zero degrees between the ultrasound beam and the direction of blood flow **(Figures 2 and 3).**[17]

The MCA-PSV is found to have a good correlation with fetal anemia. MCA-PSV diagnoses fetal anemia, even in cases of Kell sensitization in which the problem is not haemolysis but the suppression of erythroid precursor cells in the bone marrow.[18]

MCA-PSV-Based management

MCA-PSV is measured at one-two week intervals, once the diagnosis of fetal anemia is confirmed. The frequency is increased if indicated by (MoM) approaching 1.5. MCA-PSV </=1.5 MoM for gestational age is consistent with absence of moderate to severe anemia. If MCA-PSV remains at this level, delivery at 37-38 weeks should be planned.

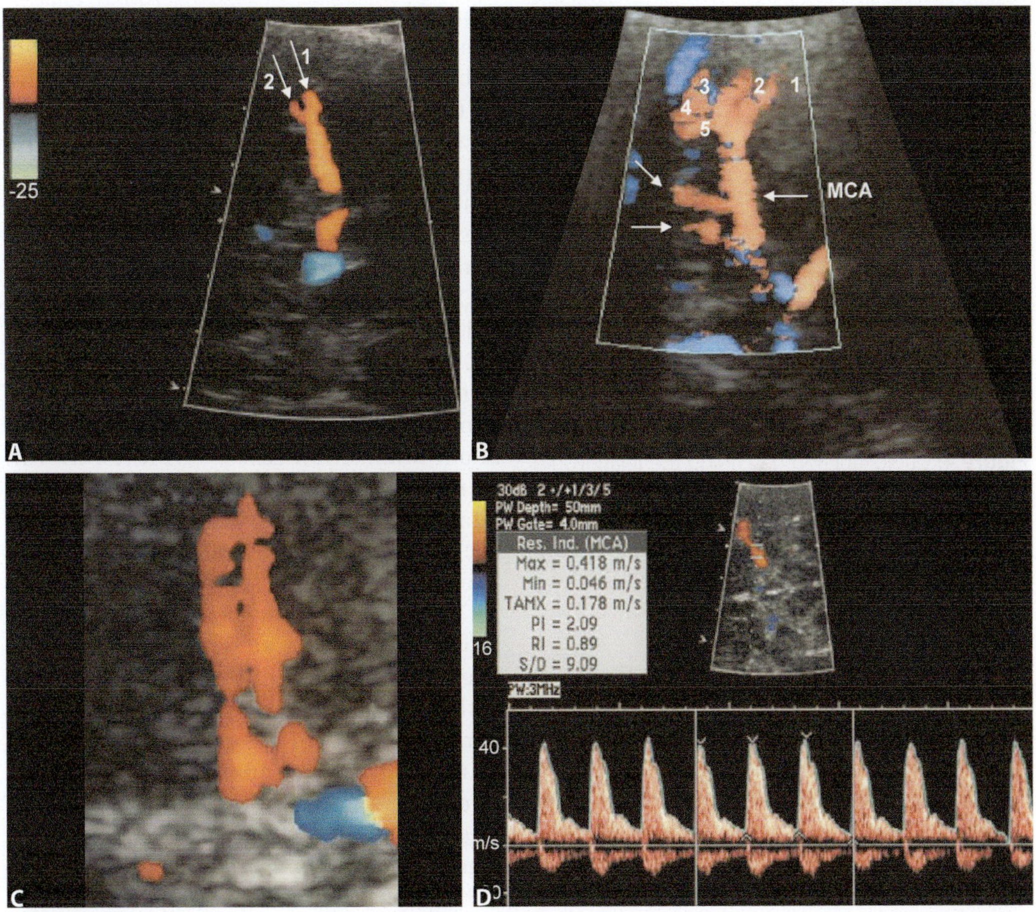

Figure 2: Color Doppler ultrasound image showing the middle cerebral artery (MCA). (A) The main trunk divides into two terminal branches (indicated by arrows 1 and 2); (B) it divides into five terminal branches (1 to 5); (C) double MCA (normal variant); (D) color Doppler of the MCA (top); flow velocity waveforms of the MCA (above the baseline) and lenticulostriates arteries (ART-LS) (below the baseline)

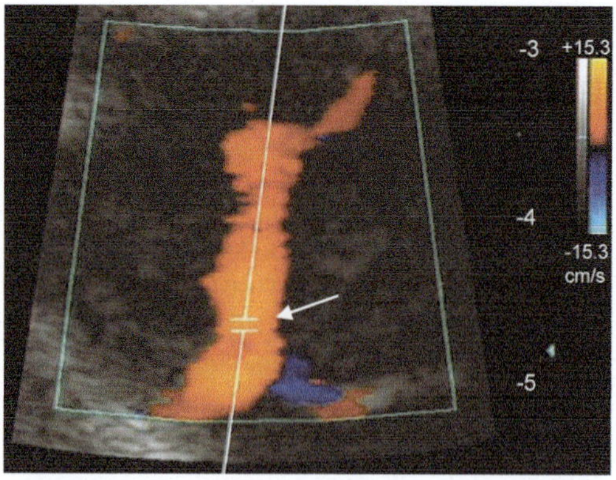

Figure 3: Color Doppler ultrasound image showing the middle cerebral artery. The sample volume (arrow) is placed in the center of the vessel after its origin from the internal carotid artery

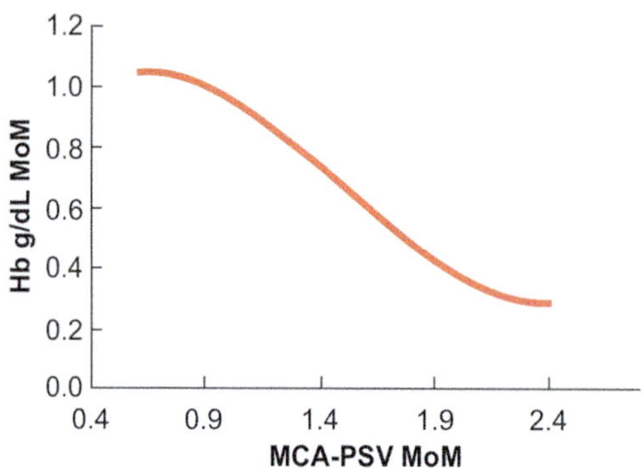

Figure 4: Cubic function describing the relationship between middle cerebral artery peak systolic velocity (MCA-PSV) and fetal hemoglobin (Hb). The values are expressed as multiples of the median (MoM). y = 0.6835 + MCA-PSV MoM × 1.2794 – 1.2885 MCA-PSV2 + 0.2861 × MCA-PSV[20]

MCA-PSV >1.5 MoM for the gestational age, fetal blood by cordocentesis is taken for assessing the hemoglobin levels and intrauterine fetal transfusion is recommended if fetal hemoglobin is two standard deviation below the mean[9]. Intrauterine transfusion is generally limited to pregnancies of 18–35 weeks, after 35 weeks intra-uterine transfusion is considered more risky than delivery followed by postnatal transfusion. At a gestational age of more than 35 weeks with MCA -PSV >1.5 MoM, delivery of the fetus should be planned.

Management of women with alloimmunization in subsequent pregnancy

A women who had a history of hydrops fetalis, intrauterine fetal transfusion or neonatal exchange transfusion for the previous child, is considered a high risk patient for development of fetal anemia in the following pregnancy. Development of severe fetal anemia is anticipated in subsequent pregnancies in these patients especially with a RhD-positive fetus and severe anemia may occur earlier than in the previous gestation.

Determine fetal RhD status using cell free DNA assessment from the mother's blood and a baseline maternal titer early in gestation would a useful guide for further comparison. Subsequent maternal titers are not informative as they may not be predictive of onset of fetal anemia. MCA-PSV monitoring of Rh D-positive fetus is initiated at 16–18 weeks of gestation. MCA-PSV assessment is done in the same way as described above for first allo-immunized pregnancies, but measurement of MCA-PSV is usually done weekly for a closer follow up.[21]

A MCA-PSV is a better test for detection of fetal anemia than amniocentesis and is considered the standard of care in red cell alloimmunization cases.[22,23] MCA-PSV can be safely used for timing cordocentesis and fetal transfusion if indicated. MCA-PSV is the more preferred method to screen for fetal anemia also because, it is noninvasive. MCA-PSV assessment should be reserved for those patients who are at risk of having an anemic fetus. Indiscriminate use of MCA-PSV without a clear indication may cause more harm than good. False-positive values may cause unnecessary anxiety and iatrogenic intervention. Hydrops is likely to develop in severe fetal anemia, but tricuspid valve regurgitation (TR) will precede the occurrence of hydrops. Combining tricuspid valve flow assessment along with the MCA-PSV can decrease the false-negative cases. If a fetus at risk for anemia has a normal MCA-PSV and TR is present, it would be important to follow that fetus very closely **(Flowchart 2).**[16]

Flowchart 2: MCA–PSV assessment

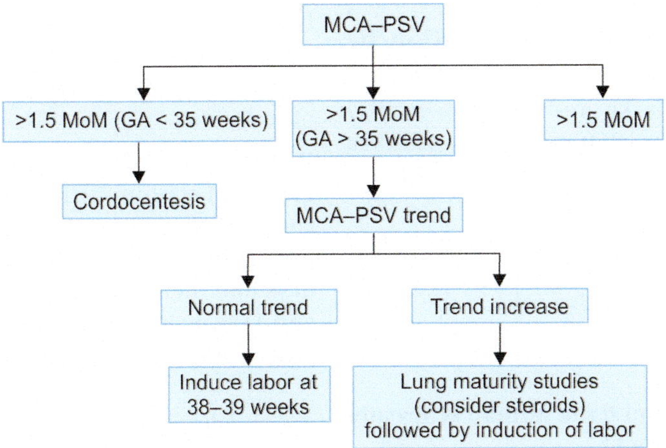

Timing of delivery of women with red cell antibodies will depend on the Rh-D antibody titers, rate of rise of antibody titers, and also whether any fetal therapy was required during pregnancy. The mode, timing and place of delivery are otherwise dependent on standard obstetric grounds.

The severity of fetal hemolysis can be predicted by:

1. Detailed history of previously affected pregnancies.
2. Maternal anti-D antibody titers.
3. Doppler study of fetal circulation which can detect changes in the flow velocity waveforms.
4. Altered morphometry of the fetus and placenta.
5. Presence of pathological fetal heart rate patterns.

Ultrasound features of fetal hydrops—Ascites, pericardial and pleural effusions, subcutaneous and scalp edema, polyhydramnios, placentomegaly.

PREVENTION OF AN AFFECTED FETUS

Each subsequent pregnancy, after the first affected pregnancy, is likely to manifest more severe hemolytic disease at an earlier gestational age, can be prevented by avoiding conception of a RhD-positive fetus in a Rh- D negative mother. (this is the ideal treatment but is practically not applicable for all noncompatible blood groups).

1. IVF with preimplantation genetic diagnosis—if biological father is heterozygous positive for Rh D. IVF with PGD can be used to identify Rh D-negative embryos and only those are considered for transfer.
2. Gestational surrogate - If the biological father is homozygous for Rh D, parents can conceive by IVF and embryos can be carried by gestational surrogate
3. Donor sperm—Sperm of Rh D-negative donor can be used for intrauterine insemination.

SPECIAL ISSUES

ART does not increase sensitivity of Rh isoimmunization, though in third party reproduction technology, care should be taken while selecting donor eggs for Rh negative pregnant women.

TWINS (Dichorionic diamniotic twins)

Maternal blood test for fetal genotyping will not differentiate between the twins.Non invasive individual monitoring of each fetus by doppler ultrasound (MCA-PSV) is the preferable method of monitoring.

Prevention of Rh isoimmunization by Anti-D prophylaxis

The work of Clarke and Finn on anti-D prophylaxis in 1960 was a landmark achievement toward reducing the incidence of severe RhD alloimmunization.[24]

Anti-D immunoglobulin, when given to a non sensitized Rh-negative person, it targets and coats any Rh positive cells in the blood stream and prevents the production of Rh antibodies.

Anti-D is not useful if the woman is already Rh sensitized (Box 1)

Indications for anti-D prophylaxis:

1. As part of routine antenatal anti-D prophylaxis (RAADP)
2. In the occurrence of potential sensitizing events
3. Postnatal anti-D prophylaxis.

RAADP: is administered as two doses of 500 IU one at 28 weeks and 34 weeks or a single dose of 1500 IU at 28–30 weeks given IM in the deltoid (**1500 IU = 300 —g)**

Box 1: Potential sensitizing events in pregnancy[25]

- Amniocentesis, chorionic villus biopsy and cordocentesis
- Antepartum hemorrhage/uterine (PV) bleeding in pregnancy
- External cephalic version
- Abdominal trauma (sharp/blunt, open/closed)
- Ectopic pregnancy
- Evacuation of molar pregnancy
- Intrauterine death and stillbirth
- In-utero therapeutic interventions (transfusion, surgery, insertion of shunts, laser)
- Miscarriage, threatened miscarriage
- Therapeutic termination of pregnancy
- Delivery—normal, instrumental or Cesarean section
- Intraoperative cell salvage

The dose of anti-D required to prevent Rh sensitisation in an Rh negative women when a sensitizing event has occurred depends on the amount of feto maternal hemorrhage that has occurred and this can be estimated by Kleihauer-Betke test.

No test for FMH is required before 20 weeks of gestation.

Postnatal anti-D prophylaxis: 1500 IU is given IM within 72 hours of delivery. In case, this deadline could not be met, some protection may still be got by giving it up to 10 days after delivery, this is in addition to any anti-D given in antenatal period, table[26] below gives summary of dose administration.

Anti-D Administration Checklist[26]

The overall survival in pregnancies complicated by red cell antibodies causing fetal anemia following treatment was reported to be 84%, with nonhydropic fetuses having better survival (94%) than hydropic fetuses (74%)**(Table 2)**.[27]

SUMMARY POINTS

- The incidence of RhD alloimmunization is decreasing.
- Genotyping of fetuses can now be done noninvasively, using maternal plasma (cfDNA).
- Serial amniocentesis to assess progression of fetal anemia is no longer necessary.
- Fetal anemia can be monitored non-invasively by using Doppler of the middle cerebral artery (MCA-PSV).
- Good neurodevelopmental outcome can be expected in treated fetuses.
- Immunotherapy may be of benefit in selected cases

NONIMMUNE HYDROPS FETALIS

Nonimmune hydrops fetalis (NIH) comprises the subgroup of cases not caused by red cell alloimmunization. The prevalence of NIHF ranges from 1/1500 to 1/3800.[28]

Table 2: Anti-D administration checklist

<table>
<tr><td colspan="2">Always confirm
• the woman's identity
• that the woman is RhD Negative using the latest laboratory report
• that the woman does not have immune anti-D using the latest laboratory report
• that informed consent for administration of anti-D Ig is recorded in notes</td></tr>
<tr><td colspan="2">Potentially Sensitising Events (PSEs) during pregnancy</td></tr>
<tr><td colspan="2">Gestation LESS than 12 weeks</td></tr>
<tr><td>Vaginal bleeding associated with severe pain</td><td rowspan="4">Administer at least 250 IU anti-D Ig within 72 hours of event.
Confirm product / dose / expiry and patient ID pre administration</td></tr>
<tr><td>ERPC / Instrumentation of uterus</td></tr>
<tr><td>Medical or surgical termination of pregnancy</td></tr>
<tr><td>Ectopic / Molar Pregnancy</td></tr>
<tr><td colspan="2">Gestation 12 to 20 weeks</td></tr>
<tr><td>For any Potentially Sensitising Event (PSE)</td><td>Administer at least 250 IU anti-D Ig within 72 hours of event.
Confirm product / dose / expiry and patient ID pre administration</td></tr>
<tr><td colspan="2">Gestation 20 weeks to term</td></tr>
<tr><td>For any Potentially Sensitising Event (PSE)
(Irrespective of whether RAADP has been given)</td><td>Request a Kleihauer Test (FMH Test) and immediately administer at least 500 IU anti-D Ig within 72 hours of event.
Confirm product / dose / expiry and patient ID pre administration</td></tr>
<tr><td>Does the Kleihauer / FMH test indicate that further anti-D Ig is required ?</td><td>Administer more anti-D Ig following discussion with laboratory</td></tr>
<tr><td colspan="2">For continuous vaginal bleeding at least 500iu anti-D Ig should be administered at a minimum of 6-weekly intervals, irrespective of the presence of detectable anti-D, and a Kleihauer / FMH Test requested every two weeks in case more anti-D is needed</td></tr>
<tr><td colspan="2">Routine Antenatal Anti-D Prophylaxis (RAADP)</td></tr>
<tr><td rowspan="5">For Routine Antenatal Anti-D Prophylaxis

(Irrespective of whether anti-D Ig already given for PSE)</td><td>Take a blood sample to confirm group & check antibody screen – do not wait for results before administering anti-D Ig</td></tr>
<tr><td>Administer 1500 IU anti-D Ig at 28 – 30 weeks</td></tr>
<tr><td>OR</td></tr>
<tr><td>Administer at least 500 IU anti-D Ig at 28 weeks and then administer at least 500 IU anti-D at 34 weeks</td></tr>
<tr><td>Confirm product / dose / expiry and patient ID pre administration</td></tr>
<tr><td colspan="2">At Delivery (or on diagnosis of Intra Uterine Death >20 weeks)</td></tr>
<tr><td rowspan="2">Is the baby's group confirmed as RhD positive ?
OR
Are cord samples not available ?</td><td>Request a Kleihauer Test (FMH Test)</td></tr>
<tr><td>Administer at least 500 IU anti-D Ig within 72 hours of delivery
Confirm product / dose / expiry and patient ID pre administration</td></tr>
<tr><td>Does the Kleihauer / FMH test indicate that further anti-D Ig is required ?</td><td>Administer more anti-D following discussion with laboratory</td></tr>
</table>

Pathogenesis

Dysregulation of the net fluid movement between the vascular and interstitial spaces leading to NIHF can be caused by various fetal disorders. Fetal disorders associated with NIHF are typically grouped into etiologic categories: chromosomal, hematologic, cardiothoracic, neoplastic, infections, structural abnormalities. Complete list is beyond the scope of this chapter. However, the following discussion will focus on the common ones.

The proportion of hydrops cases attributable to each etiologic category depends on the gestational age at presentation. NIHF prior to 24 weeks of gestation is usually related to aneuploidy, while cardiac, infections and other etiologies account for the majority of cases after 24 weeks.

Fetal Structural Anomalies

Cardiovascular Abnormalities

Fetal structural cardiac anomalies and fetal arrhythmias represent 40% cases of non-immune hydrops fetalis[29] (NIH). The most common cardiac lesions associated with hydrops are atrioventricular septal defects (AVSD), hypoplastic left or right heart syndrome, Ebstein's anomaly, cardiomyopathy, etc. Many of these lesions are also associated with aneuploidy. Most of these lesions are not amenable to intrauterine therapy and in the setting of early onset hydrops prognosis is poor with a mortality rate close to 100%.[30] Genetic counseling should be offered, as the recurrence risk is 2–5%.[31] Isolated congenital heart block is associated with maternal antinuclear antibodies (ANA), anti-SSA (Ro) antibodies and anti-SSB (La) antibodies and tends to have good outcomes.[32]

Thoracic and Lymphatic Abnormalities

These account for up to 10% of hydrops. Those lesions which increase intrathoracic pressure may obstruct venous return to the heart leading to peripheral venous congestion or may obstruct the lymphatic duct resulting in lymphedema. Interference with fluid exchange between the lung and amniotic cavity may also contribute to polyhydramnios.

Congenital cystic adenomatoid malformation (CCAM) occurs when there is an abnormal overgrowth of terminal respiratory bronchioles prior to 7 weeks; CCAM is divided into two groups: Macrocystic tumors containing cysts of at least 5 mm appear cystic on ultrasound. These are not usually associated with NIH and have favorable prognosis. Microcystic tumors contain cysts less than 5 mm, appearing solid ultrasonographically and are commonly associated with NIH. The perinatal survival rate of CCAM without hydrops approaches 100%, while the combination of CCAM and NIH and no fetal therapy is almost invariably fatal.[33]

Pulmonary sequestration (PS) is a mass of non-aerated lung tissue that receives its systemic circulation from the aorta. It is either lobar (within the pleura of the normal lung) or extralobar (out side the pleura of the normal lung). The perinatal survival rate in pure PS with or with out NIH is 80–100% respectively, and is significantly reduced by presence of other anomalies.[34]

Pleural effusion may be isolated or associated with NIH which confers worse prognosis. Persistent pleural effusion before 20 weeks of gestation can compromise lung growth and function. Thus a poor prognostic sign, the degree of pulmonary hypoplasia can not be reliably determined sonographically.

Needle aspiration of pleural effusion is not recommended as the fluid reaccumulates, in fetus with large pleural effusion placement of pleuroamniotic shunt may alleviate the increased intrathoracic pressure, thereby reducing the risk of pulmonary hypoplasia.

Aneuploidy

Aneuploidy is responsible for 7–16% percent of NIHF cases.[35] The most common aneuploidy associated with NIHF is monosomy X (Turner syndrome), which accounts for 42–67% of cases.[36] Other aneuploidies associated with hydrops include trisomy 21 (23–30% of cases); Trisomy 13, 18, and 12 (10 percent of cases); tetraploidy; triploidy; and, rarely,deletions and duplications.[29,36] The mechanism for fluid accumulation in these fetuses may involve obstruction or incomplete formation of the lymphatic system in the neck or abdomen, leading to lymphatic dysplasia. Other mechanisms include cardiac failure related to congenital heart disease (present in 15-25% of aneuploid fetuses)[37] and transient abnormal myelopoiesis, a congenital leukemia associated with Down's syndrome.[38] The prognosis is poor, with a mortality rate approaching 100%.[37]

Infections

Infections are responsible for 5–10% of NIHF.[35,39] Parvovirus B_{19} is the most common infection associated with hydrops, followed by cytomegalovirus, toxoplasmosis, and syphilis. The following infections have been associated with NIHF. Not all fetuses with these infections develop hydrops and causation has not been proven for all of the infections. In some cases, a causative organism may not be identified: Parvovirus B_{19}, TORCH pathogens (toxoplasmosis, cytomegalovirus, rubella, herpes virus [human herpesvirus 6 and 7, herpes simplex type1]), syphilis, varicella, adenovirus, coxsackievirus, leptospirosis, *Trypanosoma cruzi* [Chagas disease], *Listeria*, respiratory syncytial virus, Congenital lymphocytic choriomeningitis virus.

Sonographic signs (in addition to hydrops) that suggest in utero infection include calcifications of the brain, liver, or pericardium; microcephaly; cerebral ventriculomegaly; hepatosplenomegaly; and growth restriction. The pathogenesis for hydrops related to infection is not well understood in most cases; Parvovirus B_{19} is an exception. This virus attacks red blood cells, hepatocytes, and myocardial cells causing transient aplastic crisis, hepatitis, and myocarditis.[39-42] Since these processes are selflimited, the prognosis is generally good if the fetus is supported by intrauterine fetal transfusions until the disease remits. Platelet concentrates should also be available since some fetuses may also be profoundly thrombocytopenic. In contrast, the development of hydrops in fetuses with most other infections reflect multisystem failure (e.g.myocarditis leading to heart failure, liver involvement leading to hypoalbuminemia) and is a poor prognostic sign. Therapy, if available, is directed against the infectious agent.

Fetal Tumors

Fetal tumors and lesions that have been associated with NIHF include sacrococcygeal, mediastinal or pharyngeal teratoma; neuroblastoma; and large hemangiomas.

NIHF has also been associated with fetal tuberous sclerosis. Fetal tumors invade and obstruct the vena cava, portal vein, or femoral vessels leading to cardiac failure, hepatic failure, resulting in NIHF.

Placental chorioangiomas occur in 1% of pregnancies. Tumors of more than 5 cm function as high volume arteriovenous shunts which predispose the fetus to heart failure and/or microangiopathic hemolytic anemia.[43]

Hematological Disorders

Severe fetal anemia accounts for 10–27% of hydrops.[29] It may be due to a variety of causes, including hemorrhage, hemolysis, defective red cell production, and production of abnormal hemoglobins. Hydrops is observed when the fetal hemoglobin is less than half the median value for gestational age.[19] In general terms, fetal anemia is most likely to result in hydrops when the hemoglobin concentration is ≤5 g/dL, which approximates a hematocrit less than 30%. A presumptive diagnosis of fetal anemia is made by Doppler assessment of the fetal middle cerebral artery (MCA) peak systolic velocity (PSV) ≥1.5 multiples of the median (MoM), (sensitivity and specificity for severe anemia 75.5 and 90.8%, respectively), and can be confirmed by cordocentesis. Decision on whether to perform cordocentesis, follow MCAPSV serially, transfuse in utero, or deliver the fetus depends on the gestational age and cause of anemia. Alpha thalassemia major is the most common cause of NIHF among southeast Asians. It is an autosomal recessive condition characterized by a mutation or deletion of the hemoglobin alpha gene. Because there is no alpha globin chain production, affected fetuses cannot synthesize a functional hemoglobin molecule. Gamma chains accumulate and form gamma-4 tetramers (hemoglobin Bart's); hemoglobin Bart's binds oxygen, but cannot release it to tissues because its affinity for oxygen is much greater than that of hemoglobin A. Hemoglobin electrophoresis will show greater than 80% hemoglobin of Bart's type, while the remaining hemoglobin will be of embryonic origin, with a small component of hemoglobin H (beta 4 tetramers).[44] The fetus may be severely anemic, and a peripheral blood smear will show nucleated red cells and target cells. Profound hypoxia, acidosis and hydrops develop early in the mid-trimester, followed by intrauterine fetal demise unless the fetus is serially transfused.

Anemia secondary to massive feto-maternal transfusion, as is seen in abruptio placenta, placenta previa, trauma, twin-to-twin transfusion syndrome, is diagnosed by Kleihauer-Betke smear or flow cytometry. Transfusion or delivery can be lifesaving.

Inborn Errors of Metabolism

Inborn errors of metabolism comprise a heterogeneous group of autosomal recessive disorders that may present in the fetal period as NIHF. These account for 1–2% of these.[35] These rare genetic disorders are due to lack of specific enzymes necessary to process various metabolites within the lysosome in organs, such as the brain, heart, liver, and kidneys. The pathogenesis of hydrops is most likely related to congestion of abdominal viscera due to accumulation of these metabolites.[45] Laboratory investigations to exclude some causes of storage disorders are available. An attempt at prenatal diagnosis is an option with cases of recurrence within a family or when NIHF occurs in a structurally normal fetus and no cause has been identified after a standard workup.[35,46,47] There is no specific therapy in the antenatal period. In utero death usually occurs. It is important to make an accurate diagnosis postnatally and offer genetic counseling, as the risk of recurrence in a future pregnancy is as high as 1 in 4.

Twin Gestation

Monochorionic twin gestations are at risk for hydrops due to two disorders unique to these twin pregnancies:

Twin-twin transfusion syndrome (TTTS) and twin, reversed arterial perfusion (TRAP). Polyhydramnios/oligohydramnios sequence is the defining characteristic of TTTS. One or both twins may develop NIHF, but usually the recipient twin is affected because of hypervolemia and increased central venous pressure. In TRAP, the hydropic twin has no apparent cardiac structures. Treatment of both TTTS and TRAP involves an in utero ablation procedure.

In both monochromic and dichorionic twins, hydrops may develop in one or both twins from any of the etiologies that affect singleton pregnancies described above.

Placental and Umbilical Cord Lesions

Fetal/placental vascular tumors can lead to NIHF due to high output heart failure from arteriovenous shunting.

Chorioangiomas of the placenta greater than 4– 5 cm in diameter may lead to NIHF by this mechanism and can be difficult to treat. Intrauterine endoscopic laser coagulation of the feeding vessels has been successful, but complications, such as fetal bleeding, exsanguination, and death have also occurred.[48]

Cord lesions associated with NIHF include angiomyxoma, aneurysm, venous thrombosis, umbilical vein torsion or true knots.[35]

Ultrasound findings: NIHF may be discovered incidentally during prenatal ultrasound performed for standard obstetric indications, during a workup for decreased fetal activity or abnormal antepartum fetal test results, during a workup for uterine size greater than dates, or during monitoring of fetuses with, or at risk for disorders associated with hydrops.

Fetal findings: Two or more of the following findings should be present on ultrasound examination:

Ascites: In its early stage, fetal ascites appears as a rim of echolucent fluid just inside the abdominal wall or surrounding the bladder or liver.

Pericardial fluid: Fluid rim greater than 2 mm thick that increases on serial examinations suggests a pathologic etiology.

Skin edema: Skin edema is a late sign of fetal hydrops. Pathologic skin edema has been defined as subcutaneous tissue thickness on the chest or scalp greater than 5 mm. Fat under the scalp or in the posterior nuchal region should not be mistaken for skin edema.

NIHF may be associated with polyhydramnios and placental thickening. Polyhydramnios is generally defined as an amniotic fluid index greater than 24 cm or a maximum vertical pocket greater than 8 cm. It is present in up to 75% of pregnancies complicated by NIHF. The placenta may appear thickened due to intravillous edema. In general, a placental thickness ≥4 cm in the second trimester and ≥6 cm in the third trimester is considered abnormal and should prompt further investigation.[44,49]

PROGNOSIS

NIHF is associated with an overall perinatal mortality rate of 50–98%.[50-55] Despite advances in fetal diagnosis and therapy, the mortality rate has not changed substantially over the past 15 years. Prognosis depends upon the etiology, the gestational age at onset, the gestational age at delivery, and whether pleural effusion is present. In general, the earlier hydrops occurs, the poorer the prognosis. In particular, pleural effusions and polyhydramnios prior to 20 weeks of gestation are poor prognostic signs because of increased risk of pulmonary hypoplasia and preterm premature rupture of membranes, preterm delivery, respectively. On the other hand, absence of aneuploidy and absence of major structural abnormalities confer a better prognosis.[56,57]

MANAGEMENT

Initial Maternal Screening Tests

Indirect Coomb's test, complete blood count (CBC) with differential count and indices for infection and thalassemia.

A detailed ultrasound examination of the fetal anatomy, amniotic fluid and placenta is essential to determine coexisting major structural anomalies and signs of infection.

Amniocentesis may be performed to obtain amniotic fluid for analyzing fetal chromosomes and DNA identifying antigens of the involved organisms using PCR. Fetal blood sampling can determine fetal hemoglobin, complete blood count, organ-specific antibodies or infections.

FETAL THERAPY

Maternal administration of medications for selected fetal infections and arrhythmias may help. Invasive procedures include—thoraco-amniotic shunting to alleviate compression of fetal lungs, blood transfusion fetal anemia, close fetal monitoring is indicated as there is high incidence of fetal demise.

The timing of delivery depends on the associated conditions, gestational age and fetal growth. The mode of delivery depends on maternal condition, fetal size and fetal tolerance to labor. Fetus with NIH may benefit from a multidisciplinary approach.

Stillborns and Neonates

We recommend autopsy in all cases of fetal or neonatal death or pregnancy termination associated with NIHF. Consultation with a medical geneticist is also advisable. Storage of amniotic fluid and/or fetal cells has been suggested for future genetic testing.[58]

Recurrence Risk

The risk of recurrent NIHF depends upon the underlying etiology; therefore, every effort should be made to determine the cause. If hydrops was related to an anatomical variant the recurrence risk is minimal. Hydrops related to a specific viral exposure should not recur because the mother will develop immunity.

In contrast, the risk of recurrent NIHF can be high when hydrops has a genetic basis. Many of the times; the clinician cannot always determine the etiology of fetal hydrops. Genetics consultation can be useful in these cases as the quality of information from genetic testing continues to evolve. In cases where no cause is found, the likelihood of recurrent hydrops is low.[59-61] Since the risk of recurrence is not zero, a mid trimester sonogram in subsequent gestations is reasonable .

SUMMARY AND RECOMMENDATIONS

- Hydrops fetalis refers to abnormal fluid collections in fetal soft tissues and serous cavities. Nonimmune hydrops fetalis (NIHF) comprises the subgroup of cases not caused by red cell alloimmunization (e.g. Rh(D), Kell).
- Women carrying a hydropic fetus may have uterine size large for dates and may notice decreased fetal movement. Although hydrops is a fetal condition; in many cases, there are associated maternal findings, such as generalized edema with or without preeclampsia (i.e. mirror syndrome).
- The causes of nonimmune hydrops are heterogeneous and include aneuploidy, structural abnormalities,metabolic disorders, anemia, genetic causes and infection.
- Several etiologies can be confirmed or excluded based upon ultrasound findings.
- The cause of hydrops can be determined prenatally or postnatally in 60–85% of cases.
- Management and intervention are dictated by the underlying disease process and the gestational age at detection.
- Fetal anemia, fetal arrhythmias, and complications of monochorionic twin pregnancy are amenable to in utero intervention.
- In the absence of a lethal etiology of NIHF, weekly nonstress testing or biophysical profile testing delivery if there is evidence of fetal decompensation at a viable gestational age should be the strategy.
- Maternal-fetal medicine specialists and neonatologists should be involved in the management of these pregnancies.
- The risk of recurrent NIHF depends upon the underlying etiology.

REFERENCES

1. The fetus as a patient. The evolving challenge. 229-34.
2. The fetus as a patient .The evolving challenge, 229-34.
3. Cunningham FG etal . Williams Obstetrics, 21 st edition, MCGraw Hill Medical Publishing Division; 2001;p.1059.
4. Colin Y, Cherif- Zahar B, Le Van Kin C, Raynal V, Van Huffel V , Cartron JP. Genetic Basis of the Rh D- positive and Rh D- negative blood group polymorphism as determined by Southern analysis. Blood. 1991;78(10):2747-52.
5. Moise KJ Jr, Boring NH, O'Shaughnessy R, et al. Circulating cell-free fetal DNA for the detection of RHD status and sex using reflex fetal identifiers. Prenat Diagn 2013; 33:95.

6. Renu Mishra etal, Ian Donald's Practical obstetric problems, 6th edition , BI publications pvt Ltd. 2007;p.377.
7. Bowman JM, Pollock JM, Penston LE. Fetomaternal transplacental hemorrhage during pregnancy and after delivery. Vox Sang 1986;51:117-21.
8. Sailesh Kumar, Fiona Regan, Clinical review-Management of pregnancies with RhD alloimmunization, BMJ. 2005;330.
9. RCOG greentop guideline no 65, The management of women with red cell antibodies during pregnancy. 2014;p.11-12
10. Ahaded A, Brossard Y, Debbia M, Lambin P. Quantitative determination of anti-K (KEL1) IgG and IgG subclasses in the serum of severely alloimmunized pregnant women by ELISA. Transfusion. 2000;40:1239-45.
11. Gooch A, Parker J, Wray J , Qureshi H. Guideline for blood grouping and antibody testing in pregnancy. British committee for standards in Haematology. p.6
12. NICE clinical guideline 62, Antenatal care, Issued : March 2008 last modified : December 2014;p.23; 1.6.2.3; guidance.nice.org.uk/cg62
13. Mari G, Deter RL, Carpenter RL, Rahman F, Zimmerman R, Moise KJ Jr, et al. Collaborative Group for Doppler Assessment of the Blood Velocity in Anemic Fetuses. Noninvasive diagnosis by Doppler ultrasonography of fetal anemia due to maternal red-cell alloimmunization. N Engl J Med. 2000;342: 9-14.
14. Society for Maternal-Fetal Medicine (SMFM). Electronic address: pubs@smfm.org, Mari G, Norton ME, et al. Society for Maternal-Fetal Medicine (SMFM) Clinical Guideline #8: the fetus at risk for anemia--diagnosis and management. Am J Obstet Gynecol. 2015; 212:697.
15. Mari G, Abuhamad AZ, Cosmi E, et al. Middle cerebral artery peak systolic velocity: technique and variability. J Ultrasound Med. 2005;24:425.
16. Mari.G Opinion, middle cerebral artery peak systolic velocity for the diagnosis of fetal anaemia: the untold story, Ultrasound Obstet Gynecol. 2005;25:323-30.
17. Van Dongen H, Klumfer FJCM, Sikkkel E, etal. Non-invasive tests to predict fetal anaemia in Kell- alloimmunized pregnancies, Ultrasound Obstet gynecol. 2005;25:341-5.
18. Daniels G, Hadley A, Green CA. Causes of fetal anemia in hemolytic disease due to anti-K [letter]. Transfusion 2003;43:115-6.
19. Mari G, Deter RL, et al. Non invasive diagnosis by Doppler Ultrasound of fetal anaemia due to maternal red cell alloimmunization; N Engl J Med. 2000;342:9-141.
20. Abdel-Fattah SA, Soothill PW, Carroll SG, Kyle PM. Noninva-sive diagnosis of anemia in hydrops fetalis with the use of middle cerebral artery Doppler velocity. Am J Obstet Gynecol. 2001;185:1411-5.
21. Society for Maternal-Fetal Medicine (SMFM). Electronic address: pubs@smfm.org, Mari G, Norton ME, et al. Society for Maternal-Fetal Medicine (SMFM) Clinical Guideline #8: the fetus at risk for anemia--diagnosis and management. Am J Obstet Gynecol 2015; 212:697.
22. Mari G, Penson C, Sbracia M, Kern L, Levi D'Ancona R, Copel J. Dwlta OD450 and doppler velocimetry of the middle cerebral artery peak velocity in the evaluation of fetal alloimmune haemolytic disease, which is best? Am J Obstet Gynecol. 1997;180(Sup A):18.
23. Periera L, Jenkins TM, Berghella V. Conventional management of maternal red cell alloimmunization compared with management of Doppler of MCA PSV. Am J Obstet Gynecol. 2003;189:1002-6.
24. Finn R , Clarke CA, Donohoe WT, Mc Connell RB, Sheppard PM, Lehane D, etal. Experimental studies on the prevention of Rh haemolytic disease, Br Med J. 1961;5238:1486-90.
25. Qureshi H, Massey E, Kirwan D, Davies 3T, Robson S, White J, et al. BCSH guideline for the use of anti-D immunoglobulin for the prevention of haemolytic disease of the fetus and newborn, Transfusion Medicine. 2014; 24: 8-20.
26. Qureshi H, Massey E, Kirwan D, Davies 3T, Robson S, White J, et al. BCSH guideline for the use of anti-D immunoglobulin for the prevention of haemolytic disease of the fetus and newborn, Transfusion Medicine. 2014;24: 8-20.
27. Schumacher B, Moise KJ Jr. Fetal transfusion for red blood cell alloimmunization in pregnancy. Obstet Gynecol. 1996;88:137-50.
28. Sohan K, Carroll SG, De La Fuente S, et al. Analysis of outcome in hydrops fetalis in

relation to gestational age at diagnosis, cause and treatment. Acta Obstet Gynecol Scand. 2001;80:726.
29. Forouzan I. Hydrops fetalis: recent advances. Obstet Gynecol Surv. 1997;52:130.
30. Crawford DC, Chita SK, Allan LD. Prenatal detection of congenital heart disease: factors affecting obstetric management and survival. Am J Obstet Gynecol. 1988;159:352.
31. Hess DB, Hess LW. Fetal Echocardiography, Appleton and Lange, Stamford, CT. 1999.
32. Adzick NS,Harrison MR,Glick PL,et al. Fetal cystic adenomatoid malformation of the lung: classification and morphology. J pead surgery. 1985;20:483.
33. De santis M,Masini L,Noia G. Congenital cystic adenomatoid malformation of the lung;antenatal ultrasound findings and fetal neonatl outcome. Fetaldiag ther. 2000;15: 246-50.
34. Adzick NS, Harrison, Flake AW. Management and outcome. Amj obst gynecol. 1998;179: 884-9.
35. Society for Maternal-Fetal Medicine (SMFM). Norton ME, Chauhan SP, Dashe JS. Society for maternal-fetal medicine (SMFM) clinical guideline #7: nonimmune hydrops fetalis. Am J Obstet Gynecol 2015; 212:127
36. Machin GA. Hydrops revisited: literature review of 1,414 cases published in the 1980s. Am J Med Genet 1989; 34:366.
37. Hess DB, Hess LW. Fetal Echocardiography, Appleton and Lange, Stamford, CT 1999
38. Malin GL, Kilby MD, Velangi M. Transient abnormal myelopoiesis associated with Down syndrome presenting as severe hydrops fetalis: a case report. Fetal Diagn Ther 2010; 27:171.
39. Xu J, Raff TC, Muallem NS, Neubert AG. Hydrops fetalis secondary to parvovirus B19 infections. J Am Board Fam Pract 2003; 16:63.
40. Callen P. Ultrasonography in Obstetrics and Gynecology, 4th ed, WB Saunders, Philadelphia 2000.
41. Barron SD, Pass RF. Infectious causes of hydrops fetalis. Semin Perinatol 1995; 19:493.
42. von Kaisenberg CS, Jonat W. Fetal parvovirus B19 infection. Ultrasound Obstet Gynecol 2001; 18:280.
43. Paulaj.woodward,MD,Roya sohaye.A comprehensive review of fetaltumours with pathology correlation 1,RSNA,Radiographics, jan2005,vol1,issue1
44. Arcasoy MO, Gallagher PG. Hematologic disorders and nonimmune hydrops fetalis. Semin Perinatol 1995; 19:502.
45. Molyneux AJ, Blair E, Coleman N, Daish P. Mucopolysaccharidosis type VII associated with hydrops fetalis: histopathological and ultrastructural features with genetic implications. J Clin Pathol 1997; 50:252.
46. Gort L, Granell MR, Fernández G, et al. Fast protocol for the diagnosis of lysosomal diseases in nonimmune hydrops fetalis. Prenat Diagn 2012; 32:1139
47. Gimovsky AC, Luzi P, Berghella V. Lysosomal storage disease as an etiology of nonimmune hydrops. Am J Obstet Gynecol 2015; 212:281
48. Sepulveda W, Wong AE, Herrera L, et al. Endoscopic laser coagulation of feeding vessels in large placental chorioangiomas: report of three cases and review of invasive treatment options. Prenat Diagn 2009; 29:201
49. Chitkara U, Wilkins I, Lynch L, et al. The role of sonography in assessing severity of fetal anemia in Rh- and Kell-isoimmunized pregnancies. Obstet Gynecol 1988; 71:393.
50. Carlson DE, Platt LD, Medearis AL, Horenstein J. Prognostic indicators of the resolution of nonimmune hydrops fetalis and survival of the fetus. Am J Obstet Gynecol 1990; 163:1785.
51. Castillo RA, Devoe LD, Hadi HA, et al. Nonimmune hydrops fetalis: clinical experience and factors related to a poor outcome. Am J Obstet Gynecol 1986; 155:812.
52. Ismail KM, Martin WL, Ghosh S, et al. Etiology and outcome of hydrops fetalis. J Matern Fetal Med 2001; 10:175.
53. Heinonen S, Ryynänen M, Kirkinen P. Etiology and outcome of second trimester non-immunologic fetal hydrops. Acta Obstet Gynecol Scand 2000; 79:15.
54. Wy CA, Sajous CH, Loberiza F, Weiss MG. Outcome of infants with a diagnosis of hydrops fetalis in the 1990s. Am J Perinatol 1999; 16:561
55. Santo S, Mansour S, Thilaganathan B, et al. Prenatal diagnosis of non-immune hydrops fetalis: what do we tell the parents? Prenat Diagn 2011; 31:186.
56. McCoy MC, Katz VL, Gould N, Kuller JA. Non-immune hydrops after 20 weeks' gestation:

review of 10 years' experience with suggestions for management. Obstet Gynecol 1995; 85:578

57. Iskaros J, Jauniaux E, Rodeck C. Outcome of nonimmune hydrops fetalis diagnosed during the first half of pregnancy. Obstet Gynecol 1997; 90:321.
58. Désilets V, Audibert F, Society of Obstetrician and Gynaecologists of Canada. Investigation and management of non-immune fetal hydrops. J Obstet Gynaecol Can 2013; 35:923.
59. Schwartz SM, Viseskul C, Laxova R, et al. Idiopathic hydrops fetalis report of 4 patients including 2 affected sibs. Am J Med Genet 1981; 8:59.
60. Cumming DC. Recurrent nonimmune hydrops fetalis. Obstet Gynecol 1979; 54:124.
61. Etches PC, Lemons JA. Nonimmune hydrops fetalis: report of 22 cases including three siblings. Pediatrics 1979; 64:326.

Index

Page numbers followed by *f* refer to figure and *t* refer to table.

T